COMPLEMENTARY
MEDICINE

For Rhianne

COMPLEMENTARY MEDICINE
A Research Perspective

Charles Vincent
and
Adrian Furnham
Department of Psychology,
University College London, UK
with a contribution by
Phil Richardson
UMDS, University of London, UK

JOHN WILEY & SONS

Chichester • New York • Weinheim • Brisbane • Singapore • Toronto

Copyright © 1997 John Wiley & Sons Ltd,
Baffins Lane, Chichester,
West Sussex PO19 1UD, England

National   01243 779777
International (+44) 1243 779777
e-mail (for orders and customer service enquiries): cs-books@wiley.co.uk.
Visit our Home Page on http://www.wiley.co.uk
or http://www.wiley.com

Other Wiley Editorial Offices

John Wiley & Sons, Inc., 605 Third Avenue,
New York, NY 10158-0012, USA

VCH Verlagsgesellschaft mbH, Pappelallee 3,
D-69469 Weinheim, Germany

Jacaranda Wiley Ltd, 33 Park Road, Milton,
Queensland 4064, Australia

John Wiley & Sons (Asia) Pte Ltd, 2 Clementi Loop #02-01
Jin Xing Distripark, Singapore 129809

John Wiley & Sons (Canada) Ltd, 22 Worcester Road,
Rexdale, Ontario M9W 1L1, Canada

Library of Congress Cataloging-in-Publication Data

Vincent, Charles, Dr.
    Complementary medicine : a research perspective / Charles Vincent
and Adrian Furnham.
       p. cm.
    Included bibliographical references and index.
    ISBN 0-471-96645-2 (paper)
       1. Alternative medicine. 2. Alternative medicine—Evaluation.
    3. Alternative medicine—Research. I. Furnham, Adrian. II. Title.
       [DNLM: 1. Alternative Medicine. 2. Research. WB 890 V769c 1997]
    R733.V53 1997
    615.5—dc21
    DNLM/DLC
    for Library of Congress   97–4321
                                                                  CIP

British Library Cataloguing in Publication Data

A catalogue record for this book is available from the British Library

ISBN 0-471-96645-2

Typeset in 10/12pt Palatino from authors' disks
by Mayhew Typesetting, Rhayader, Powys
Printed and bound from postscript disk in Great Britain
by Biddles Ltd, Guildford and King's Lynn

This book is printed on acid-free paper responsibly manufactured from sustainable forestation,
for which at least two trees are planted for each one used for paper production.

Contents

Acknowledgements

We would like to thank Phil Richardson for contributing Chapter 7 and allowing us to draw on his encyclopaedic knowledge of placebo effects in both orthodox and complementary medicine. Pam La Rose was, as ever, splendidly calm and efficient in coping with re-writes, references and the eccentricities of the authors.

Any academic book relies on the efforts of many other researchers for the raw material. However, particular mention must be made of Jos Kleijnen, Paul Knipschild, Gerben ter Riet and their colleagues at the University of Limburg. Without their comprehensive reviews of several complementary therapies the two chapters on evaluation would have presented immense problems and the book could not have taken its present form.

Publishers Note

The authors and publishers wish to thank the following for permission to use copyright material: In the Introduction, *The Independent* for the article by Penelope Dening, 16 September 1992.

In Chapter 2, Butterworth-Heineman Ltd for text extracts from Helman, C. 1990. *Culture, Health and Illness*; and Routledge Ltd for text extracts from Sharma, U. 1992. *Complementary Medicine Today: Practitioners and Patients*.

In Chapter 3, BMJ Publishing Group for text extracts from Dennison, J.A.G. 1989. Conventional and complementary treatment for cancer. *British Medical Journal* **298**: 1583.

In Chapter 6, Tavistock Publications for text extracts from Taylor, R. 1985. Alternative medicine and the medical encounter in Britain and the United States. In: Salmon, W. ed. *Alternative Medicine*.

In Chapter 12, BMJ Publishing Group for text extracts from Briskman, L. 1987. Doctors and witchdoctors: which doctors are which? *British Medical Journal* **295**: 1108–10.

Introduction

Complementary medicine is now widely used in Australasia, Britain, Europe and the United States. In 1983 Fulder estimated that in Britain one medical consultation in ten was with a complementary practitioner of some kind (Fulder and Munro, 1985). Since then interest in complementary medicine has grown and the number of complementary patients and practitioners has dramatically increased. In the United States an estimated one in three people used an unconventional therapy in 1991, and the number of visits made to unconventional therapists exceeded those to all US primary care physicians (Eisenberg, Kessler and Foster, 1993). Complementary medicine encompasses an enormous range of diagnostic techniques and therapies. Some, for instance osteopathy, are gradually being incorporated into conventional health care. Homeopathy is available in the National Health Service, in spite of the former's underlying philosophy being quite at odds with orthodox scientific explanations of the action of drugs on the body. Other forms of complementary medicine, such as radionics, remain very much on the fringe and are regarded with scepticism.

The reaction of the medical profession to complementary medicine has been varied. Some have sought to embrace complementary therapies and incorporate them into their own practice. Others dismiss the whole range of techniques as, at best, offering harmless comfort to sick people and, at worst, as dangerous quackery that may deprive those people of effective medical treatment. Critics point to the lack of supporting evidence for the efficacy of most of these therapies and the reluctance of complementary practitioners to subject their therapies to formal evaluation. Medical practitioners may also express exasperation with their patients for rejecting empirical science in favour of mysticism. Complementary therapists counter by pointing to the obvious demand for their therapies and their patients' reports of the benefits of complementary forms of treatment.

The fact that so many people choose to attend complementary practitioners in a country where health care is largely free at the point of delivery suggests that they are receiving something that is important to them. Some complementary techniques may, as we will discuss, be of direct therapeutic benefit. However, whatever the benefits of the specific therapies, we believe that the phenomenon of complementary medicine has a great deal to teach us about the ingredients of a successful therapeutic relationship and the factors that assist or delay recovery from illness.

As a way of introducing some of the themes of this book, consider this wry account of a woman's experience of the treatment of recurrent cystitis by both orthodox and complementary treatment (Penelope Dening, *The Independent*, 16 September 1992).

I was seventeen when I first experienced the misery embodied in the word 'cystitis': the dreadful urge to pee every five minutes and the ghastly pain and burning. I was rapped over the knuckles by my GP for being promiscuous and packed off to the local VD clinic—despite being a virgin. So began an intimate relationship with my urinary tract that was to last a quarter of a century. Self-help routines such as peeing after sex and drinking gallons of water laced with bicarb limited the attacks to between four and six a year. But when push came to shove, antibiotics were the only answer.

Last winter I went down with pneumonia. Seven weeks and three courses of antibiotics later, I was just beginning to stagger up and down stairs when there it was, the unmistakeable dragging pain; the cystitis bacteria were back in business. I struggled on with the usual over the counter remedies—most of them variations on 'pot.cit.' (potassium citrate)—but it was no good, my resistance was too low. Ten days later my GP reluctantly prescribed the old standby, more antibiotics. But no sooner came relief than a relapse. This time no effect at all.

As well as the physical symptoms the sense of unease that always accompanied my attacks was by now verging on paranoia. I found myself seriously depressed and weeping hysterically over a boyfriend's illusory love affair; clearly I was in a bad way. A hospital appointment was made. The consultant was as sympathetic as anyone can be who has never been there. His diagnosis, if lacking in tact, was graphic: camel bladder, he called it. Over the years mine had stretched, and like an old balloon had lost its elasticity. As a result it never completely emptied but left that little soupçon behind, bursting with bacteria, all ready to infect the next intake of pee. He could offer no cure, but a prophylactic dose of antibiotics would keep the bacteria at bay, he said. Four times a day. For ever. Desperation overrode scepticism and I did as I was told. Then, two months later, a different set of symptoms broke cover. Same nether region, but this time the raw, dry itching of thrush. Thanks to the effectiveness of the antibiotics, candida yeasts were now up and at it and driving me mad. I stopped the pills. Within hours the cystitis was back.

A friend who believes antibiotics should carry a health warning persuaded me to try homeopathy. The first consultation cost £50, subsequent visits £25. Each time produced lots of chat, a new remedy, but no change.

By now I was completely incapacitated. My hot water bottle came with me everywhere. I even drove the car with it stuffed down my trousers. The thrush was back and, just to put the boot in, I had piles now, too. A full house. What about acupuncture, another friend asked. He could put me in touch with someone really good. Well, why not? I was at the end of the road.

Janine spent an hour going through my medical history. She took my pulses (each organ has its own, apparently) and found that the lower part of my body was colder than the rest. Had I noticed? Well, yes. The hot water bottle. It's what acupuncturists call damp heat, she told me, a significant cause being antibiotics. The cystitis, thrush, even the piles—everything was connected. All that was needed was a simple adjustment of my thermostat.

I don't know where she put the needles, I didn't watch. Somewhere on my left arm, I think. But, bizarre and irrational though it all was, I left feeling calm and well. That was in early November. Since then I have not had the slightest ache, twinge, sting or itch. It has gone. Just like that.

I have suffered too long to advise anyone to throw caution (i.e. pot.cit., yogurt or bicarb) to the wind. But if any of this nightmare rings bells, then it might be worth putting conventional medicine on hold. It is important not to forget that this is just **my** story and **my** happy ending. All I can say for sure is that for me it was without a doubt the best £35 I have ever spent, even though my fingers are still firmly crossed.

As Ms Dening says, this is just her story and her happy ending. One cannot draw any definite conclusions about the general efficacy of either orthodox or complementary treatment for cystitis, impressive though the final treatment seems to be. Her route to complementary medicine, essentially out of desperation, is only one possible pathway to using complementary medicine. Her account contains a number of important themes, however, which will recur throughout this book.

First, the content and tone of this account challenges various obstinate stereotypes that are sometimes invoked of the patient who seeks complementary treatment. Ms Dening does not appear to be stupid, naïve, credulous or dismissive of orthodox medicine. Nor does she appear to be neurotic by nature, though as she admits, the continual incapacitating attacks made her depressed.

Second, the complaint, cystitis, is chronic but not life threatening. In this instance conventional medicine was not effective, and this was an important factor in the decision to seek alternative forms of therapy. Chronic problems, usually requiring sustained and sympathetic treatment, are probably the most common ones encountered by complementary practitioners, just as they are for general practitioners. Failure to obtain relief of symptoms by conventional means and dissatisfaction with orthodox medicine or with orthodox practitioners may underlie a move to complementary medicine for some people.

Third, the account is a warning not to equate all forms of complementary medicine, either in terms of underlying philosophy, methods or the behaviour of practitioners. Homeopathy is clearly dismissed in this instance, while acupuncture, scepticism notwithstanding, appears to have been at least temporarily effective.

Fourth, there is the mystery of why one or two sessions of acupuncture proved effective after years of antibiotics and a course of homeopathic treatment. The natural progress of disease, 'tincture of time', is sometimes invoked as the explanation of the apparent success of complementary treatments. Here this seems improbable; the improvement is too rapid, and the history too long. It is possible that the acupuncture had some specific physiological effect, though the mechanism by which it might act is entirely unknown. Alternatively, some other concurrent factor or advice from the acupuncturist might have been responsible; reducing antibiotics, taking more rest or whatever.

Fifth, we can consider what other aspects of the therapeutic encounter might have provided a stimulus towards change. The initial session with the acupuncturist was long, the history appears to have been detailed, and there was a careful physical examination. The acupuncturist was sympathetic and attentive. Yet the consultant is also described as 'as sympathetic as anyone can be' and the homeopath provided 'plenty of chat', but neither led to recovery. Paying for treatment is sometimes thought to lead to the patient being more likely to value the treatment and be more ready to report improvements. However, homeopathy was also, in this instance, much more expensive but no more effective for all that.

Sixth, there is the actual system of medicine and the explanation it provides for the patient. The acupuncturist asks whether Ms Dening had noticed that part of her body was colder than the rest, and links various previously largely unconnected symptoms to a single basic imbalance. Understanding a variety of symptoms in terms of a single concept is, of course, equally a part of orthodox medicine; the suggestion is simply that it is important, not unique, to complementary medicine.

Finally, the sessions with the acupuncturist left her feeling 'calm and well'. The immediate experience of the treatment was positive, providing hope for the future and perhaps also indicative of enduring change.

The purpose of this book is to explore these and other themes from a research perspective. We consider why and how patients seek out various forms of complementary medicine and discuss the benefits they experience. Other academic books have already considered patients' experiences of complementary medicine (Sharma, 1992), and its historical context and relationship to orthodox medicine in both the United States and the United Kingdom (Salmon, 1985; Saks, 1992). While we draw on some of this work, our primary focus is on the empirical literature, particularly on that relating to the evaluation of complementary medicine and to studies that have examined the characteristics of the patients, practitioners and the encounters between them. We have limited discussion of the evaluation of complementary medicine to the major systems—acupuncture, osteopathy and chiropractic, homeopathy, herbalism and naturopathy. It is not feasible to review all the outcome literature in a single volume, which attempts to present a broad range of research from a number of perspectives, rather than focus exclusively on evaluation.

The literature on complementary medicine is scattered through many medical, psychological, and sociological journals, and in the growing number of specialist complementary medical journals. Several major reviews have been published of the efficacy of complementary therapies, and there are many other relevant and important studies. One of the primary purposes of this book is to draw this scattered literature together to acquaint the reader with the general features of this enormous literature.

While one of us has some personal experience of practising a form of complementary medicine, we do not consider ourselves experts on the philosophies, methods and practice of the various complementary therapies which, apart from anything else, would require a lifetime of study. There are already a considerable number of useful introductory books on complementary medicine (e.g. Stanway, 1986) and many books written for practitioners on the therapeutic techniques and underlying philosophy of individual therapies. However, these books do not tend to review or evaluate the empirical literature in any detail. It is our aim to provide a critical, comprehensive and balanced review of the current literature in this diverse field.

This book begins with an overview of the major therapies, their methods and philosophies. We then discuss the reasons people turn to complementary therapies, the characteristics of people who seek complementary treatment and the wide range of conditions which are treated. Chapter 4 reviews the relationship of complementary medicine with mainstream or orthodox medicine. We then move to the heart of the book: an evaluation of the major therapies according to criteria used in the scientific evaluation of new treatments within conventional medicine. By way of an introduction to the evaluation of therapies, Chapter 7 discusses the ubiquitous nature of the placebo effect in therapies of all kinds, whether complementary or orthodox. After addressing the very real methodological problems involved in the evaluation of complementary medicine, we review the evidence for the efficacy of each of the major therapies. Chapters 8 and 9 address psychological themes, the attitudes and beliefs of patients receiving

complementary treatment and the nature of the consultation with complementary practitioners. Finally we draw together the arguments developed
throughout the book to consider the appeal of complementary medicine, its
safety and efficacy and the direction that research into this fascinating topic
might take in years to come.

Chapter 1
████████████

Theories and Therapies

The term 'complementary medicine' embraces a wide range of therapeutic practices and diagnostic systems that stand separate from, or in some cases opposed to, conventional scientifically based modern, Western medicine. Previous terms used to describe these therapies have included fringe medicine, unconventional medicine, unorthodox medicine, natural medicine and, the most widely used, alternative medicine. In the last decade practitioners of many of these therapies have become less willing to be seen as providing an alternative to orthodox medical care, and certainly less willing to be seen as fringe practitioners, with its connotations of 'lunatic fringe'. Many now believe that they can work alongside doctors as independent practitioners with specialist knowledge. There has therefore been a gradual shift away from the use of unconventional, unorthodox and alternative towards the term 'complementary' medicine, which implies that the therapies are seen as supplements to orthodox medical treatment that enhance and strengthen the overall care offered to sick people.

In parallel with this development many doctors, particularly those in general practice, have shown an interest in and acceptance of many complementary therapies. 'The apparent success of many of the currently popular alternative strategies could be of great value to many of the patients seen in general practice. This is more likely if such strategies are seen as alternative treatments within the context of primary health care teams rather than "alternative medicine". The emergence of the concept of "complementary medicine" rather than "alternative medicine" bodes well for the future' (Freer, 1985).

In this book we have chosen, for the reasons given above, to use the term 'complementary medicine' rather than 'alternative medicine'. A less easy task has been to choose a phrase that suitably describes the treatment available in modern systems of health care, which is variously referred to as conventional medicine, scientific medicine, technical medicine, modern medicine and orthodox medicine. Technical medicine and modern medicine are too narrow in their scope. Scientific medicine seems both to overstate the dominance of science in medicine and also, in this context, to imply that complementary medicine could never be scientific (although complementary medicine is undoubtedly not science based). The central importance of the scientific method does indicate that the definition of medicine is not simply conventional or cultural, and so we have opted to describe modern, scientific medicine as 'orthodox medicine', while recognizing that this, too, is not entirely satisfactory.

Many complementary therapies are, of course, only considered to be complementary or alternative in countries where orthodox, Western medicine is the dominant mode of practice. In China, for instance, acupuncture is very much part of mainstream medicine with both Western-trained and traditional medicine doctors undergoing an extensive and largely parallel training. Although attitudes to, and beliefs about, acupuncture vary considerably, it is so widely used in hospitals that it could never be considered an alternative to Western medicine. Similarly, the World Health Organization is encouraging the use of medicinal plants and herbs in many poor, underdeveloped areas of the Pacific Rim, where drugs are simply not available. In such a situation one would not want to use the term 'complementary medicine' to describe such treatment.

THE VARIETIES OF COMPLEMENTARY MEDICINE

The British Medical Association report on alternative therapy (BMA, 1986) listed 116 different types of therapy and diagnostic aid, though the subsequent report (BMA, 1993) concentrated on the much smaller number which are both widely used and represented by professional organizations. The history, philosophy and methods of these different practices are extremely diverse. The origins of some, for example acupuncture, are ancient while others have been developed comparatively recently. Some, such as traditional acupuncture and homeopathy, constitute complete systems of medicine, others are restricted to diagnosis alone (iridology) or to a specific therapeutic technique (massage). Some styles of practice attempt a whole person view, while others are content with the treatment of specific symptoms. Some complementary practitioners have had no formal training whatever, while others (e.g. osteopaths) have attended rigorous full-time courses to degree level, which include a thorough grounding in human anatomy and physiology. While they all differ to some extent from orthodox medicine in both philosophy and practice, there is no sharp dividing line: 'The philosophies of radionics or healing are utterly at odds with conventional medical principles but the bases of osteopathy or herbalism are quasi-scientific and could be incorporated into conventional medicine without stretching its scientific model to breaking point' (Fulder, 1984).

Pietroni (1986) presents a useful classification of the different approaches in complementary medicine. He distinguishes:

1. Psychological approaches and self-help exercises, such as breathing and relaxation, meditation, exercise regimes and visualization.
2. Specific therapeutic methods, such as massage, reflexology, aromatherapy and spiritual healing.
3. Diagnostic methods, such as iridology, kinesiology and hair analysis.
4. Complete systems of healing, such as acupuncture, herbal medicine, osteopathy, chiropractic, homeopathy and naturopathy.

This book focuses predominantly on the last category, complete systems of medicine which offer distinct approaches to the diagnosis and treatment of a wide range of complaints and disorders. These therapies are the most frequently used in Europe, North America and Australasia and are the most developed in terms of philosophy, research and professional status. They constitute the heart of complementary medicine, which is not necessarily to say that other complementary approaches do not have value and status. However, discussion and research on complementary medicine frequently involves reference to an enormous range of practices and so the other approaches are also briefly described.

PSYCHOLOGICAL APPROACHES AND SELF-HELP

Fulder (1984), in his valuable *Handbook of Complementary Medicine*, specifically excluded psychological therapies 'in order to keep the book within manageable proportions'. He cited President Carter's commission on mental health which listed 140 separate psychotherapies. We agree that most psychological therapies should not be considered within the rubric of complementary medicine. There is certainly a kind of complementary psychotherapy, encompassing a variety of humanistic and Eastern approaches, even though there is not yet agreement about what should constitute orthodox psychotherapy. Many of these approaches are practised outside orthodox medicine and have unusual philosophies and methods of treatment. Examples are psychosynthesis, developed by Roberto Assagioli, a pupil of Freud's; bioenergetics, the creation of Wilhelm Reich; the Gestalt therapy of Frederick Perls; autogenic relaxation techniques, encounter groups and co-counselling. However, most are not primarily aimed at the treatment of medical conditions, and therefore should not really be considered as medicine, whether orthodox or complementary. There are borderline cases, such as hypnotherapy which is employed in the alleviation of specific medical symptoms and is frequently listed as a complementary medical technique. Many practitioners, both orthodox and complementary, also suggest to their patients that they take courses in relaxation or meditation as an aid to recovery and may recommend particular psychological exercises, such as visualization, as an adjunct to treatment. Many see these as preferable to tranquillizers and antidepressants, which may be addictive, do not encourage patients to address the underlying cause of anxiety and depression or empower them to help themselves. Because these techniques are primarily used as adjuncts to the main treatment, we consider them as only having subsidiary status in complementary medicine. We have also followed Fulder (1984) in distinguishing between techniques used in the healing or treatment of sick people and those used by healthy people for physical, psychological or spiritual development. Yoga, T'ai Chi, sport, prayer and meditation as a spiritual practice all fall outside our definition of complementary medicine.

SPECIFIC THERAPEUTIC METHODS

In contrast to the psychological therapies, the methods described in this section undoubtedly qualify as complementary techniques. They are often allied to a theory or philosophy but lack the development of the systems that underlie acupuncture, homeopathy and so on. The following are some examples:

Massage Techniques

Massage is, of course, widely used by physiotherapists and others, in orthodox medicine as well as outside medicine, as a treatment for minor ailments and for relaxation. Complementary forms of massage are distinguished by being allied to distinct philosophies and systems of diagnosis. Reflexology, for instance, concentrates on massage of the feet and is based on a system of relationships in which each organ of the body corresponds to a particular area of the foot; tender areas on the feet are both signs of imbalance elsewhere in the body and foci for treatment of these disorders. Rolfing is a deep, whole body massage technique aimed at breaking down abnormal connective tissue and restoring proper posture and balance. Shiatsu therapy is massage based on the acupuncture system of meridians, energy flow and acupuncture points.

Sense Therapies

Both sound and colour are used for therapeutic purposes in many systems of medicine and religious traditions. Sound and colour therapy are available in Britain, but the most popular sense therapy (Fulder, 1984) is aromatherapy, in which plant oils, vapours and essences are massaged into the skin or sometimes inhaled or taken internally. Aromatherapists match oils to the person and their condition, using several different diagnostic methods.

Healing

Healing, whether at a distance or by laying on of hands and therapeutic touch, is widely used for all manner of medical conditions. Healing can mean marshalling the will-power and faith of the patient, but more commonly implies an active transmission of some kind of therapeutic energy between healer and patient. This may or may not be associated with particular religious beliefs. All major religions have pre- and proscribed ways of healing, nearly all of which require touch. Although we do not discuss healing *per se* in any detail, it is important to note that many complementary practitioners consider that some form of healing occurs during treatment. Most doctors, and probably all psychologists, would agree that the relationship between patient and practitioner is an extremely important component of treatment. However, some, acupuncturists for instance, also believe that the attitude and intention of the practitioner during the treatment has a direct effect on the energy change they are seeking to produce within their patient. Healing could in this sense be seen as integral to complementary medicine.

DIAGNOSTIC METHODS

All the major complementary systems of medicine have their own diagnostic methods, but some complementary approaches are primarily systems of diagnosis which may be used in the context of a number of different forms of treatment. Some of the better known methods are listed below:

Iridology

A technique in which detailed, microscopic observation of the eye, often from photographs, is used to diagnose illness and disorder. Each organ and body system is held to be reflected in the patterns and colours of the iris. The idea that the state of the whole body is mapped on to a particular part is found elsewhere in complementary medicine; in reflexology it is the foot and in auricular acupuncture each area of the body has a corresponding point on the ear.

Radionics

A system of diagnosis and treatment in which a hair or blood sample from the patient is assessed using a pendulum, or special instrument, with the radionics practitioner mentally posing questions and sensing the answer. The pendulum and instruments appear to help the practitioner focus on the patient (who is not necessarily present). Treatment, often homeopathic remedies, minerals or tissue salts, can be selected on this basis.

Kirlian Photography

This system uses photography in which the subject is placed in a high frequency alternating electric field. The photographs show an aura or energy body around any living tissue which, in the case of humans at least, changes shape and colour according to emotional state and in the presence of disease.

COMPLEMENTARY SYSTEMS OF MEDICINE

The therapies considered in this section are the main complementary ones practised in Europe, North America and Australasia today. Each therapy is associated with a coherent and systematic theory of the functioning of the body and the mode of action of the therapy, which is not to say that the theory is necessarily correct or that it has been subjected to any kind of empirical testing. Practitioners of these therapies usually belong to professional associations and have undertaken a course of professional training. The therapies discussed—acupuncture, herbalism, homeopathy, osteopathy, chiropractic and naturopathy—are by no means the only complementary approaches which could be described as systems of medicine. The anthroposophical medicine of Rudolph Steiner, for instance, is also a complex and well-elaborated system but it has not attained the same prominence. However, these are the major systems actually practised and those that have been most researched. The sketches of each therapy are only intended to highlight the principal ideas underlying each approach and the main therapeutic methods. For more detail the reader is referred to Fulder (1984), Stanway (1986), or books on the individual therapies cited in the text.

Acupuncture

Traditional Chinese medicine, which uses a combination of acupuncture, herbs, diet and exercise, dates from about 3000 BC. Acupuncture is now the most widely used component, although many acupuncturists also use herbs in their work. The essential idea underlying acupuncture is that the human body is an energy system which reflects health, disease and emotional states. The task of the traditional acupuncturist is to detect subtle changes in the energy flow, correct any deficiencies or excesses, and so restore health and harmony to the individual. The energy flows through channels known as meridians, each associated with a particular organ or function of the body. The acupuncture points, places where the energy may be manipulated, are located along the meridians. Treatment is carried out by inserting and manipulating needles at acupuncture points, or sometimes by heating or massaging the points.

In diagnosis the acupuncturist takes a careful history, but also observes the colour of the face, the sound of the voice, the odour of the body and the person's emotional disposition. Particularly important are the twelve pulses, six on each wrist, each associated with one of the main meridians. The diagnosis can be made in terms of the eight principles of acupuncture, in which disease is classified as strong–weak, yin–yang, internal–external or hot–cold, or as one of the five elements, or fundamental forms of energy: fire, earth, metal, water or wood. Whichever conceptual system is employed, the diagnosis points to the meridians that are out of balance and the acupuncture points that should be treated to restore health. From this perspective any disease or malaise can be assessed and a diagnosis offered, even if the symptoms are slight or do not conform to any recognized orthodox diagnosis. In practice, most acupuncturists recognize that many disorders do not respond to acupuncture and that acupuncture should sometimes only be given as a supplement to orthodox treatment (O'Connor and Bensky, 1981; Lewith and Lewith, 1983; Vincent and Richardson, 1986).

Herbalism

Plants have been used for medicinal purposes for at least 5000 years. A number of modern drugs (digitalis, for example) derive from plant material, although the active ingredients are now almost always extracted or synthesized. Modern Western herbalists use much the same terminology and concepts and many of the same diagnostic methods as orthodox medicine, but they are interested in detecting imbalance and restoring normal function rather than acting to reverse pathology. Herbalists are strongly impressed by the ability of the body to correct its own imbalances, and see themselves as supporting the action of the vital adaptive energy of the body. Herbal remedies can provoke protective reactions within the body, act to stimulate the elimination of toxins and in some cases are seen as foods that provide the body with a balance of nutrients and minerals. Remedies may contain a complex mixture of constituents: a dozen would not be unusual. Herbalists consider that complex combinations of actual plant material are generally more effective in promoting health than the specific isolated compounds used in modern pharmacology. However, they would acknowledge the importance of drugs in acute or severe conditions. Herbal medicine comes into its own in treating chronic functional conditions where the aim is a gradual return to full health using gentler remedies which stimulate the body to heal itself (Mills and Fulder, cited in Fulder 1984; Mills, 1993a).

Homeopathy

Homeopathy was formulated by Dr Samuel Hahnemann, who published the first textbook of homeopathy in 1810. Like herbalists, homeopaths view the body as being sustained by a vital energy. The task of the homeopath is to stimulate this vital force and allow healing to take place. A skilled homeopath can detect imbalances and dysfunctions before a disease actually manifests. Diagnosis takes account of changes that may be physical, sensory, emotional, mental or even moral. Diagnosis is expressed not as the name of a disease, but as the name of the remedy that corresponds to it. The fundamental principle of treatment is to give a remedy which would provoke an identical symptom complex in the patient on the principle that like should be cured by like. The use of vaccines to stimulate the production of natural antibodies could be seen as a parallel approach. However, the aspect of homeopathy which has caused most controversy is Hahnemann's observation that minute doses were more effective in stimulating healing than conventional doses. Homeopathic remedies are frequently, but not always, diluted to the point where it seems inconceivable that any single molecule of the original substance could be left. Various explanations are given for the action of these remedies: one is that a dissolved substance leaves an imprint in water after high dilution. Others consider that homeopathic remedies operate at a subtle level not amenable to scientific investigation. Homeopathy is used in many minor acute conditions and in a wide range of chronic problems (Fulder 1984; Ullman, 1991).

Manipulative Therapies: Osteopathy and Chiropractic

An osteopath is a practitioner who is skilled in the examination, treatment and interpretation of abnormalities of function of the musculo–skeletal system. The first school of osteopathy was founded in 1892, based on a theory developed by Andrew Still some twenty years earlier. Osteopathy has evolved considerably since Still's time, but the fundamental principle is that a wide variety of problems can be traced to disorders of the musculo–skeletal system, particularly the spinal vertebrae. Back pain is the most frequently treated problem, though many osteopaths see their role as being wider than this and will also treat respiratory problems and other chronic conditions. In diagnosis the osteopath uses many orthodox techniques but also carefully observes the patient walking, sitting and at rest and carries out a detailed physical examination. Like many complementary therapists, the osteopath is looking for minor areas of dysfunction that may be a prelude to later problems, as well as searching for the cause of the presenting complaint. The final diagnosis is formulated in terms of mobility, muscle tone or altered posture. Treatment consists of massage of soft tissue, the manipulation of joints and muscle and a number of other techniques. Some osteopaths also practice cranial techniques, in which a patient's head is held, with little or no movement being made. This extremely gentle intervention could be considered a form of direct healing, and is at the other extreme from the popular image of the osteopath as cracking or popping joints and bringing instantaneous relief.

Chiropractic was also developed towards the end of the last century and similarly holds that many common conditions are caused by, or at least aggravated by, misalignments or excessive strain placed on the vertebrae or other joints. Although we will generally consider the techniques together, as therapies based on manipulation, both osteopaths and chiropractors are adamant that there are important differences in technique and theory. Chiropractic lays more emphasis on the joint itself, while osteopathy lays equal emphasis on the joint and adjacent muscles, fascia (fibrous supporting tissues) and ligaments that make up each spinal vertebra. In diagnosis chiropractors place major emphasis on X-ray evidence, whereas osteopaths may be more concerned to diagnose by physical examination and touch. The methods of manipulation also differ. Chiropractors use sharp, short, thrusting pressure on the spine, whereas osteopaths tend to use more rhythmical and gentler pressure on the whole body including the spine.

Naturopathy

Naturopathy, more than any other complementary therapy, is a system which holds that healing depends on a vital curative force within the human organism. The guiding principle is that the body is capable of healing itself, given the proper conditions. Although such ideas can be traced back to Hippocrates, the basic naturopathic concepts were formulated in the early part of the twentieth century by an American doctor named Henry Linlahr. Naturopathy is first and foremost a preventative system of medicine aimed at maintaining and promoting full health.

Naturopaths use many conventional diagnostic techniques, such as blood tests, but will also rely upon iridology and hair analysis. Their diagnosis attempts a formulation of the patient's total state of health, with the presenting symptom being seen as only an aspect of the overall picture. Treatment consists of prescribing a therapeutic regime for the patient to follow, which will enable him or her to regain full health. The naturopath is more of a guide or teacher than a therapist and it is essential that the patient take an active and responsible part in the treatment. Nutritional and dietary measures are fundamental. If the patient is very debilitated, a wholefood diet, vitamin and mineral supplements, together with rest, relaxation, exercise and gentle manipulative procedures may be recommended. With conditions where there is an accumulation of toxins, dietary restriction, fasting and hydrotherapy may be instituted. Many naturopaths also consider the psychological and social aspects of illness and practise other complementary therapies in addition; naturopathy is almost always multidisciplinary in nature (Newman-Turner, 1990a).

THE PRACTICE OF COMPLEMENTARY MEDICINE

How do orthodox and complementary medicine practitioners differ in their diagnosis and consultation?

Diagnosis and Consultation

Diagnosis in orthodox medicine begins, as in complementary medicine, by taking a careful history and with a physical examination. Thereafter tests of various kinds become important in an effort to confirm or disconfirm the hypotheses that constitute a tentative diagnosis: blood tests, X-rays of various kinds, scans and perhaps biopsy may be employed. These tests can be invasive, painful and distressing, and some patients may be reluctant to have them, or even be suspicious of 'high-tech' medicine.

Diagnosis within complementary medicine also consists of taking a careful history, although more information of a personal and psychological nature may be sought. Observation, touch and sensitive palpation are given a high priority in most systems. Fulder (1984) uses the oriental diagnosis used in traditional acupuncture as an example, as it contains most of the procedures used in other systems:

> The key to oriental diagnosis is that inner states are projected onto a screen. Oriental pathology is highly complex and systemised, classifying diseases by means of qualities of body function (such as hot/cold, damp/dry) and qualities of the various body energies (such as stagnant energy, withdrawn) . . . These qualities can be read by a sensitive and trained practitioner. The colour and texture of the tongue and skin, the timbre of the voice, the distribution of hot or cold patches, the responses and actions, the smell and appearance of the urine and body secretions and above all the qualities and strengths of the twelve pulses.

Other complementary therapists use similar methods. Osteopaths naturally pay particular attention to posture and to tensions and pressures the patient describes or shows. Naturopaths may in addition use some of the diagnostic techniques described earlier, such as iridology.

Leaving aside the question of the value of these techniques, we can ask what difference a complementary approach makes to the patient. The patient will probably be questioned more widely about their lifestyle and values, more personally (about issues not immediately relevant to the problem) and at a considerably greater length than in the average general practice consultation. Few private patients in orthodox medicine, who always get more time and attention than National Health Service patients, would be given the time that most complementary patients receive at a fraction of the cost. The physical examination, whatever form it takes, will probably be more leisurely, gentler and more soothing than the National Health Service allows most doctors to be. The most striking aspect of the complementary diagnosis is that it provides a radically different explanation of the patient's symptoms than an orthodox diagnosis. General practitioners are faced with a large number of patients who are by no means well, but who have no clearly diagnosable condition. This 'undifferentiated illness' has been considered to be especially fertile ground for complementary medicine by both sceptics and adherents (Lewith, 1988). As we have seen, a diagnosis can be made by a complementary practitioner whatever the malaise in question. This in itself may provide hope, comfort and legitimization for the patient—just as, of course, a diagnosis from a doctor will.

Treatment

A wide variety of therapies and treatment techniques come under the umbrella of complementary therapy. Murray and Rubel (1992) divide them into four categories:

1. Spiritual and psychological techniques ranging from faith healers, paranormal healing and divination, visualization and hypnosis.
2. Nutritional therapies, including some herbal treatments, vitamin and mineral supplements and specific dietary regimes, such as macrobiotics.
3. Biological and pharmacological: herbal remedies, drugs, serums and vaccines and, although they do not really fit here, homeopathic remedies.
4. Physical interventions: manipulative therapies, massage, acupuncture.

Common themes are difficult to discern in this mixture. Indeed, one attraction of complementary medicine to general practitioners is the fact that a wide range of additional skills and interventions is on offer. Freer (1985) has commented that for general practitioners faced with chronic problems, the ultimate skill is not to run out of therapeutic choices, so additional skills and interventions may be very welcome. Complementary practitioners, although usually having one major specialty, may use, comment on and recommend a very wide range of different treatment methods in routine clinical practice. The most widely used supplementary regimes are diet, exercise, vitamins, herbal remedies, massage and relaxation. These are core treatments drawn on by many practitioners. Referral to other complementary and orthodox practitioners is also not unusual, so that many patients will have seen several practitioners of different kinds for their current problem (Canter and Nanke, 1989).

Different patients will be attracted to different forms of complementary medicine, both because they view them as particularly suitable for their condition and because of the nature of the therapy. In osteopathy, chiropractic, massage and, to a lesser extent, acupuncture, the patient is touched a great deal, which may be particularly important to some people. Herbal remedies and homeopathy are medical in style, in that little may be required of the patient other than that they take the remedy. Other patients may value a therapy that encourages a change in lifestyle. Patients of complementary practitioners appear to be treated more as partners in the treatment process and are encouraged to take an active part in their treatment where possible (Aakster, 1989). Many patients attending complementary therapy may be attracted by a greater involvement in the treatment process, and it is probable that this greater involvement and sense of responsibility is itself beneficial.

A DIVERSITY OF THEORIES, PHILOSOPHIES AND THERAPIES

Complementary medicine is often treated as a single entity in the orthodox medical literature. Questions such as, 'Why do patients turn to complementary medicine?' or 'Should complementary medicine be available on the NHS?' all imply that the various complementary therapies have similar philosophies and are of equal value. It must now be clear that this is far from the truth. Origins, philosophies, extent of empirical backing vary widely.

The origins of the various therapies are extremely diverse: acupuncture has its roots in traditional Chinese medicine several thousand years ago, homeopathy in Germany in the early nineteenth century, osteopathy and chiropractic in the United States in the late nineteenth and early twentieth centuries. The theoretical frameworks employed vary in coherence, complexity, underlying philosophy and the degree to which they could be incorporated in current scientific medicine. Complementary practitioners vary enormously in their attitude to science and orthodox medicine, the extent of their training and their desire for professional recognition. The range of treatments given is equally diverse: diet, plant remedies, needles, minuscule homeopathic doses, mineral and vitamin supplements and a variety of psychological techniques. Canter and Nanke (1991) give some examples:

> Iridologists with their arcane diagnostic system have virtually nothing in common with osteopaths who spend a number of years in training studying human anatomy in great detail. The bizarre, pseudo-scientific explanations of gem therapy bear no relationship to the carefully articulated but virtually science free accounts of homeopathy. The use of plants and infusions by naturopaths make some pharmacological sense but is antithetical to the very small, virtually non existent, doses of homeopathy. The list is endless as to the forms of treatment and associated diagnoses that are used by complementary practitioners and the variety of ways in which they contradict each other.

The diversity found within complementary medicine may not be generally perceived either by doctors or by the general public who make use of complementary practitioners. People may perceive complementary medicine as having certain attributes, desirable or not, whether or not all the associated practices actually have these features. They may believe, for instance, that all complementary therapies treat the whole person, although individual therapies may vary considerably in the meaning they give to 'the whole person' and the extent to which this ideal is important.

Although there is considerable variation, the complementary therapies do share some common features which can be approached from two distinct viewpoints. The first is essentially a view from within, from the perspective of complementary medicine itself. Are there any defining features in theory, philosophy or practice? The second is a view from outside, from the perspective of orthodox medicine. This is the position usually taken by the writers of editorials in medical journals discussing, like us, the appeal of complementary medicine. From this second viewpoint, complementary medicine is usually defined by the ways it differs from orthodox medicine, essentially by an absence of some of the characteristic features of orthodox medicine. This latter perspective is discussed in Chapter 3.

COMMON THEMES IN THE PHILOSOPHIES OF COMPLEMENTARY THERAPIES

In this section we consider the viewpoint from within complementary medicine. What common features do the various therapies have in terms of their underlying theory, philosophy and approach to health and illness? We will primarily consider the major systems of complementary medicine: acupuncture, herbalism, homeopathy, osteopathy, chiropractic and naturo-pathy, which constitute in our view the heart of complementary medicine.

Vitalistic Philosophy

Many systems of complementary medicine embrace the idea that the body and emotions, mental and spiritual life, are all maintained by an underlying energy or vital force. Some kind of vital energy is postulated by acu-puncturists, herbalists, homeopaths and naturopaths. Health and disease are a reflection of balance and imbalance within this system, or viewed as an interaction between positive life-enhancing forces and negative destructive forces. In naturopathy the positive force is described as the principle of Vis Medicatrix, that is, a natural curative power which is activated by any injury or disease (Newman-Turner, 1990a; Ullman, 1991).

The Body is Self-healing

The belief in an underlying vital force or energy is closely associated with the view that the body is essentially self-healing, and the task of the practitioner is to assist the healing process—a fundamentally gentler approach to treatment than orthodox medicine. This belief and approach to treatment is expressed well by Fulder (1984) who, while acknowledging the immense diversity within complementary medicine, states that there is a 'common bond':

> They all attempt, in varying degrees, to recruit the self-healing capacities of the body. They amplify natural recuperative processes and augment the energy upon which the patient's health depends, helping him to adapt harmoniously to his surroundings. Symptoms are sometimes treated at the outset, as in osteopathy or chiropractic, or can be left to clear up by themselves as the individual progresses towards health, as in traditional acupuncture. In all cases, however, the symptoms are used as tools or guides to the nature of the patient's imbalance.

The emphasis on self-healing has a corollary which is important psychologically, and affects the relationship between the complementary practitioner and patient. Because the patient's body is viewed as healing itself, rather than being acted upon by drugs or surgery, the patient must do what they can to help themselves. Many of the therapies are partly instructional and many therapists take the view that improper eating habits, impure food or an unhealthy lifestyle are powerfully implicated in the genesis of disease (Newman-Turner, 1990a). The patient is encouraged to discover why they are sick and to work for their own cure, with the therapist as a partner in the enterprise. In some cases the journey to health is also seen as a journey to self-discovery (Fulder, 1984).

A General All-encompassing Theory of Disease

Complementary therapies tend to have a single, all-encompassing theory of disease. Fulder's remark that symptoms are used as guides to the nature of the general imbalance leads us to another defining feature: specific symptoms are seen as the most obvious manifestation of a general imbalance or dysfunction affecting the whole system. Any doctor views symptoms as indicating an underlying disorder, but a complementary practitioner seeks to diagnose in a more general sense. Specific symptoms are seen as the most obvious manifestation of a general imbalance or dysfunction affecting the whole system. For instance, in the energy systems of traditional acupuncture, disease is always a manifestation of energy imbalance. Similarly, Reckeweg, a prominent German naturopath, theorized that all disease is caused by homotoxins, autotoxic or useless residues, and that elimination of such homotoxins will clear the body of the disease. A corollary of these theories is the claim by some complementary practitioners to be treating the whole person rather than just the specific symptoms.

Prevention and Positive Health

An ideal state of mental and physical health is implicit in many of the theories. Newman-Turner (1990a) begins his book on naturopathy with a discussion of the nature of health before discussing the naturopathic conception of disease. Acupuncturists hope to correct minor imbalances in the energy system before they manifest as actual illness. Poor vitality and low resistance to infection are seen as treatable conditions by homeopaths (Ullman, 1991), whereas a general practitioner would only consider treating more serious fatigue and actual infections as they occur. Much complementary medicine aims to be preventative in nature, as exemplified by the ancient Chinese, who were supposed to pay their physician only when they were well! If they fell ill, their physician had failed in his duty.

Being maintained in good health is an immensely attractive idea, and important if it has any validity. It is interesting that a criticism that is sometimes made of Western medicine, that many ordinary events in life have been over-medicalized (Illich, 1976), applies especially powerfully to complementary medicine. Complementary medicine tends to draw more emotional and physical malaise into the medical arena. The psychological effects of considering any slight malaise as something that requires treatment are not necessarily beneficial, an issue which is discussed further in the final chapter.

IS COMPLEMENTARY MEDICINE HOLISTIC?

Complementary medicine is sometimes equated with holistic medicine, and the idea that complementary medicine is inherently more holistic than orthodox medicine might be considered a further way of defining the attraction of the complementary approach.

Holistic medicine is not an easy term to define. Pietroni (1987) considers it to involve:

1. Responding to the person as a whole (body, mind and spirit) within the context of his environment (family, culture and ecology).
2. Willingness to use a wide range of interventions, from drugs and surgery to meditation and diet.

3. An emphasis on a participatory relationship between doctor and patient.
4. An awareness of the impact of the 'health' of the practitioner on the patient (physician heal thyself).

Pietroni (1987) describes a clinician who, for many people, would be the ideal practitioner (whether orthodox or complementary)—sensitive to psychological and social issues, non-authoritarian, trying to guide the patient towards the most appropriate treatment and so on. It is clear from his definition that a holistic approach derives more from the practitioner than the kind of medicine they practise. A surgeon might be a holistic practitioner, while an acupuncturist might not. It is an open, and essentially empirical, question whether the styles of practice and consultations of complementary and orthodox practitioners vary to any great extent. The notion that complementary practitioners are inherently more holistic has been indignantly attacked by some doctors:

> It seems to me that complementary therapists, and others interested in these approaches, have hijacked the idea of holism. It is true, of course, that there are doctors who are not very good at their job who do not handle their patients and their illness in a holistic manner. Doubtless the same is true of complementary therapists, but it must be refuted as sheer nonsense to say that conventional medicine is not holistic in its outlook. (Baum, 1987)

While there seems no doubt that a doctor can practice in a holistic way, the daily pressures and the increasingly specialized and technical nature of modern medicine may conspire to prevent the doctor providing the kind of care that he or she would wish. Whorton (1989) has argued that under these circumstances patients may turn to alternative, more holistic practices. His account of alternative medicine in the nineteenth century has many parallels with the position of complementary medicine in the late twentieth century. The need for patients to take personal responsibility for their health, the emphasis on more natural methods of treatment, a greater reliance on the body's own healing powers and a concern with iatrogenic illness (e.g. the effects of bleeding, blistering and other therapeutic assaults) and the battle with the medical profession are familiar themes. While having no particular sympathy with the alternative practices (some of which were distinctly unpleasant) he does point out that:

> The introduction of naturopathy reminds us that while there were still more 19th century alternative systems (magnetic healing, eclecticism, chrono-thermalism and others), each with a unique theory and practice, all were linked by their reverence for nature and their reliance on natural recovery. Preisnitz and other irregulars may have deserved the 'quack, quack, quack' japery of allopaths. At the same time, however, their repeated demonstrations of the strength and resilience of the human body have tempered scientific medicine's urge to treat every ailment aggressively.

Holism can be considered in another way, as a property of the theory or philosophy underlying an approach to medicine. Many complementary theories do emphasize the importance of a person's emotional and sometimes spiritual state in the assessment and treatment of disease. In practice, this will mean that many complementary practitioners will routinely enquire about emotional issues, whether or not a psychological problem is a presenting symptom. An orthodox practitioner may also enquire about emotional problems where it seems relevant, but it is not an integral part of every diagnosis. In this sense, some complementary systems might be said to be more holistic, though in practice the clinical manner and approach of individual complementary therapists probably varies considerably. Nevertheless, the emphasis on emotional factors may encourage an empathy and sensitivity in complementary practitioners which may be a very important aspect of their appeal.

COMPARING COMPLEMENTARY AND ORTHODOX MEDICINE

Just as a holistic approach cannot clearly define the boundaries between complementary and orthodox medicine, so most of the defining features we have discussed are a matter of degree rather than absolute standards. Some complementary practitioners aspire to be scientific in their approach, much orthodox medicine is preventative, work on the evaluation of quality of life is a move towards a broader view of health and so on. Any doctor will recognize that a physician can only assist in the healing process, and may also resist the charge that drugs interfere with the body's natural healing capacities.

> Many homeopathic practitioners choose to stigmatize drugs such as cimetidine as powerful allopathic repressive therapy that poisons the natural reparative capacity of the body. I choose to look upon this group of drugs as restoring the natural harmony between the sympathetic and parasympathetic nervous systems, following which established mucosal ulcers will heal under the natural stimuli of local cellular growth factors and hormones. (Baum, 1987)

Although there is no absolute dividing line on clinical, theoretical or professional issues, there are nevertheless differences of emphasis between orthodox and complementary approaches. Many of these have been discussed, but they are helpfully summarized by Aakster (1989) in his comparison of two textbooks, one on orthodox medicine and one edited book on complementary medicine (Table 1.1).

Table 1.1 Comparison of orthodox and complementary medicine

Dimension	Orthodox medicine	Complementary medicine
Model of thinking	'Classical': causality, linearity, specialization, differentiation, materialization, short-time perspective	'Perspectivistic': regulation (feedback), interaction development, connectedness, wholeness, learning
Definition of disease	Organ-specific, accent upon lesion	Functional status, imbalance
Epidemiology	Secondary in interest	General interest in relation to environment
Causation	Linear causality, priority with material factors	Interactive development
Natural history	Accent upon full grown clinical pathology	Interest in (early) development of disease
Pathology	Of central importance	Second in priority
Clinical features	Accent upon organ-bound signs	Interest in complete picture of dysfunctions
Diagnostic procedures	Organ-specific measurement, technical approach, accent upon material	Whole person context, also psychology and energetic, soft methods
Treatment	Organ-specific, technical, accent upon material	Directed at regulation, self-correcting measures, also psychology and energetic aspects
Complications	Secondary in interest, high tolerance for harmfulness	Excluded by choice, low tolerance for harmfulness
Rehabilitation	Secondary in interest, accent upon elimination of disease	Of central importance, orientation upon restoration of health
Care organization	Hospital oriented, differentiated care	Ambulant care, direct access to comprehensive care
Prevention	Secondary in interest, technical and individualized measures	Of central importance, awareness and behaviour of the patient, societal/environmental measures
Doctor–patient relationship	Secondary in interest, detached concern	Often of prime interest, condition in therapeutic process, education of the patient
Position of patient	Passive, dependent	Active, partner, responsible
Cost and burdens	Secondary interest	Certain awareness

(From Aakster, 1989. Reproduced by permission of Elsevier Science Inc.)

While some of Aakster's conclusions are rather extreme and the dimensions too obviously polarized, the different perspectives of orthodox and complementary medicine do emerge. Many of these dimensions, however, are only likely to be of direct relevance to practitioners, whether orthodox or complementary. The philosophical underpinnings may not be relevant, or even apparent, to many patients. What will matter more to them and determine whether they attend and later recommend complementary medicine, is the nature of the treatment and consultation and whether it appears to help them. In other words, how the theory and philosophy translate into practice. The next chapter considers why patients seek out complementary medicine and the complex paths they take through the various therapies.

Chapter 2

Pathways to Complementary Medicine

When people feel unwell they have a considerable number of therapeutic options. They may consult a home medical encyclopaedia, a family member, a friend who has suffered from the same complaint, their local general practitioner, or a complementary practitioner. In practice, people may follow a quite complex path, reaching a complementary therapist only after consulting a number of other people, both lay and professional.

Helman (1990), following Kleinman (1980), divides health care into three sectors: the folk sector, the popular sector, and the professional sector. Each sector has its own individual approach to health and illness, its own methods of treatment and characteristic relationship between patients and practitioners. The professional sector refers to what we have described as orthodox medicine. Folk medicine includes all forms of complementary medicine, together with both sacred and secular forms of healing. The popular sector encompasses all forms of self-medication, advice or help given without payment from any lay person, self-help groups and support organizations. Helman (1990) describes the folk and popular sectors, which provide the major part of medical care, as the 'hidden health care system'.

FOLK MEDICINE

The extent to which folk medicine is perceived as antithetical to orthodox care varies considerably from country to country, especially when the technique is rooted in the culture of the country. In some societies folk medicine is both well established and highly regarded. For instance, in Finland Vaskilampi (1990) has noted that many folk medical techniques are widely accepted, in fact embedded, in the culture and yet might be seen as alternative or complementary therapies in other European countries. Finnish folk medicine includes manipulative methods, such as massage and bone-setting, herbs, and naturopathic techniques, such as hydrotherapy and shamanistic healing. Vaskilampi in fact separates these folk techniques from complementary systems of medicine, such as chiropractic, osteopathy, homeopathy and herbalism, on the grounds that the complementary therapies are of generally more recent development and have different roots from the traditional folk methods.

THE POPULAR SECTOR

Some people avoid health professionals if at all possible, preferring to treat themselves and ask family members and friends for help, advice and therapy. According to Helman (1990) there are certain individuals, though, who tend to act as a source of health advice more often than others. These include:

1. Those with long experience of a particular illness, or type of treatment.
2. Those with extensive experience of certain life events, such as women who have raised several children.
3. Doctors' wives or husbands, who share some of their spouses' experience if not training.
4. Individuals such as chiropodists and hairdressers, who sometimes act as lay confessor or psychotherapist.
5. The organizers of self-help groups.
6. The members or officiants of certain healing cults or churches.

All of these people may be considered as sources of advice and assistance on health matters by their friends or families. Their credentials are mainly their own experience rather than education, training or social status. A woman who has had several pregnancies, for example, can give informal advice to a newly pregnant young woman, telling her what symptoms to expect and how to deal with them. More worryingly, a person with long experience of a particular medication may 'lend' some to a friend with similar symptoms.

Even within the popular sector there are a considerable number of thera-peutic options. Helman (1990, pp. 56–57) notes:

> Among these options are: self-treatment or self-medication; advice or treat-ment given by a relative or friend, neighbour or workmate; healing and mutual care activities in a church, cult or self-help group; or consultation with another lay person who has special experience of a particular disorder, or of treatment of a physical state. The main arena of health care is the family; here most ill-health is recognized and then treated. It is the real site of primary health care in any society. The popular sector usually includes a set of beliefs about health maintenance. These are usually a series of guidelines, specific to each cultural group, about the 'correct' behaviour for preventing ill-health in oneself and in others. They include beliefs about the 'healthy' way to eat, drink, sleep, dress, work, pray and generally conduct one's life. In some societies, health is also maintained by the use of charms, amulets and

religious medallions to ward off 'bad luck', including unexpected illness, and to attract 'good luck' and good health. Most health care in this sector takes place between people already linked to one another by ties of kinship, friendship, co-residence or membership or work or religious organizations.

It seems likely that non-professionals are consulted more for psychological or mildly chronic disorders. Certain individuals often build up a reputation in a small community for knowledge or even 'special powers' and are hence frequently consulted.

Self-medication

People who become ill typically follow a 'hierarchy of resort' (Helman, 1990) beginning with self-medication, leading onto consultation with others, which perhaps leads to further self-treatment or to consulting a doctor or other professionals. One should not, however, assume that people always follow a logical, linear path from self-medication to orthodox medical consultation. Patients may return to earlier methods if one fails, or different methods are tried simultaneously. Indeed, this is one factor which often makes testing the efficacy of certain treatments so difficult.

Self-treatment may encompass proprietary drugs, patent remedies, herbal or homeopathic remedies, as well as changes in diet or other regimes or rest, exercise, staying warm and so on. In the United Kingdom, despite a free National Health Service, about 75% of abnormal symptoms are dealt with outside the formal health-care system. The general practitioner sees only 20% of those with symptoms, 16% take no action, 63% self-medicate and 1% go directly to hospital. Helman (1990) gives some examples of the range and scope of self-treatment, and the range of people involved in a decision about choice of treatment:

> The idea of using a particular . . . medicine came from a variety of sources, including: spouses (7%), parents and grandparents (18%), other relatives (5%), friends (13%) and the doctor (10%). Fifty seven percent of people thought the pharmacist a good source of health advice for many conditions. This is confirmed in Sharpe's study of a London pharmacy where, in a 10-day period 72 requests for advice were received, especially for skin complaints, respiratory tract infections, dental problems, vomiting and diarrhoea. In another study in a working class housing estate two thirds of people interviewed were taking some self-prescribed medication, often in addition to a prescribed drug. Laxatives and aspirin were most commonly self-prescribed. The aspirins, and other analgesics, were used for many symptoms including arthritis and anaemia, bronchitis and backache, menstrual disorders and menopausal symptoms, nerves and neuritis, influenza and insomnia, colds and catarrh, and of course for headaches and rheumatism.

Many people also take regular vitamin and mineral supplements, which might be described as complementary self-medication. Annual sales of over-the-counter medicines amount to £1 billion (US $1.5 billion) in the United Kingdom, with vitamin and mineral preparations in the United Kingdom being estimated at more than £120 million (US $180 million) (Newman-Turner, 1990). A recent survey of vitamin and mineral intake in the western half of the United States found that more than half of those surveyed used some kind of supplement (Medeiros et al, 1989). Self-treatment then is by far the main source of health care in the United Kingdom for minor or persistent chronic conditions. Self-treatment is frequently continued alongside conventional treatment and, very probably, alongside complementary treatment.

THE PROFESSIONAL SECTOR

While the achievements of orthodox medicine are undoubtedly impressive, many commentators have pointed out the adverse consequences of an increasingly technological approach to medicine and suggested that this might underlie the popularity of more traditional, less technologically based therapies. We will briefly consider some of the main characteristics of the professional sector in order to understand some of the factors that might influence a person choosing between different therapeutic options.

In most Western countries the orthodox medical system is well established, regulated and controlled, but also subject to criticism. Common criticisms are that orthodox medicine has become too technical and has tended to reduce patient autonomy, making them dependent on drugs or surgery. Pfifferling (1980) considers that modern medicine has become too physician-centred in that the doctor, and not the patient, defines the nature and boundary of the patient's problem; diagnostic and intellectual skills are valued above communication skills; settings for health care, such as doctors' offices, are often located for the benefit of doctors, far from their patients' homes.

The experience of being in hospital may also be disturbing for some people, over and above any pain or distress associated with their illness. From an anthropological perspective, Helman (1990) describes the key characteristics of the experience of hospital:

> In most countries, the main institutional structure of scientific medicine is the hospital. Unlike in the popular and folk sectors, the ill person is removed from family, friends and community at a time of personal crisis. In hospital they undergo a standardized ritual of 'depersonalization', becoming converted into

a numbered 'case' in a ward full of strangers. The emphasis is on their physical disease, with little reference to their home environment, religion, social relationships, moral status or the meaning they give to their ill-health. Hospital specialization ensures that they are classified, and allocated to different wards, on the basis of age (adults, paediatrics), gender (male, female), condition (medical, surgical or other), organ or system involved (ENT, ophthalmology, dermatology) or severity (intensive care units, accident and emergency departments). Patients of the same sex, similar age range and similar illness often share a ward. All of these have been stripped of the props of social identity and individuality, and clothed in a uniform of pyjamas, nightdress or bathrobe. There is a loss of control over one's body, and over personal space, privacy, behaviour, diet and use of time. Patients are removed from the continuous emotional support of family and community, and cared for by healers whom they may never have seen before. In hospital, the relationship of health professionals—doctors, nurses, technicians—with their patients is largely characterized by distance, formality, brief conversation and often the use of professional jargon. Patients in a ward form a 'temporary community of suffering', linked together by commiseration, ward gossip, and discussion of one another's condition. However, this community does not resemble, or replace, the communities in which they live; and unlike the members of self-help groups, their afflictions do not entitle them to heal others, at least not within the hospital setting.

Bakx (1991) has also argued that an increased general awareness of 'green' issues, the rejection of 'modernism' in all its forms, and various reforms in public health policies in industrialized countries has meant an increasing dissatisfaction with traditional, orthodox biomedicine. Bakx believes that orthodox biomedicine is losing its actual and ideological hegemony for three reasons: by culturally distancing itself from its consumers; by its failure to match its propaganda promises of various 'breakthroughs'; and through the alienation experienced by patients of orthodox medicine. Bakx suggests that the emergence of medical pluralism combined with some dissatisfaction with orthodox medicine has allowed an expansion of folk and complementary therapies throughout Western society, especially the complementary medicines.

MAKING THERAPEUTIC CHOICES

The therapeutic choices facing a sick person are complex. Helman (1990) stresses that ill people make choices, not only between different types of healer, but also between diagnoses and advice that make sense to them and those that do not. A doctor's treatment is evaluated in the light of his or her past performance, compared both with other people's experience and with what the person expected the doctor to do. If the advice does not make sense, a further consultation may be sought. Different practitioners may be consulted according to the patient's previous experience, the advice of those around them and their experience with other kinds of medical and lay practitioners. One cannot, indeed should not, assume that there are two kinds of patients/clients: those that visit an orthodox medical practitioner and those that consult an alternative practitioner. Patients may mix and match their chosen therapy (and therapies) depending on a whole range of factors such as the chronicity of their complaint, demographic factors like age, sex and class, and the recommendations and advice of friends and family about both therapist and therapy. 'In general, ill people move freely between the popular and the other two sectors, and back again, especially when treatment in that sector fails to relieve physical discomfort or emotional distress' (Helman, 1990, p. 58).

The question 'Why do people choose complementary medicine?' is therefore more complex than it first appears. First, it depends on the particular branch of complementary medicine under consideration. The reasons and motives may differ according to whether the person is consulting an aromatherapist, a homeopath or an osteopath. Patients consider a range of therapeutic options including self-medication, complementary medicine and conventional treatment and will make use of different forms of medicine on different occasions (Thomas et al, 1991; Eisenberg, Kessler and Foster, 1993). The decision may be made out of curiosity or depression, spontaneously or long considered, with the advice and blessing of friends and relatives or in direct contradiction to their wishes, and the reasons for using complementary medicine may vary between individuals. Some patients are positively attracted to complementary medicine, others may be sceptical but nevertheless turn to complementary therapies when orthodox medicine proves ineffective. Even then we should not assume that patients are necessarily turning away from orthodox medicine, though they may have exhausted the orthodox remedies available for a particular condition. As we shall see in the next chapter, patients tend to seek complementary medicine treatment as a supplement to, not a substitute for, traditional, orthodox health care (Rasmussen and Morgall, 1990; Thomas et al, 1991). In fact it is becoming clear that it is rare for complementary patients to abandon orthodox medicine altogether.

Prospective patients of any practitioner, be they from orthodox or complementary medicine, usually have certain criteria for choosing first a particular specialty, and second a particular practitioner. Criteria for the latter frequently include accessibility, perceived clinical competence, communication skills and professional values. Presumably one of the major criteria of the former, namely the choice between orthodox and complementary, or indeed, different branches of complementary medicine, is perceived efficacy for a particular problem. Both lay and professional people acknowledge that different therapies appear particularly able to 'cure' particular problems, and are more or less acquainted with the associated risks and side-effects.

The decision to consult a general practitioner, for instance, is often only taken after a number of informal consultations with family or friends. This advice may then be discussed with others, before a doctor's opinion is finally sought. Elliott-Binns (1973, 1986) found that 96% of people consulting a general practitioner had received some advice beforehand, averaging 2.3 sources each or 1.8 excluding self-treatment; 55.4% of patients had treated themselves before going to the doctor.

What reasons do patients give for visiting a complementary medical practitioner and whom have they previously consulted? Budd et al (1990) studied 197 British patients: 90 visiting an acupuncturist and 107 an osteopath; 58% of the acupuncture and 83% of the osteopathy patients said that the treatment was suggested by a doctor, while 13% and 12% respectively said that a family member or friend had suggested it. Few said they were interested in the treatment *per se*, but 20% of acupuncture and 26% of osteopathy patients said that it was their choice because it was readily available. The only major difference between the two groups was that only 3% of the osteopathy patients said they sought the treatment 'as a last resort', as compared with 27% of the acupuncture patients. Clearly the recommendations of family, friends and the doctor played a major part in the initial decision to consult a complementary practitioner.

Given the complexity of the problem it is not surprising that a considerable number of reasons have been advanced for patients turning to complementary medicine. Some patients may have become dissatisfied with orthodox medicine, rejecting its reliance on high technology and being wary of the dangers of invasive techniques and the toxicity of many drugs. Others may retain a belief in the value and effectiveness of orthodox medicine, at least in certain areas, but find some aspects of complementary medicine attractive. They may regard it as especially efficacious for some conditions, as dealing more with the emotional aspects of illness, or as having a spiritual dimension that is not seen as important in orthodox medicine. Complementary patients may also be distinguished by having a stronger belief in the ability of the body to heal itself, given gentle therapeutic encouragement, or be distinguished by 'greener' lifestyles and different beliefs and values. Such factors, discussed in detail later in the book, might concern beliefs about science and medicine, the prevention of illness, perceived susceptibility to illness, biological knowledge and the control that one has over one's health. Finally, some have suggested that the move towards complementary medicine represents a 'flight from science' (Smith, 1983) or credulous faith in occult or paranormal phenomena (Skrabanek,

1988; Baum, 1989). This latter assertion will be discussed before we move on to studies that actually assess the reasons patients of complementary practitioners themselves give for their choices.

Credulity and Illusory Belief: The Sceptic's View

Patients using complementary or unconventional therapies tend to be those with relatively more education and higher incomes. At first glance, these facts are 'not compatible with a picture of a patient unable to understand the medical possibilities or to make discriminating choices' (Fulder and Munro, 1985), which in turn might argue against them being naïve and credulous. Nevertheless, a higher level of education is no guarantee against credulity. Sutherland (1992) has reviewed numerous examples of illogical thinking culled from a very wide range of human endeavour and numerous highly educated professional groups. Some of the more common arguments put forward for the credulity of complementary patients are as follows.

Many illnesses are cured by the body's own healing processes without assistance from medical science (spontaneous remission). Even a pointless therapy can therefore look effective when the base-rate of success is so high. By trying a treatment (bogus, real, placebo), a patient cannot learn what would have happened if another treatment (or indeed, no treatment) had been attempted. With other illnesses that do not self-heal, decline is not uniform and linear, but erratic with periods of deterioration, improvement and further deterioration. We rarely plot this carefully, so when improvement does occur it is sometimes hard to determine whether this is due to the action of the therapy or to natural recovery. Sutherland (1992) points out that people generally are very poor at calculating the chances of a coincidence, and we may easily attribute improvement to the therapy rather than the passage of time. People tend in any case, and in many spheres of activity, to be unrealistically overconfident in their own judgements and abilities. For instance, the majority of drivers think that they are of above average ability.

There will also always be some truth in a set of vague predictions and, if you are a believer or want to believe, you are likely to seize upon the few predictions that happen to be correct. Moreover, if the prediction is sufficiently vaguely worded, you will distort its meaning to suit your own situation (Sutherland, 1992). Some complementary therapists do not specify in any detail the precise benefits of the cure, except vague phrases like 'wellness', 'togetherness' or 'better integration'. They know that the more ambiguous the criterion, the easier it is to detect evidence of success.

Similar criticisms have been levelled against astrologers and graphologists. Vague, ambiguous criteria of cure can be exploited by those wishing to promote complementary therapies, but more importantly, they can impede genuine efforts to understand whether the therapy has really worked. Without specific predictions of success (and hence failure), people's often desperate hopes and expectations lead them to detect more support for the therapy than is warranted. The wish to believe is said to be especially strong for serious illnesses for which no conventional treatment exists. Thus, ineffective remedies are particularly prevalent for medical problems like arthritis, ageing, cancer and back pain, for which medicine can do so little. It is important to distinguish between genuine belief and desperate actions. But the comfort in believing that there are cures for various afflictions can seriously and dramatically affect how people evaluate information about the remedies, philosophy and effectiveness (Gilovich, 1991).

Can these and other ways of 'irrational thinking' be used to explain the attraction of complementary medicine as Gilovich (1991), Skrabanek (1988) and others suggest? Certainly there are grounds for thinking that many people's assessment of the efficacy of complementary medicine could be mistaken, but this does not necessarily show that they are generally credulous. The problem with the argument for the greater credulity of complementary patients is that such irrational thinking seems to pervade every human activity, applying to orthodox medicine as well as to complementary medicine. Sutherland's examples of irrationality involve doctors, psychologists, lawyers, civil servants, business people. There is no evidence to suggest that patients attending complementary practitioners are any more prone to irrational thinking than anyone else. The importance of these factors lies elsewhere. It is undoubtedly true that it is very difficult to assess the efficacy and value of a therapy in a small number of people without knowing what would happen if no therapy was administered and what would happen if another treatment was given. In addition, ethical factors do not permit one always to test most easily the efficacy of certain treatments. The history of medicine is littered with examples of discredited therapies which were later found, when larger systematic studies were conducted, to be without any benefit. The human tendency to irrational thinking and an incomplete assessment of evidence does point to the need for systematic research on complementary medicine, as personal testimony can easily be mistaken and based on unsound foundations.

Some cynics have argued not for credulity but for instability. They suggest that it is only the mentally unstable people that are attracted to complementary medicine, particularly the more avant-garde areas of practice. There is some evidence that patients attending homeopaths have a slightly higher level of minor psychological disturbance than general practice patients. Furnham and Smith (1988) gave the Langner 22 measure, an index of psychological disturbance, to two groups of homeopathic and general practice patients. Patients visiting the homeopath scored higher than those visiting their general practitioner, who, in turn, scored slightly higher than the general population. Similar results were reported by Furnham and Bhagrath (1993), also in respect of patients of homeopaths and general practitioners. The basic finding, however, does not provide very strong evidence for the neuroticism of complementary medicine patients. In the first place, the differences are only slight, and there is no real evidence of a higher rate of serious psychiatric problems. More importantly though, complementary patients tend to be suffering from more chronic illnesses than general practice patients, and so might well be more prone to suffer from sleep disturbance, worry, despondency, fatigue, aches and pains and other symptoms of mild psychological disturbance. The symptoms are probably simply a consequence of a chronic illness. While the chronicity of the illness might be a factor in the move to complementary medicine, the psychological consequences of the illness might not be relevant as a motivating factor.

REASONS FOR TURNING TO COMPLEMENTARY MEDICINE

There have been some empirical attempts to understand the popularity of complementary medicine. Moore et al (1985) carried out a small survey of 56 patients attending the Centre for Complementary Medicine in Southampton, where doctors and other therapists provide a range of complementary treatments. The failure of orthodox medicine for their current problems was almost always the principal reason given. Most of these people had a good relationship with their general practitioner and thought that they had received satisfactory orthodox treatment. Of these, 19 thought they were rushed by their general practitioner, but 18 also claimed to be rushed by the doctor at the Centre (which has a high volume of patients). More importantly, about half the patients thought that their general practitioner did not understand their problems, whereas the doctor at the Centre did. Most of the patients said that they would return to orthodox medicine for future problems.

In an interesting and perhaps unique study Finnigan (1991) reviewed 38 patients in depth from the 300 or so visiting a general centre specializing in complementary medicine. From the demographic information that he collected, he found support for the generally held view that a high proportion of the patients had long-term chronic ailments, had been unable to find a conventional diagnosis for their symptoms and seemed unresponsive to conventional treatment. In other words, the primary motivation was the failure of conventional medicine to bring about a satisfactory improvement in their condition. He found evidence for two distinct types of patient: those who turned to complementary medicine as a last resort and were not interested in its philosophy, and those who were more committed to belief and ideology than the alleviation of their personal suffering. What would be of considerable interest in future studies is whether these two types showed any difference in their progress.

In an effort to provide some more substantial empirical data after almost a decade of speculation about patients' motives for seeking complementary treatment, we carried out a study of 268 patients of complementary practitioners (Vincent and Furnham, 1996). Three of the main systems of complementary medicine were contrasted, as reasons could vary according to the type of treatment and problem concerned.

A total of 268 patients, 201 (74.9%) female, took part in the study; 89 were attending the British School of Osteopathy, 92 a large acupuncture centre in South London, and 87 the Royal Homeopathic Hospital. Each completed a questionnaire covering three broad areas:

1. Basic demographic information
2. History of present complaint, previous treatment, and other health problems
3. Reasons for seeking complementary treatment.

Twenty reasons for seeking complementary treatment were derived from preliminary interviews with patients and from the literature on complementary medicine (e.g. Sharma, 1992), each being rated on a five-point scale.

Patients attended for a variety of different complaints, which varied with the therapy in question. Over 90% of the osteopathy patients had musculoskeletal problems and over a quarter of the homeopathic patients had allergies or skin disorders. Over a fifth of acupuncture patients were seeking treatment for psychological or stress-related problems, and over a quarter of the total sample had received some help for emotional problems in the past. This does not necessarily mean a high incidence of psychological or psychiatric disorders, but may show the importance that complementary medical patients attach to the emotional aspects of their problems and to counselling aspects of treatment.

Of the 20 reasons they were presented with, the patients agreed strongly with almost a third. The reasons most strongly endorsed were: 'because

I value the emphasis on treating the whole person'; 'because I believe complementary therapy will be more effective for my problem than orthodox medicine'; 'because I believe that complementary medicine will enable me to take a more active part in maintaining my health' and 'because orthodox treatment was not effective for my particular problem'. There was little difference between the groups on their rating of the most important reasons. The least important reasons rated by the groups included 'because complementary treatment is less expensive than orthodox private medicine' and 'because I value a form of therapy that involves actually touching me'. Patients did not perceive orthodox medicine as generally ineffective, indicating that they were not suffering from a wholesale disillusion with medicine. Orthodox medicine was only seen as ineffective for their specific problem. (See Tables 2.1 and 2.2.)

The factor analysis of the 20 reasons (Table 2.1), gave fairly clear results which underpinned many speculations from researchers in this field. Two stood out as being more important than the others. The first, most important, factor labelled 'Value of complementary medicine' included items that stressed that complementary treatment was more natural, effective, relaxing, sensible and that one could take an active part in it. The second, with almost equal importance, was the specific failure of orthodox medicine to bring them relief. The third factor concerned the adverse side-effects of orthodox medicine, the fourth concerned communication between patients and orthodox medicine practitioners. The fifth, relatively unimportant, factor stressed the easy, cost-effective and available nature of complementary therapies. Clearly these different factors, although not strongly distinguished between the three complementary therapies, are likely to differ in importance for each individual according to their specific medical history, personal beliefs and temperament.

This was an exploratory study which only provided the beginnings of a complete account of why patients turn to complementary medicine. Other aspects of the complementary consultation (the role of explanations, etc.) need to be explored in more detail. It would have been valuable to have included more questions on the role of discussion of emotional aspects of illness in the questionnaire, in an effort to delineate more precisely those aspects of complementary therapies that patients find most important. The study also failed to separate clearly the reasons for beginning treatment with complementary medicine, from the reasons for continuing it. It is possible, for instance, that the failure of orthodox medicine is the strongest motive for seeking complementary treatment, but that once treatment has been experienced other, more positive factors, become more important. A more detailed medical history, including information about previous

Table 2.1 Reasons for having complementary treatment

Value of complementary medicine
1. Because I have a more equal relationship with my complementary practitioner than with my doctor.
2. Because I believe complementary therapy will be more effective for my problem than orthodox medicine.
3. Because I believe that complementary medicine enables me to take a more active part in maintaining my health.
4. Because I value the emphasis on treating the whole person.
5. Because I feel so relaxed after complementary treatment sessions.
6. Because the explanation of my illness that I was given by my complementary practitioner made sense to me.
7. Because I value a form of therapy that involves actually touching me.
8. Because I feel that complementary treatment is a more natural way of healing than orthodox medicine.

Orthodox medicine ineffective
1. Because orthodox medicine was not effective for my particular problem.
2. Because I am desperate and will try anything.

Adverse effects of orthodox medicine
1. Because the orthodox treatment I received was too distressing.
2. Because the orthodox treatment I received had unpleasant side-effects.
3. Because I believe that orthodox medicine generally has too many unpleasant side-effects.

Communication between patient and practitioner
1. Because my doctor did not understand my problem.
2. Because I found it difficult to talk to my doctor.
3. Because my doctor did not give me enough time.
4. Because I believe that orthodox medicine is generally ineffective.

Cost and availability
1. Because I was persuaded to come by a friend or relative.
2. Because it was easier to get an appointment with a complementary practitioner.
3. Because complementary treatment is less expensive than orthodox private medicine.

(From Vincent and Furnham, 1996. Reproduced by permission of The British Psychological Society)

orthodox treatment, might also shed light on the initial move to complementary forms of treatment. The nature of the complaint and the previous history of treatment do seem to be very important precursors and predictors of the initial complementary consultation. For instance, Furnham, Vincent and Wood (1995) found that, as compared with general practice patients, patients of complementary practitioners were more likely to have had a serious illness in the last five years and more likely to have suffered from some kind of psychological problems, osteopathy patients excepted (see Table 2.3).

Table 2.2   Reasons for having complementary treatment

Factor	Acupuncture	Homeopathy	Osteopathy	Mean
Value of complementary medicine	3.92	3.88	3.98	3.90
Orthodox medicine ineffective	3.51	3.95	3.52	3.66
Poor doctor communication	2.85	2.95	2.89	2.90
Adverse effects of orthodox medicine	3.05	3.01	2.67	2.91
Availability of complementary medicine	2.18	2.37	2.91	2.49

(From Vincent and Furnham, 1996. Reproduced by permission of The British Psychological Society)

Table 2.3   Medical history of complementary and general practice patients

Item	General practice	Osteopathy	Homeopathy	Acupuncture
Length of time with complaint (years)	9.3	14.7	21.3	21.6
Consulting other practitioner (%)	18	48	47	62
Serious illness in last 5 years (%)	7	12	13	35
Chronic illness or problem (%)	21	37	48	53
Psychological problems in last 5 years (%)	16	11	24	40

(From Furnham, Vincent and Wood, 1995. Reproduced by permission of Liebert Inc)

PATHWAYS TO COMPLEMENTARY MEDICINE

Sharma (1992) conducted a number of detailed interviews with people attending complementary practitioners, revealing many important themes which were later confirmed in our larger scale survey. However, the detailed discussions she had with her interviewees allowed an additional longitudinal perspective and showed how health choices evolved over time, changing according to personal circumstances, fluctuation in health and disease and an evolving understanding of both orthodox and complementary medicine. Sharma argued that the decision to consult a complementary practitioner should be studied as part of a process and, as Helman (1990) also suggests, in the context of the entire range of resources which a user has at their disposal in making decisions about health care. Few would disagree with this position. She discerned both pathways to an initial contact with complementary medicine, and endeavoured to track the evolving health choices of her interviewees.

All Sharma's interviewees, bar one, had used complementary medicine for the first time in order to cure some condition for which orthodox medicine had been either unable to offer any relief at all, or unable to offer a cure which was deemed satisfactory by the patient. Complaints were of musculo–skeletal problems, allergies, skin conditions, asthma, chest conditions, migraine and stress-related problems. Many of the accounts quoted by Sharma mirror the account given by Ms Dening quoted in the Introduction in that the initial stimulus was the failure of orthodox medicine to bring relief from their symptoms. For instance, one interviewee is quoted as saying:

> Before, I was a very fit person. I could swim, play squash, run and suddenly I just keeled over. I went to the doctor but nobody could tell me what it was. My GP said it was glandular fever and gave me antibiotics which gave me terrible thrush. Then he kept saying that he did not know what it was either . . . I went through all the tests. I was really very poorly. It went on for six months. I was still ill and they still did not know what it was.

Other common concerns were the side-effects of drugs, in that many of the patients described their orthodox treatment as effective, but only at the cost of unpleasant side-effects. Others had been offered orthodox treatment which they regarded as too drastic or invasive to be acceptable. Waiting for hospital treatment was another factor, especially when people were worried about the length of time they had been off work. These are all, of course, familiar complaints to anyone who uses the National Health Service in its present embattled state. Such factors, however, provide the background and some of the motivation for turning to other forms of therapy.

The great majority of Sharma's interviewees first heard about their complementary practitioner through personal recommendation, though a few responded to advertisements. Sharma comments that the more chronic the problem the more effort seemed to be invested in preliminary 'homework'—that is, making efforts to inform themselves about the range of treatments available, the complementary practitioners in their area and, most importantly, the experiences of friends and acquaintances who had already been treated. For most of the people in Sharma's study, the first time they used complementary medicine was not the last; the majority had used at least one complementary technique before. Evidence from studies also suggests that once a person has tried one form of complementary therapy, they may be more willing to try another. Canter and Booker (1987) studied the consultation patterns of 202 patients, finding that those

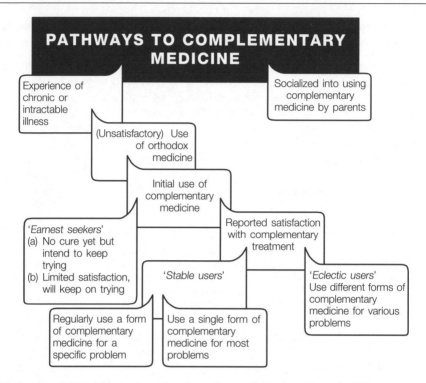

Figure 2.1 Motivation and exploration of complementary therapies (*Source*: Sharma, 1992. Reproduced by permission of Routledge)

who had used complementary medicine had visited an average of 5.4 practitioners each.

Sharma grouped her interviewees into different categories according to their motivation and the stage they had reached in their exploration of complementary therapies. The categories she used, and an indication of their route to complementary medicine, are shown in Figure 2.1.

The largest group of Sharma's interviewees were the 'stable users', people who had had an initially favourable experience with complementary medicine, made regular use of a particular system and had a relationship of trust with the practitioner concerned. 'Earnest seekers' had received limited benefit, or in some cases no help at all, from complementary medicine but equally had received no help from orthodox medicine for their particular problem but were determined to find a solution. In contrast the 'eclectic' group were those who, after their initial experience, had become enamoured of complementary medicine in general and tended to 'shop around' for what they felt was the best form of treatment, whether orthodox or complementary. Sharma comments that some of these had an explicitly consumerist approach:

> We don't talk about health a lot, but I think there is this thing . . . you go to the doctor and if you think the treatment is a bit much, or does not work, you look around for the right kind of alternative. I tend to try things, and if they work—great! (Sharma, 1992, p. 50)

And from another interviewee:

> I am not criticizing people but very often they just accept what the doctor says. Perhaps there are some who can't afford it, but they will happily spend £15 on a meal when for the same money you could have alternative medicine as a second opinion. I am far more healthy than I was twenty years ago. I would advise anybody, yes, go to the doctor and get the best you can from there, but you can always get a second opinion from alternative medicine. (Sharma, 1992, p. 50)

Sharma comments that these categories are, of course, not fixed; an earnest seeker might evolve into a stable user of one particular form of treatment that they eventually found to be effective. There is also no way of knowing how these patterns of use are distributed in the general population of users of complementary medicine.

> This section of this group of interviewees was probably biased in favour of those whose experience of it is prolonged and conclusive and who therefore have more of a 'story' to tell. A large random sample might well net a number of transient 'one-off' users and would probably include more of the 'earnest seekers' as well. There may even be other patterns of usage which were not represented in my relatively small group, and others may emerge in future; this typology is no more than a summary of what I found at a particular time.

Evolving Choices

The strength of Sharma's approach is that, while the sample is small, the interview method allows a longitudinal approach to health-care decisions and some assessment of the evolution of the choices people make. Sharma (1992) says:

> If we want a full answer to the question 'why do people use non-orthodox medicine?' then we must be prepared to study not isolated decisions, but chains of decisions taken over quite a long period. The considerations that prompted the initial use may not be the same as those which contribute to the second, third or subsequent occasions. . . .

Complementary medicine is almost always used in the first place to deal with a specific, generally chronic, illness which orthodox medicine has not resolved satisfactorily, but to have said this is not to have said very much for 'what happens next' is quite as interesting as 'what happened in the first place'. Evidently many people are in the process of changing their approach to medical authority and to family healthcare, and the decision to consult a non-orthodox practitioner may represent only one moment in a series of connected shifts in practice. (pp. 51–3)

My interviewees' accounts of their experiences over time suggest that the initial visit to a complementary practitioner is almost always motivated by a straightforward and pragmatic desire to cure some intractable problem. Subsequent decisions will be influenced by the outcome of the first encounter, by interaction with practitioners' ideas and methods, perhaps also by the degree of encouragement they receive from family members . . . In the area of health and illness—as in most others—ideas and values are constantly being re-worked in the light of personal experience, interaction with others, exposure to the media and a myriad other influences. (p. 69)

At present no longitudinal studies of evolving attitudes to a complementary treatment have been carried out and for the most part we cannot say which factors are likely to be uppermost at any particular time. It seems likely though that the opinions and experience of others, and perhaps attitudes to orthodox medicine, will be most important in the initial decision to try complementary medicine. However, the studies of both Vincent and Furnham (1996) and Sharma (1992) suggest that other factors may play a part in the decision to continue with complementary treatment. An assessment of both the treatment and the practitioner is involved. Many patients agreed that the willingness of their practitioner to discuss emotional factors, the explanation given for their illness and the chance to play an active part in their treatment were all important reasons for receiving complementary treatment. A belief in the efficacy of the treatment is clearly significant, whether gained from personal experience or, prior to beginning treatment, from the personal recommendation of friends. More general beliefs about health and illness, such as the extent to which disease can be controlled by one's own efforts, may also play a part. Although particular beliefs, behaviour and expectations may be important in choosing the type of treatment, they could also equally be the result of that treatment. Furthermore, they may, quite simply, have nothing to do with their reasons for seeking out treatment in the first place. Clearly these various factors are not mutually exclusive and several may operate simultaneously. It is quite possible that different patterns exist for clients of the different branches of complementary medicine, particularly those from the more well-established branches versus those from the more fringe areas. The sparse literature on patients' use and experience of complementary medicine is reviewed in Chapters 4 and 5.

Chapter 3

The Use of Complementary
Medicine

Complementary medicine is now widely used in Australasia, Europe and
the United States. In this chapter various national differences will be
examined, together with how patients with particular problems use complementary medicine. We will describe the use of complementary medicine
in the United Kingdom in some detail and provide a broad indication of
the extent of its use in Europe and North America, before discussing its
use in chronic and life-threatening illnesses such as arthritis, AIDS and
cancer.

COMPLEMENTARY MEDICINE IN THE UNITED
KINGDOM

This summary of the use of complementary medicine in the United
Kingdom will draw on two particularly comprehensive studies (Fulder
and Munro, 1985; Thomas et al, 1991). Fulder and Munro (1985) interviewed all complementary practitioners working in the Oxford and
Cambridge areas in 1980. In 1981 the study was extended by postal
questionnaire to other areas of the country which differed in level of
industrialization and social structure. Thomas et al (1991) focused on a
particular type of non-orthodox care—that provided by qualified, non-
medical practitioners belonging to national professional associations. In
1987 they contacted all 2152 practitioners of 11 national registers covering
the disciplines of acupuncture, chiropractic, homeopathy, medical herbalism, naturopathy and osteopathy—the therapies that we have described
as systems of complementary medicine. Fulder and Munro's sample of
practitioners was broader, but they excluded purely psychological therapies, those who were primarily teachers (e.g. yoga teachers) and those
who did not regard their work as primarily therapeutic (e.g. masseurs).
Both studies extrapolated from their results to provide estimates of the
availability and use of complementary medicine across the United
Kingdom.

Table 3.1 Complementary practitioners in the United Kingdom: membership of professional associations*

Main treatment	Registered practitioners (%)	
Acupuncture	507	(27)
Chiropractic	290	(15)
Homeopathy	93	(5)
Medical herbalism	115	(6)
Naturopathy with osteopathy	128	(7)
Osteopathy	680	(36)
Membership of more than one association	96	(5)
Total	1909	(100)

* Sample size 1575 questionnaires returned

(From Thomas et al, 1991. Reproduced by permission of the BMJ Publishing Group)

Complementary Practitioners

Fulder and Munro (1985) found that the number of lay practitioners varied from 11% of the number of general practitioners in Cardiff to 91% in Cambridge. The mean number was 12.1 per 100 000 population, equivalent to 26.8% of general practitioners. When the overall count was restricted to the main professional groups (i.e. complementary systems of medicine), there were 6.1 per 100 000 population, equivalent to 14% of general practitioners. In 1987 Thomas et al (1991) identified 2152 practitioners in the main professional groups, and estimated that 1909 were actively practising, representing about four practitioners per 100 000. However, not all practitioners (e.g. Chinese acupuncturists) belong to a British professional association, so this did not mean that the number of practitioners was declining. Table 3.1 shows the proportion of practitioners belonging to each professional group.

In 1980 Fulder and Munro found that just under half the practitioners were working full time, and they had been in practice for an average of 7.5 years. Half of the practitioners had been to college for a full- or part-time course. The rest had learned by apprenticeship, group work or correspondence course. Virtually all acupuncturists, Alexander teachers, chiropractors and osteopaths had been formally educated, compared with less than half the naturopaths and hypnotherapists, and few of the healers and homeopaths. By now, over a decade later, the proportion of practitioners who have attended formal courses is probably very much higher. The courses are longer and more comprehensive, and some osteopathic colleges are now able to award degrees after three years' full-time study.

Table 3.2   Consultation rates by practitioner, by specialty, and by population in the United Kingdom

Specialty	Mean consultations /wk/practitioner	Consultations/yr in UK (× million)
Acupuncture	42	1.7
Alexander	12	0.15
Chiropractic	64	1.8
Herbalism	30	0.47
Homeopathy	21	0.4
Hypnotherapy	26	0.7
Manual therapy*	19	3.1
Naturopathy	103	1.2
Osteopathy	53	2.2
Radionics	121	1.1
Others		0.88
Total		12.7
New patients**	4.5	

* Manual therapy covers therapeutic massage, applied kinesiology, polarity therapy, shiatsu and reflexology
** For all therapies

(From Fulder and Munro, 1985. Reproduced by permission of The Lancet Ltd)

Consultations

Fulder and Munro (1985) showed that practitioners averaged 40 consultations per week, less than half the average number of consultations per general practitioner (21 per day at that time). Annual consultations per 100 000 people averaged 19 500 for all study areas, and 25 700 for Oxford and Cambridge (where virtually all practitioners were identified); these figures are 6.5% and 8.6% of general practice consultations. Acupuncture, chiropractic and osteopathy were the most popular specialties, with about 2 million consultations per year each. Overall, about 1.5 million people (2.5% of the population) were receiving courses of treatment in a single year. Table 3.2 shows the consultation rates for individual therapies.

In 1987 Thomas estimated that her more restricted group of professionally registered complementary practitioners undertook four million consultations, roughly one for every 55 patient consultations with an NHS general practitioner.

Fulder and Munro (1985) noted that the first diagnostic visit lasted an average of 51 minutes and subsequent visits an average of 36 minutes. The average number of treatments in a course was 9.7, high compared with orthodox medicine. Chiropractors and osteopaths gave fewer linked treatments, presumably reflecting the predominance of patients with acute musculo–skeletal problems. Acupuncturists, hypnotherapists and homeopaths gave longer consultations than naturopaths, osteopaths and chiropractors. Consultations of complementary practitioners were six times longer than the average general practice consultation. The fees, however, were low. In 1981 the average fee for a diagnostic visit was £10 and for a subsequent visit £7. Prices in 1992 were probably about two and a half times 1981 prices and currently three times the figure 15 years ago. Moreover, complementary medical fees were, in 1981, roughly half the total cost (including drugs) per consultation in the family practitioner services, even though consultations were six times longer. This ratio is probably still approximately correct. The fees of complementary practitioners are generally very much lower than their orthodox counterparts in the private sector.

Patients

As in general practice, proportionately more patients of complementary practitioners are female; 67% in Thomas's sample and 65% in Fulder and Munro's. All social classes are represented, but social classes I and II are predominant; they presumably have the opportunities to research and explore the possibilities of complementary medicine (Fulder and Munro, 1985). They also have more disposable income, necessary to pay the relatively modest fees of complementary practitioners. The great majority of patients are between 21 and 60 years of age; compared with general practitioners complementary therapists see very few children and old people. New patients make up about 10% of the patients seen in an average week, with two-thirds of these never having used complementary medicine before (Thomas et al, 1991).

Fulder and Munro (1985) offer the following comment on the characteristics of patients attending complementary practitioners:

> It has been suggested that complementary medicine thrives as a last resort for frustrated and gullible individuals attracted by its media-expanded promises. However, a simple analysis of complementary medical patients showed that two-thirds were women and that they were drawn largely from the upper social classes. Both Dutch and Australian surveys have found that complementary medical patients were somewhat more likely to have had tertiary education than general practice patients. These results are not compatible with a picture of a patient unable to understand the medical possibilities or to make discriminating choices.

Illnesses for which People seek Complementary Treatment

Fulder (1984) points out that establishing the precise conditions for which people seek complementary therapy is more difficult than it might seem, as practitioners may diagnose in complementary medical terms rather than using orthodox diagnostic categories. Most surveys have therefore concentrated on patients' descriptions of their own symptoms, sometimes aided by the patient's recollection of the diagnosis given them by a medical practitioner. In the mid-1970s, a survey of over 17 000 patients was carried out by the University of Queensland which was later used as evidence to a parliamentary enquiry on complementary medicine. At about the same time the British Naturopathic Association carried out a survey of 1000 recent patients seen by its members. The results of these surveys are shown in Table 3.3.

Table 3.3 shows that patients who sought complementary treatment in the 1970s were primarily suffering from chronic complaints, particularly musculo–skeletal problems, for which orthodox medicine could probably only provide palliative treatment. The primary motivation might well have been, as Fulder suggests, that orthodox medicine had failed to provide effective treatment. Patients with chronic conditions may also be more prepared to make the changes in diet and lifestyle that complementary medicine often demands.

In 1987 in the United Kingdom Thomas et al (1991), using the International Classification of Primary Health Care, also found that musculo–skeletal problems were by far the most common problem, accounting for 78% of the principal presenting complaints. Neurological problems (5.6%), psychological (4.6%), respiratory (1.9%), digestive (1.6%), skin complaints (0.9%) and metabolic (0.9%) and urinary (0.6%) were the main other specified reasons for seeking treatment. A general check-up, with no specific symptoms, was also sought by 3.7% of people. The preponderance of musculo–skeletal symptoms is partly accounted for by the large proportion (51%) of osteopaths and chiropractors in her sample.

The 1976 survey in Australia (Bowen et al, 1977, cited in Fulder, 1984) also presented a breakdown of symptoms according to the type of comple-mentary treatment. Chiropractors treated mostly musculo–skeletal prob-lems, with acupuncturists seeing a wider spread of more chronic conditions, more like those seen in general practice. It is interesting that in this 1976 survey, acupuncturists and naturopaths dealt with many more psychologically based problems than doctors in general practice. Fulder suggests that this may have reflected a growing realization by patients of

Table 3.3 Health problems presented to complementary practitioners

Naturopaths and osteopaths—British Naturopathic and Osteopathic Association (1976)		Chiropractors plus some other therapists—University of Queensland Survey (1977)	
Diagnostic area	Percentage of patients	Diagnostic area	Percentage of patients
Back	46	Aches and adhesions in back, limbs	35
Neck, shoulders, arms	18	Neuralgia, sciatica	11
Arthritis and spondylitis	14	Postural and joint problems	10
Hips, legs, feet	9	Migraines, headaches	8
Headaches and migraine	6	Respiratory, nutritional and digestive	7
Anxiety and depression	2	Sprains and strains	7
Asthma, bronchitis, hay fever	2	Muscular problems	5
Sinusitis, tinnitus, ménières, facial pain	1	Arthritis, bone disease	5
Skin conditions	1	Nervous and mental disorders	2
Angina, hypertension, chest pain	1	Skin conditions	1
		Others	9

(From Fulder and Munro, 1985. Reproduced by permission of The Lancet Ltd)

the psychological aspects of illness. It is unfortunate that Thomas's data do not permit a similar analysis 15 years later in the United Kingdom.

Use of Orthodox Medicine by Patients using Complementary Therapies

Fulder & Munro (1985) reported that about 10% of complementary patients were referred by doctors and a similar proportion of patients were referred to doctors by complementary practitioners. Most patients (59%) sought complementary treatment because of personal recommendation (probably to a specific practitioner), while 15% were referred by practitioner organizations and 10% from other complementary practitioners. From these figures we can see that at least a proportion of complementary patients had either recently seen their doctor or were receiving concurrent orthodox treatment.

Thomas and her colleagues (1991) specifically set out to discover whether complementary patients had turned their backs on orthodox medicine. The majority of patients in this sample (64%) reported having received orthodox treatment for their main problem from their general practitioner or a hospital specialist before receiving their present complementary treatment; just under a quarter of those who had received orthodox treatment continued it while receiving complementary treatment (Table 3.4). The remaining 36% had not received any orthodox treatment, but they may have received advice on their condition from their general practitioner who may also have suggested complementary therapy. It is also noteworthy that 3% of the patients were recommended to visit their general practitioner by the complementary therapist whom they had consulted.

Thomas and her colleagues found that the use of prior orthodox treatment was, not surprisingly, dependent on the type of problem for which patients were seeking help. As Table 3.4 shows, patients reporting atopic conditions, headaches and arthritis were more likely to report a combination of previous and concurrent orthodox treatment, usually drugs. Thomas rejected the view that patients attending complementary therapists do not understand or appreciate the benefits of orthodox medicine or that the popularity of complementary medicine represents a 'flight from science'.

> Overall our findings suggest that the patients seeking non-orthodox health care from this group of practitioners have continued to make use of orthodox medicine; almost a quarter of all patients had visited their general practitioner in the two weeks preceding the surveyed consultation and two thirds had received conventional treatment for their main problem . . . A substantial minority, however, seems to have sought help directly from a non-orthodox

Table 3.4 Use of orthodox medical care by patients consulting United Kingdom complementary practitioners

	% of patients with each complaint		
Patient defined problem	No previous or concurrent orthodox care	Previous orthodox care only	Previous and concurrent orthodox care
Neck	47	46	7
Back	35	50	15
Low back	38	55	6
Arthritis	31	42	27
Fatigue/unwell	32	61	7
Headache/migraine	18	61	21
Anxiety/stress/depression	39	44	17
Atopic conditions	3	44	53
Digestive system disorders	4	86	10
Other	33	49	17
All patients (% of total)	35	50	15

(Adapted from Thomas et al, 1991. Reproduced by permission of BMJ Publishing Group)

practitioner and most of this group did not report any contact with their general practitioner in the two weeks preceding the survey. (Thomas et al, 1991)

They go on to suggest that complementary medicine is not deflecting appreciable demand away from the National Health Service, partly because of the limited range of problems treated and the scale on which care is provided, but mainly because the patients concerned have not turned their backs on orthodox care. Complementary medicine is generally a supplement to rather than a substitute for conventional care. Indeed, this is the finding of nearly all researchers in this area. Thomas did not specifically ask patients why they had turned to complementary medicine, although the chronic conditions they suffered from and the fact that they continued to receive conventional care suggests at least that orthodox medicine was not meeting all their needs.

COMPLEMENTARY MEDICINE IN THE UNITED STATES

In a very comprehensive review, Levin and Coreil (1986) looked at what they called 'new age' healing, which encompasses complementary medicine. This described the rising costs and risks of conventional medicine in the United States, the 'medicalization' of non-medical social institutions, the proliferation of holistic health alternatives as well as the burgeoning interest in self-care, self-help in health and traditional healing. Alternative healers were consulted for a very wide range of physical complaints, from sexual dysfunction and general malaise to serious medical complaints. There was a great heterogeneity among new age therapists, some dealing primarily with bodily complaints, others having a psychological or spiritual orientation. Those that emphasized the mind followed Western esoteric teachings; those concentrating on the soul/spirit used contemplative, ritualistic, Eastern religious methods. People calling themselves alternative or complementary medical practitioners could be found in each group. While describing the general themes, however, Levin and Coreil did not present data about the actual usage of complementary medicine.

A comprehensive survey of the use of complementary medicine was carried by Eisenberg, Kessler and Foster (1993), who completed telephone interviews with 1539 adults (67% response rate) throughout the United States. Respondents were asked about serious or troublesome medical conditions, and their use of both conventional and unconventional medical services. Unconventional medical services were widely defined as 'commonly used interventions neither taught widely in US medical schools nor generally available in US hospitals'. This definition included all the major complementary therapies, vitamin and mineral supplements, and other complementary remedies. Also included, however, were taking exercise and relaxation techniques—hardly unconventional techniques. Important though the results are, they perhaps exaggerate the use of truly unconventional therapies.

One in three respondents (34%) reported using at least one unconventional therapy in the past year, and a third of these saw providers of unconventional therapy. The latter group had made an average of 19 visits during the previous year, with an average charge per visit of $27.60 (£20). The highest use was reported, as in other studies, by people with relatively higher education and income. Extrapolating the results to the population of the United States suggested that more visits are made to providers of unconventional therapy than to all US primary care physicians (general practitioners). The expenditure on unconventional therapies ($13.7 billion) was comparable to that spent on all hospitalizations in the United States ($12.8 billion).

Unconventional therapy was generally used for chronic conditions. When unconventional therapies were used for serious conditions it was almost always as an adjunct to conventional treatment, rather than as a replacement for it. The vast majority of people with serious medical conditions (83%) also sought treatment from a doctor; however, 72% of them did not tell their doctor about the concurrent unconventional therapy. People with serious medical conditions were far more likely to see a doctor (65%) than a provider of unconventional therapy (10%); only 3% saw solely a provider of unconventional medicine. In contrast to some studies on cancer patients (see below), no cancer sufferers reported seeing a provider of unconventional therapy without also seeing a doctor. Eisenberg, Kessler and Foster (1993) point out that all doctors are likely to see a great number of patients using unconventional treatments (28% of those with medical conditions in their study), the majority of which will probably not be discussed with them. The highest rates of concurrent use of unconventional therapies were for anxiety (45%), obesity (41%), back problems (36%), depression (35%) and chronic pain (34%), though the fact that anxious people might be using relaxation is hardly a surprise, nor a cause for concern. More detail about the overall use of unconventional therapies for these conditions is given in Table 3.5.

The interest and growth in complementary medicine has led to calls for proper funding and investigation of the various therapies. In 1992 the United States Senate Appropriations sub-committee for the National Institute of Health (NIH) added the following statement to its budget plans:

UNCONVENTIONAL MEDICAL PRACTICES

The Committee is not satisfied that the conventional medical community as symbolized by the NIH has fully explored the potential that exists in unconventional medical practices. Many routine and effective medical procedures now considered commonplace were once considered unconventional and counter indicated. Cancer radiation therapy is such a procedure that is now commonplace but once was considered to be quackery. In order to more adequately explore these unconventional practices the committee requests that the NIH establish within the Office of the Director an office to fully investigate and validate these practices. The committee further directs that the NIH convene and establish an advisory panel to screen and select the procedures for investigation and to recommend a research programme to fully test the most promising unconventional medical practices. The Committee has added $2,000,000 for this purpose.

The Office of Alternative Medicine has now been established and attracted a phenomenal public and media response (Monckton, 1993). It has several functions, including serving as a broker between the orthodox and complementary medical communities, developing research expertise among complementary practitioners, evaluating complementary therapies and providing research grants. In terms of the overall funding of the NIH it is a tiny organization, but it has already provided a great stimulus to research into complementary medicine.

Table 3.5 Use of unconventional therapy in the United States for the ten most frequently reported medical conditions

Condition	% reporting condition	% used unconventional therapy last 12 mo	% saw provider in last 12 mo	Therapies most commonly used
Back problems	20	36	19	Chiropractic, massage
Allergies	16	9	3	Spiritual healing, lifestyle diet
Arthritis	16	18	7	Chiropractic, relaxation
Insomnia	14	20	4	Relaxation, imagery
Sprains or strains	13	22	10	Massage, relaxation
Headache	13	27	6	Relaxation, chiropractic
High blood pressure	11	11	3	Relaxation, homeopathy
Digestive problems	10	13	4	Relaxation, megavitamins
Anxiety	10	28	6	Relaxation, imagery
Depression	8	20	7	Relaxation, self-help groups
10 most common conditions	73	25	10	Relaxation, chiropractic, massage

From Eisenberg, Kessler and Foster, 1993. Unconventional medicine in the United States. *New England Journal of Medicine* **328**: 246–52. Copyright © 1993 Massachusetts Medical Society. Reprinted by permission of *The New England Journal of Medicine*.

COMPLEMENTARY MEDICINE IN EUROPE

Between 1988 and 1990 a series of papers were published in *Complementary Medical Research* summarizing the available information on the use of complementary medicine in Europe, and later published in book form (Lewith and Aldridge, 1991). An overview of these and other studies was presented by Fisher and Ward (1994).

The papers give little information on sample sizes or survey methods, but it is possible to give some indication of the scale of use of complementary medicine in several European countries, although the figures should only be taken as a rough guide to actual usage. Since definitions of complementary medicine and the questions asked vary considerably between studies, no precise comparison is possible. Tables 3.6, 3.7 and 3.8 summarize some of the more important statistics. Although the information provided varies between countries, it suggests that between a third and a half of the adult population in most of the countries listed have used complementary medicine at some time. Where self-medication with homeopathic and herbal remedies is included in the definition (for studies in Belgium, Finland and France), approximately a third of people have had complementary treatment in the last year. Menges (1994) reported that data from the Dutch Central Office of Statistics showed that in 1990 5.9% of the Dutch population visited an alternative healer, but 15.7% called on a doctor who also used alternative therapies. This represents 1.2 million first patient contacts per annum and a total of 13 million annually. He estimates that there are 4000 alternative healers in The Netherlands.

The popularity of complementary medicine is growing rapidly. Fisher and Ward (1994) give several examples of the trends.

> For instance, in 1981, 6.4% of the Dutch population attended a therapist or doctor providing complementary medicine, and this increased to 9.1% by 1985 and 15.7% in 1990. In the United Kingdom the proportion of members of the Consumers Association who had visited a non-conventional practitioner in the preceding 12 months rose from one in seven in 1985 to almost one in four in 1991. Homeopathy is the most popular form of complementary therapy in France—its use rose from 16% of the population in 1982 to 29% in 1987 and 36% in 1992.

As regards patient characteristics, the findings are broadly comparable with those from the United Kingdom and the United States. In France, Belgium, Finland and Denmark patients of complementary practitioners are more often female, tend to be well educated, of higher than average social class and between the ages of 30 and 60. Similarly, most conditions are minor or chronic, with musculo–skeletal problems being the most

Table 3.6 Use of complementary medicine in Europe

Country	Date	Period of survey	Complementary medicine %	Acupuncture %	Homeopathy %	Manipulation %	Herbal %
Belgium	1986	1 year	31	5.8	17.5	12.2	9.5
Denmark	1988*	1 year	6 (M) 12 (F)	1.5	3.6**	2.3	—
Finland	1989	1 year	32	—	—	—	most popular
France	1985	Ever	49	21	32	7	12
Netherlands	1987	1 year	11.8	0.9	1.6	—	—

Figures are expressed as percentages of total adult sample over specified period of time
* Date of paper, not survey; ** Including natural remedies

(From Fisher and Ward, 1994. Reproduced by permission of the BMJ Publishing Group)

Table 3.7 Percentage of public reporting use of complementary medicine

Country	Any form of complementary medicine	Acupuncture	Homeopathy	Manipulation (including osteopathy and chiropractic)	Herbalism
Belgium	31	19	56	19	31
Denmark	23	12	28	23	ND
France	49	21	32	7	12
Germany	46	ND	ND	ND	ND
Netherlands	20	16	31	ND	ND
Sweden	25	12	15	48	ND
United Kingdom	26	16	16	36	24
United States	34	3	3	30	9

ND = data not available

(From Fisher and Ward, 1994. Reproduced by permission of the BMJ Publishing Group)

Table 3.8 Use of complementary medicine in The Netherlands: proportions
consulting complementary practitioners

Therapy	% of sample of 689	% of Dutch adult population
Homeopathy	37.7	6.9
Healing	35.5	6.5
Naturopathy	18.9	3.4
Herbalism	16.7	3.0
Chiropractic and osteopathy	13.2	2.4
Acupuncture	11.6	2.1
Yoga therapy	6.1	1.1
Anthroposophical medicine	2.9	0.5
Others	3.8	0.7

Notes
1. 689 people out of the 3782 adult members of the public polled at random had been to see a complementary practitioner.
2. The figures add up to more than 100% as some people have seen more than one kind of practitioner.

(From Fisher and Ward, 1994. Reproduced by permission of the BMJ Publishing Group)

common presenting symptom. Headaches and unspecified nervous conditions were also common and, in Denmark, a small but significant number of people with diabetes sought help from complementary practitioners. Otherwise acute or serious chronic conditions were seldom mentioned. Common reasons for seeking complementary treatment were frustration or dissatisfaction with orthodox medicine (at least in relation to its effect on a particular complaint), the absence of iatrogenic effects in complementary medicine and the more positive patient–practitioner relationship. There are no details on the relative importance of these different reasons.

USE OF COMPLEMENTARY MEDICINE BY PATIENTS WITH SPECIFIC DISEASES

The surveys discussed above have generally recorded the presenting complaints of patients attending complementary practitioners, but have not attempted to relate the use of complementary medicine to the type of illness reported. The use of complementary medicine by patients suffering from serious illnesses, such as cancer and acquired immuno-deficiency syndrome (AIDS) is of particular concern, as one of the main charges levelled against complementary practitioners is that they may, intentionally or not, deprive patients of potentially lifesaving orthodox treatment.

Acquired Immuno-deficiency Syndrome (AIDS)

Hand (1989) reported that 36% of 50 AIDS patients were using some form of unorthodox therapy, as compared with 5% of general medical patients. Patients were using acupuncture (15 people), imagery (12), massage (11), megavitamins (10), acupressure (8), unapproved medicines (8) and a high cereal diet (1). All of the patients who used these complementary therapies thought they were of value, but none expected the treatments to be curative. Similar results were reported by Anderson et al (1993), but their patients had generally higher expectations of complementary treatments, with almost half hoping for a delayed onset of symptoms, or 'better immunity', and some hoped, at least in conjunction with conventional treatment, for a cure.

Greenblatt et al (1991) studied 197 AIDS patients from the University of California clinic and found that 29% of patients were using some form of unorthodox medicine, mostly herbal remedies and Vitamin C in very high doses. There is no indication of how many patients were using the main systems of complementary medicine. Use of unorthodox remedies was associated with a more advanced stage of illness and greater educational attainment. The authors suggest that the use of such compounds could create an increased risk of adverse drug reactions, and might affect clinical drug trials, but it is not clear how real these dangers are.

Arthritis and Rheumatism

Visser, Peters and Rasker (1992) carried out a survey of 101 Dutch rheumatologists and 1466 of their patients. Of these patients, 43% had visited a complementary therapist at some time, 26% in the last year; visits to spas were included as complementary therapy. Healing (16% at some time), homeopathy (15.5%) and acupuncture (13.8%) were the most popular therapies. Rheumatologists were generally not very enthusiastic about their patients' use of complementary medicine, although the majority were quite positive about visits to spas. Manipulative therapies, acupuncture and homeopathy were seen positively or neutrally by the great majority. Rheumatologists seldom practised complementary medicine themselves, but 42% had referred a patient for complementary treatment at some time. Surprisingly, few patients realized that their doctors did not approve of their having complementary treatment. Although many patients visited a complementary practitioner because orthodox medicine was not helping them, their satisfaction with complementary medicine was not markedly different from their satisfaction with orthodox medicine. It is noteworthy that rheumatologists who were more accepting of their patients trying complementary medicine were rated more highly on various indices of satisfaction, especially on communication—whether or not these patients were actually visiting complementary practitioners. Visser, Peters and Rasker (1992) comment that: 'this implies that having an open mind towards complementary medicine might have something to do with a doctor–patient relationship in which not only somatic aspects of disease have a place'.

In Australia, Gray (1985) carried out a series of detailed interviews with 76 arthritis sufferers assessing their knowledge and beliefs about arthritis and their treatment strategies. In general, the longer the period since onset, the younger the patient and the more rapid the onset, the wider the range of treatments employed. Almost a quarter of the sample had used complementary medicine, mostly chiropractors and acupuncturists. Chiropractors were seen by patients as providing effective relief of symptoms, but treatment by acupuncturists and naturopaths was considered to be less effective. In a later Australian study, Vecchio (1994) found that 40% of rheumatology outpatients had attended one or more complementary practitioners at some stage in their illness, with acupuncture being the most common supplementary treatment. In Canada, Boisset and Fitzcharles (1994) found that 60% of rheumatology patients had used some complementary treatment (mostly herbs and vitamins, or relaxation and meditation), but only 13% had actually attended a complementary practitioner.

Interestingly, Gray found a lack of correspondence, albeit in a very small sample, between the explanatory models of illness of chiropractors and their patients. Patients of chiropractors had little awareness of chiropractic theory and they were chiefly regarded as specialized physiotherapists. This suggests that the implausibility of the underlying theories of complementary medicine, so often targeted by medical critics, may not be of such great concern to patients who appear to take a more pragmatic view. This topic warrants further research.

Asthma

The use of complementary medicine in 128 Australian families of children with asthma, and 110 families of children with minor surgical complaints, was investigated by Donnelly, Spykerboer and Thong (1985). It was found that 45% of the asthma families and 47% of the others had used complementary medicine at some time, though as they did not give information about which, or how many, family members were treated it is not possible to estimate the proportion of individuals who had used complementary medicine. In asthmatic families, chiropractic was the most commonly used treatment (21.1%), followed by a combination of homeopathy and naturopathy (18.8%), acupuncture (9.4%) and herbal remedies (4.7%). Use of complementary medicine was not associated with any demographic variables.

The main interest of the study lies in the assessment of overall satisfaction with complementary medicine and orthodox medicine. The majority of families using complementary medicine (76%) were satisfied with both forms of medicine, a small percentage (4.5%) were dissatisfied with both, and only 2.7% were dissatisfied with orthodox medicine yet satisfied with complementary. This argues against the idea that general dissatisfaction with orthodox medicine is a primary stimulus to seeking complementary treatment in this patient group. Use of complementary medicine seems more a wish to improve on existing treatment. There seem to be no grounds for the authors' suggestion that the use of complementary medicine represents a 'part of a general fascination with the occult and the paranormal'.

Gastroenterology

Smart, Maybury and Atkinson (1986) carried out a questionnaire study on 96 patients with irritable bowel syndrome, 143 patients with organic upper gastrointestinal tract disorders and 222 patients with Crohn's disease. Significantly more patients with irritable bowel syndrome (16%) had consulted a complementary practitioner, would consider consulting one (41%) or were currently using complementary remedies (11%) than either of the other two conditions. Only about 5% of the other patients had ever used complementary therapies. Herbalists and homeopaths were the most frequently consulted complementary practitioners. The authors point out that irritable bowel syndrome does not respond well to orthodox treatment, which could partly explain the increased use of complementary medicine in these patients. Some features of Crohn's disease are also not well controlled, however, and they also suggest that patients with irritable bowel syndrome have an 'attention-seeking attitude' to their disorder. Why this should be is not considered; the implication seems to be that this disorder has a stronger psychological component to which complementary practitioners have the time and ability to respond.

A similar conclusion was reached by Verhoef, Sutherland and Brkich (1990) after a survey of 395 patients attending a gastroenterological clinic. Of these, 9% had consulted a complementary practitioner for the problem that had brought them to the gastroenterologist and a further 18% had sought complementary treatment for some other reason. Almost half (46%) of the complementary medicine users had consulted more than one practitioner. Patients with a functional disease were more likely to seek complementary treatment than those with an organic disorder (in which an underlying pathology has been diagnosed). The authors suggest that this may be because patients with functional diseases become dissatisfied as they realize how difficult it is to diagnose and treat their diseases. Fewer alternative medicine users (54%) than non-users (85%) were satisfied with conventional medicine. Furthermore, fewer users of complementary medicine felt that their orthodox practitioners answered their questions about their problems (77% versus 91%). Users of complementary medicine were more satisfied with complementary than with orthodox medicine, though not significantly so. Users of complementary medicine were, however, significantly more sceptical of orthodox medicine (49% versus 13%).

Cancer and Complementary Medicine

The use of complementary medicine in the treatment of cancer has attracted particular attention because of the fear among oncologists, radiologists and cancer surgeons that patients may be denied effective and potentially lifesaving treatment because of a reliance on unproven fringe techniques.

This issue naturally arouses strong feelings among both orthodox and complementary practitioners and their patients. There are certainly some persuasive and alarming anecdotes from opponents of complementary medicine:

> I have . . . my own anecdotes of patients with early breast cancer who have put themselves in the hands of alternative practitioners who allowed the disease to progress in an uncontrolled manner. I have witnessed a very nice middle class lady whose screen-detected subclinical cancer was treated by homeopathy, and I was allowed to observe its natural history over a four-year period, during which time it progressed to a 3cm diameter mass with involved axillary lymph nodes. I have recently cared for two elderly women whose breast cancer had been treated for four or five years by diet and carrot juice. They ultimately arrived for a tertiary opinion with huge ulcerating cancers with their skin a deep orange tint from the carrot juice. Even more remarkable was the daughter of a family practitioner whose hideous growth of neglected breast cancer should be on the conscience of some guru who went on prescribing potions made up of a filtrate of her own urine! And finally, perhaps the worst example of faith masquerading as science, was when I was called upon to administer the last rites to a beautiful young West Indian girl who died in agony with a huge fungating breast cancer which had ulcerated through her brachial plexus, leaving a paralysed swollen arm and uncontrollable pain from nerve root infiltration. The Christian Scientist

responsible for this outrage showed no contrition but blamed the family for not praying hard enough, or ascribed the outcome to God's will. Which, if any, of these practices can be condoned when the quality of life of these poor women could have been infinitely enhanced by the application of medical science? (Baum, 1991)

The harm that can result from the misuse of complementary medicine (and of orthodox medicine) will be discussed in more detail in Chapter 11. For now it is sufficient that we understand why the use of complementary medicine in the treatment of cancer has attracted so much attention; to begin with we will briefly review the historical background.

History of Unorthodox Cancer Care

Cassileth (1986) gives a succinct overview of unorthodox cancer care in the United States from the early nineteenth century until the present day. Thomsonianism, popular in the early nineteenth century, was based on the belief that all disease resulted from one general cause (cold) and encompassed Thomson's opposition to 'mineral' drugs and the 'tyranny' of doctors. Cassileth then notes the growth in the nineteenth century of homeopathy, naturopathy and osteopathy respectively, though it is not clear how often these therapies were used to treat cancer. In the early years of the twentieth century, specific tablet and ointment cancer cures became popular, such as Chamlee's Cancer Specific Purifies-the-blood Cure and a host of others. The 1920s and 1930s saw the introduction of 'energy' cancer cures by Abrams (radio waves), Brown (radiotherapy), Kay (cosmic energy) and Ghadiali (spectro-chrome therapy). Koch's glyoxylide (distilled water) cure of the 1940s was followed by the Hoxsey treatment in the 1950s, by injectable Krebiozen during the 1960s and in the 1970s by laetrile. Today the most popular unorthodox treatment is metabolic therapy, usually a combination of special diets, detoxification and high-dose vitamins and minerals.

Cassileth notes that today's unorthodox cures differ in three important ways from their major twentieth century predecessors, which were cancer targeted medicines:

> First contemporary cures are not pills or potions, but lifestyle oriented remedies. Second, they are not secret formulae known only to their manufacturers, but activities of daily living understood and accomplished by the patient himself. Finally, they carry an aura of respectability, even a hint of conventional medicine's blessing, because they are not far removed from orthodox medicine's concerns with diet, lifestyle, environmental carcinogens, and the reciprocal relationship between many emotional and physiologic responses. (Cassileth, 1986)

To Cassileth and to some other writers in this area (e.g. McGinnis, 1991) unorthodox cancer cures are clearly anathema. McGinnis goes as far as to consider the terms 'unproven', 'unconventional', 'complementary', 'ineffective', 'fraudulent', 'dubious', 'disproven' and 'questionable' to be more or less equivalent. However, even from Cassileth's own comments we can see that at least some aspects of the current complementary treatment offered to cancer patients cannot be simply equated with quack medicines; changes in diet and lifestyle are of concern in both orthodox and complementary medicine. Danielson, Stewart and Lippert (1988, p. 1009) have observed that:

> Patients who have been influenced by the speculation that cancer is largely the result of stress or toxic environmental factors and who place a high value on personal responsibility and control are more likely to turn to unconventional therapies when confronted with the diagnosis of cancer.

This orientation, together with the promise of reduced, or at least controlled, suffering and added pressures from family, friends and the media and difficulties with the existing doctor/patient relationship, may all be influences on the choice of complementary medicine.

Lammes (1988) noted that patients sometimes give occasionally accurate, detailed reports of apparently miraculous cures after unconventional treatment. However, the following alternative explanations should always be considered:

1. The tumour was removed in total at the moment of diagnosis.
2. The tumour/mestases grows extremely slowly.
3. Spontaneous regression of a tumour does occur.
4. The first surgical treatment was effective.
5. The diagnosis of malignancy was not correct in the first place.

He argues that, whereas one should not preclude other explanations, it behoves the doctor, in helping science and the patient, to rule out all other explanations before accepting the effectiveness of unconventional treatment. The same strictures should, of course, apply to conventional treatment.

The Use of Complementary Medicine by Cancer Patients

The first major study in this area was carried out by Cassileth et al (1984). They interviewed 304 patients from the University of Pennsylvania cancer centre and, after considerable difficulty, managed to persuade 34 local complementary practitioners and 11 complementary clinics to ask their cancer patients to take part. They eventually interviewed 356 patients with cancer, who were contacted through complementary practitioners. Of the total of 660 patients, 282 were using conventional therapy alone, 325 a combination of orthodox and complementary medicine and 53 were only receiving complementary treatment at that point—which is not to say that they had not already received conventional treatment. They found that 13% of the cancer centre patients had used or were using an unorthodox regime. The most common unorthodox regime in Cassileth's study was metabolic therapy, which differs according to practitioner, but includes detoxification, through some form of cleansing regime, special diets, vitamins and minerals. The next most common therapies were, in descending order of frequency: diet, (often macrobiotic), megavitamins, mental imagery, spiritual or faith healing, and immune therapy (interferon). Over 40 additional therapies, mostly herbal treatments, were used by at least one patient.

In 1988 the American Cancer Society (ACS) commissioned a telephone interview survey of 5047 cancer patients indicating a 9% usage of complementary treatments, with imagery and diet regimes predominating (McGinnis, 1991). A study in New Zealand, Clinical Oncology Group, 1987 (Anon, 1987), found that 32% of cancer patients had been advised about complementary medicine, with about 20% indicating that they were intending to follow the advice, at least in part; only one of 463 patients questioned had decided to rely entirely on complementary treatment. In Britain, Downer et al (1994) found that 16% of cancer patients had used complementary therapies.

> The most popular were healing, relaxation, visualisation, diets, homeopathy, vitamins, herbalism, and the Bristol approach. . . . Three quarters used two or more therapies. Therapies were mostly used for anticipated antitumour effect. Ill effects of diets and herb treatments were described. Satisfaction with both conventional and complementary therapies was high, although diets often caused difficulties. Patients using complementary therapies were less satisfied with conventional treatments, largely because of side effects and lack of hope of cure. . . . Patient satisfaction with complementary therapies, other than dietary therapies, was high even without the hoped for anticancer effect.

Cassileth and colleagues (1984) found that most patients used complementary treatments in the belief that it would control their disease: 41% expected the therapy to effect a cure or remission; 18% anticipated prevention or halt of metastatic growth. Only 6% of patients turned to complementary medicine because their physicians had told them that their condition was terminal. Cassileth comments sardonically that 'these expectations were less than fully realized'. However, 22% of patients using imagery, 43% on megavitamins, 53% on immune therapy and 61% on metabolic regimes believed that these treatments were effective (in bringing about cure or remission, augmenting other treatments, or preventing spread of the disease). Chemotherapy was also judged to be efficacious by 56% of patients, radiation therapy by 59% and surgery by 72%. British cancer patients appear to have similar expectations of complementary therapies and to be generally satisfied with the complementary treatment they receive (Downer et al, 1994).

Cassileth considers that it is intrinsic to the belief in unorthodox therapies that conventional cancer treatments weaken the body's reserve, inhibit the capacity for cure, and misguidedly address the symptom (cancer) rather than the underlying systemic disorder (Cassileth et al, 1984). It is perhaps understandable that cancer patients enduring the rigours of chemotherapy and radiotherapy have some sympathy with this point of view. When asked what attracted them to complementary medicine, the most frequent response (39%) was the 'natural, non-toxic' qualities of the complementary regimes. British cancer patients reported feeling more hopeful when using complementary therapies, being attracted to the non-toxic, holistic nature of the therapies and the emphasis on patient participation in the treatment (Downer et al, 1994).

The two American surveys found that there is wide knowledge of complementary therapies, both through word of mouth and the media. A third of patients who sought complementary treatment were supported by their physician in their decision (not necessarily an oncologist) and 12% were actively encouraged. Half of the patients used complementary medicine after using orthodox medicine, about 20% used both simultaneously and 17% used complementary medicine before orthodox medicine. Most patients used complementary methods in the hope of some improvement, but with little hope of a cure with these methods alone. Two-thirds of patients reported some beneficial effect. There was little distress or disillusionment and, in the ACS survey, 98% of patients continued to receive standard therapy. The proportion of cancer patients relying on complementary medicine alone appears to be small, though this may still represent a substantial number of people. Even those relying only on complementary medicine may well have previously received orthodox treatment. Average expenditure was modest—less than $1000 per annum; patients did not seem concerned about the cost of complementary therapies.

Characteristics of Cancer Patients Seeking Complementary Medicine

Comparisons between cancer centre patients who did and did not use complementary medicine (Cassileth et al, 1984) revealed no differences in terms of diagnosis, sex, race, education, religion, marital status, history of cancer in the family or stage of disease at diagnosis, although patients using imagery treatments were somewhat better educated. Many were asymptomatic and in the early stages of the disease. Only 25% initiated alternative regimes while under conventional care. Patients did not fit the stereotype of desperate people in the terminal stages of their illness.

Cancer patients using complementary medicine differed substantially in their beliefs about illness and treatment from patients using only conventional therapy. Patients using complementary medicine were more likely to believe their cancer was preventable, primarily through diet (32%), stress reduction (33%) and environmental changes (26%). They were also more likely to believe that disease in general is caused mainly by poor nutrition, stress and worry; that chemotherapy and radiation therapy are useless or more harmful than helpful; and, not surprisingly, that unorthodox treatments are beneficial. Almost 100% believed that patients should take an active role in their own health, as compared with 74% of patients having conventional therapy only. Cancer patients receiving conventional treatment only were more likely to report having a good relationship with their physician, better relationships with previous physicians and to have a generally more positive attitude to the medical profession than those who were also receiving complementary treatment.

Themes of Complementary Treatment for Cancer

Within the various types of complementary treatment, two underlying themes can be discerned. On the one hand, there are alternative forms of medicine being offered (vitamins, diets, herbal remedies, etc.) and, on the other, a variety of psychological interventions, support, imagery, counselling, meditation and so forth. In many complementary centres, these two types of intervention are presented as a total package, whereas their value and appropriateness may be very different. Weir (1993), a former director of the Bristol Cancer Help Centre (a centre for the complementary treatment for cancer), noted that, while he now has less confidence in metabolic therapies, he remains convinced of the need for a holistic approach in the prevention and treatment of cancer that takes account of the psychological, and even spiritual, dimensions. A discussion of the possible adverse effects of this regime and the furore over its evaluation at the Bristol Cancer Help Centre in the United Kingdom is contained in Chapter 11. From the orthodox side, a realization of the need for psychological support for cancer patients has led to some oncology clinics incorporating a cancer counsellor or psychotherapist with special training in the psychological problems and communication difficulties that arise with cancer (Cosh and Sikora, 1989).

Downer et al (1994) found that cancer patients using complementary therapies were more anxious, but not more depressed, than other cancer patients. This result must be treated cautiously, as the difference was slight and the measure quite basic (Hospital Anxiety and Depression scale). They nevertheless put forward an interesting interpretation of this finding:

> One reason could be that this group of patients scored higher on the cancer locus of control questionnaire's dimension of internal control over cause/ origin. Patients who attribute the cause of their illness to something within themselves may carry an undue burden of responsibility for their illness and thus become anxious. It may also be assumed that patients who attribute the cause of the disease to one of their own activities may be more likely to think that if they change their lifestyle in some way—through diet or stress reduction, for example—they may influence the outcome of their disease. (Downer et al, 1994)

The value or otherwise of complementary therapies in cancer is largely unknown, but its emphasis on dealing equally with the disease and the person suffering from it, and taking full account of the emotional consequences of such a diagnosis, certainly seems to fulfil an important need in many patients. The distinction between the medical and psychological aspects of complementary medicine is well drawn in this letter from a cancer sufferer to the British Medical Journal:

> As a cancer patient I would like to think that support services for cancer patients stand a good chance of success . . . Such services are very much needed.
>
> Increasing openness leaves many patients fully aware of the limitations of surgery, drugs, and radiotherapy. They turn to complementary medicine seeking not only the cure doctors cannot promise them but also care and recognition of their own role in maintaining their health, which is sadly lacking in many hospital regimens.
>
> I found some of what is offered as complementary treatment very helpful. Emotional support, counselling, and a little assertiveness training allowed me to overcome my shock and accentuate the positive aspects of my illness. Changing my lifestyle through healthy eating, exercise, and techniques for relaxing and reducing stress has improved the quality of my life immensely. Perhaps they have lengthened it as well. I also found, however, several remedies, sometimes backed by quite bogus scientific claims, which are truly 'alternative'—faith healing, herbal concoctions, megadoses of vitamins, and rigorous diets to name but a few. I can joke about refusing to live on organically grown carrots, but I was deeply distressed by the bewildering choices and contradictions. I resented the stamina needed to extract common sense from the fringe.
>
> . . . I question why the aspects of compassionate care that are fully compatible with orthodox medicine have to be packaged along with the unconventional. Why should cancer patients have to go outside the health service for psychological support and encouragement of self-help. But I feel that glossing over the broad range of practices covered by the term 'complementary' and

refusing to acknowledge that some practices are and should remain alternative is to lessen the chances of integrating the others into conventional care. The debate will centre, mistakenly, on the question of scientific verification not on the need to offer patients both care and cure. That is unfortunate because both cancer doctors and cancer patients have much to gain from rethinking their roles and strategies. (Dennison, 1989)

Few would not agree that offering emotional support is helpful to many patients and improves their quality of life and if complementary practitioners can provide such support this can only be beneficial. The more contentious issue is the stronger claim, hinted at by Dennison, that psychological processes and interventions may have some impact on the course of the disease. Cassileth (1989) makes an interesting point about claims that the 'mind has the power to heal'. She points out that: 'we do not say this about tuberculosis or syphilis or any illness that can be treated and cured. We do not say that where we have the comfortable sense of comprehension and control now missing to a large degree in cancer medicine.'

There is, nevertheless, some fascinating preliminary evidence for support increasing survival time (Spiegel et al, 1989), and that the approach taken by cancer patients to their disease may influence survival (Greer, 1991). In the late 1970s, David Spiegel, a psychiatrist, conducted a randomized trial in which a group of women with metastatic breast cancer attended weekly support groups. The original purpose of the intervention was simply to improve the quality of life of the patients and support them through the rigours of cancer treatment. Compared with women receiving standard care alone, the women receiving support showed less anxiety, confusion, fatigue and mood disturbance a year later. Spiegel, highly sceptical of the 'mind over matter' community, followed up these women 10 years later. After numerous analyses and attempts to explain the results as an artefact, he finally concluded that patients who had been in the experimental group had survived 18 months longer than patients receiving standard care only.

This study has, of course, attracted much attention, as it appears to validate at least some of the claims of those who believe that cancer patients are, to some extent at least, responsible for their health and can powerfully influence their chance of recovery. Spiegel's attitude is very different, however. He regards the results as a preliminary finding, which may or may not be confirmed by later studies that are currently under way (e.g. Richardson et al, 1990; Fawzy et al, 1993). Spiegel's paper was published in the *Lancet* and accompanied by a thoughtful abstract, noting that what distinguishes unorthodox from standard medical treatment is not so much the treatment itself, which varies from culture to culture, but rather the nature of the proof offered that the treatment is efficacious (Spiegel et al, 1989, p. 901).

Perhaps the sometimes vociferous arguments between the proponents of orthodox and complementary cancer care will resolve into a constructive collaboration. It is abundantly clear that the complementary approach has some vital ingredients which are badly neglected in orthodox care. What these ingredients are and whether they improve the quality of life or actually prolong it is not yet clear, but they are certainly highly valued by considerable numbers of cancer sufferers.

Chapter 4

Complementary Medicine and Medical Profession

The attitudes of doctors towards complementary medicine vary widely, ranging from hostility bordering on paranoia to an all-accepting embracing of complementary medicine as representing the way forward towards holistic medicine and the antidote to an all too prevalent, impersonal and ultimately life-denying high technology medicine. These are, of course, the extreme positions; most doctors, whether in general practice or hospital medicine, adopt an intermediate stance. They are perhaps sceptical, rather than cynical, of most forms of complementary medicine, but acknowledge its importance to patients and the possible benefits of some techniques.

There is also considerable interest in complementary therapies among nurses, midwives, physiotherapists and other professions allied to medicine (Wright, 1995). Some physiotherapists, for instance, have trained in acupuncture to provide an additional therapy to help chronic pain patients. Many nurses are interested in therapeutic touch, a form of healing, not as a separate therapy but as something that can be incorporated into the nursing process in order to 'bring the heart into nursing' as Wright puts it. While nurses and others have written about complementary therapies and the way they might be incorporated into routine practice there is, as yet, little formal research on nurses' attitudes and their relationship with complementary therapists. This chapter, focusing as it does on research, mainly discusses the relationship of the medical profession with complementary medicine, while acknowledging the growing interest and enthusiasm from other professions. Doctors exert, in any case, a much more powerful influence on the referral of patients to complementary therapists and on the political processes affecting legislation governing complementary medicine.

THE EMERGENCE OF THE PROFESSION OF MEDICINE

The organization of medicine during the nineteenth century was much more pluralistic than today, in the sense that no one professional group minated others (Baer, 1989). Homeopathy, and, later in the century, osteopathy and chiropractic, all had their adherents, their training colleges and competed for patients. Interestingly, the establishment of the profession of medicine in the early and mid-nineteenth century preceded the establishment of scientific medicine, although many great scientific advances that would become crucial to medicine (for example, the discoveries of Virchow and Pasteur) were taking place at the time. The orthodox doctors, although hardly any of their practices would be recognizable as orthodox today, joined together to form professional groups whose members were bound by a common set of beliefs and principles, or at times simply a common set of vested interests. The British Medical Association (BMA) was founded in 1832, and the American Medical Association (AMA) in 1847.

Qualification as a medical practitioner in the first half of the nineteenth century was a haphazard and perfunctory affair. The usual way to qualify as a medical or surgical practitioner was to serve an apprenticeship, which was quite unstructured, and to set up in practice either with or without passing some sort of examination set by the Royal Colleges of Surgeons or Physicians. After several attempts at legislation the first Medical Act was passed in 1858, setting up the General Medical Council (GMC) which was to regulate entry to the profession by the establishment of a medical register. In 1867 the GMC produced a formal curriculum, establishing that each doctor should have a certain basic knowledge of medicine and the medical sciences (Smith, 1978). The duties of a doctor and the responsibilities of the profession are thus enshrined in law whereas, in the United Kingdom at least, most complementary therapies have neither the same legal duties, nor the same professional status.

REGISTRATION OF COMPLEMENTARY PRACTITIONERS

The fortunes of the main complementary therapies have fluctuated considerably over the last 100 years with the demise of homeopathy, for instance, being regularly predicted. The last 20 years have seen a flowering of unconventional therapies. Inglis (1985) estimated a figure of over a hundred (if fringe psychological therapies are included) compared with 20 at the time he wrote *Fringe Medicine* in the late 1960s.

Inglis (1985) concluded that there was a need both for the registration of complementary practitioners, and for formal courses which would provide a basic education. Chiropractors had already put themselves forward in Britain for designation as one of the 'Professions Supplementary to Medicine' (such as physiotherapy), but been rebuffed. Their ability as spinal manipulators was apparently accepted, but their claims to treat asthma and other complaints not obviously related to the condition of the spine was not. As Burton (1990) pointed out, a clash with orthodox medicine is likely if the complementary therapy is truly presenting an alternative point of view.

Cant and Calnan (1991) examined how complementary practitioners saw their role; how they believed it should develop; how they felt they should exist within an orthodox medical framework; and their thoughts about the future. These practitioners resisted being lumped together in a homogeneous group. Overall, they believed patients turned to them as a last resort, not because they reject the 'medical model' but rather the 'system', which has delayed and frustrated them. The results showed that while most practitioners sought collaboration with the medical profession, they did not seek integration, preferring to keep their identity. Most groups wanted to establish associations and training standards so that they should not be subordinate to orthodox medicine but form a separate and autonomous domain. Most sought validation and legitimation by the government in order to gain credence in the medical field. Most seemed optimistic, envisaging themselves as expanding and accruing credibility and acceptability.

Wardwell (1994) has summarized the great advances in status and professional independence made by chiropractors in the United States in the past 25 years. In the 1930s officials of the AMA attempted to destroy the profession of chiropractor. By 1974, however, they had gained licensure in all states, a commission to accredit colleges. In 1976 a massive anti-trust lawsuit was organized by chiropractors against a number of medical organizations alleging a criminal conspiracy to prevent doctors associating and accepting referrals from chiropractors.

> After two court trials, two appeals, and two petitions to the United States Supreme Court, in 1990 (only the AMA not having settled out of court), the AMA was conclusively found guilty of criminal conspiracy, required to have its Judicial Council change its official 'opinion' regarding professional association of MDs with chiropractors, formally change its code of medical ethics (which it had actually done in 1980), pay chiropractors' legal expenses and damages, and inform each of its members about the court's findings and the revised AMA policies.
>
> As a result, 50,000 chiropractors now have the right to consult professionally (to and from) with MDs; use hospital diagnostic facilities; and apply for appointment to hospital staffs for the purpose of co-admitting patients (as dentists do), administering chiropractic treatments, and ordering tests, diets, and physical therapy. At least 60 hospitals or ambulatory surgical centers now have chiropractors on staff. (Wardwell, 1994)

Finally, however, after 60 years of trying, osteopaths have achieved statutory registration in the United Kingdom (Warden, 1993). At the seventh attempt a bill passed though parliament, with government support, and reached the statute book in July 1993. A General Osteopathic Council (GOC) was created, along the lines of the GMC, but actually with wider powers. The GOC will, under the heading 'unacceptable professional conduct', be able to investigate incompetent practice. The GMC has had little power to discipline a doctor for incompetence, 'serious professional misconduct' being more usually applied to serious moral or ethical breaches. Critics of the GMC would like to see a similar council (with greater lay involvement) established for doctors, to bring greater accountability to the medical profession (e.g. Simanowitz, 1985), but this has only recently become a reality. It is ironic that, after orthodox medicine's attempts to control complementary practitioners and make them accountable, the registration of osteopaths has paved the way for greater accountability and control of the medical profession.

In the United Kingdom and the Republic of Ireland there is no direct regulation of non-medically qualified practitioners: they can practise freely, subject to minor limitations imposed by various laws. Many other European countries restrict the practice of complementary medicine to doctors, though the laws are not always strictly enforced (Box 4.1 and Figure 4.1).

Box 4.1   Legal status of complementary medicine in Europe

In most member states of the European Union, including Belgium, France, Spain, Italy, and Greece, the practice of medicine, except by statutorily recognized health professionals, is illegal. This is also technically the situation in The Netherlands, but the Dutch government has stated that it will not prosecute non-medically qualified practitioners unless there has been malpractice. A comprehensive reform of the law governing medical practice in The Netherlands is under way. This will create a system of statutorily regulated registers and protected titles. In Denmark non-medically qualified practitioners may practice, but the scope of their activities is restricted by law.

Germany has the unique *Heilpraktiker* (health practitioner) system. Originally introduced in 1939, it licenses practitioners who are not members of recognized health professions to practise provided they have passed an examination in basic medical knowledge and are registered. The system is administered by the *Länder* (provincial governments), and standards vary considerably between regions. *Heilpraktikers* are specifically prohibited from practising obstetrics, dentistry, and venereology. Non-medical psychotherapists are regulated by the same system.

(From Fisher and Ward, 1994. Reproduced by permission of the BMJ Publishing Group)

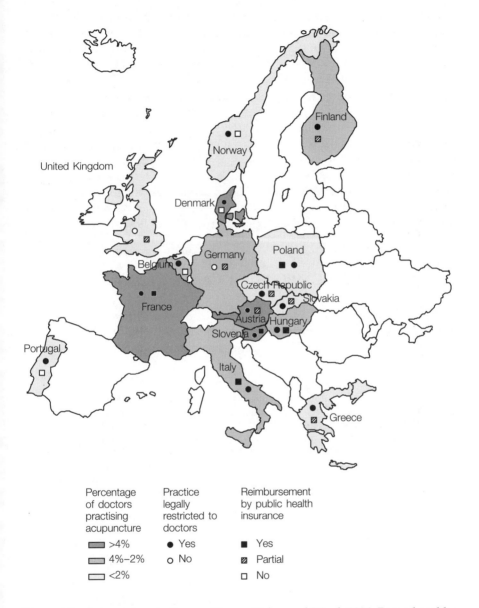

Figure 4.1 Acupuncture in Europe (*Source*: Fisher and Ward, 1994. Reproduced by permission of the BMJ Publishing Group)

The GOC is only the second statutory complementary medicine authority in Europe, the first being the United Kingdom's Faculty of Homeopathy. There are signs, however, that other European countries may follow suit. In April 1994, the Committee on the Environment, Public Health, and Consumer Protection of the European parliament adopted a proposal on the status of complementary medicine. This called for provision of complementary medicine within social security systems, . . . demanded an end to prosecutions of non-medically qualified practitioners in countries such as France and Spain, and for a pan-European system of regulation of non-medically qualified practitioners along the lines of the British Osteopaths Bill. This proposal was to be debated by a full session of the European parliament on 6 May 1994, but its opponents had it removed from the agenda on procedural grounds. Its sponsor, Belgian Green MEP Paul Lannoye, has vowed to revive it (Fisher and Ward, 1994).

EDITORIALS ON COMPLEMENTARY MEDICINE

A number of surveys of doctors' attitudes to complementary medicine have been conducted, but it is also interesting and illuminating to consider some of the editorials written about complementary medicine in medical journals.

> Modern medical science can be proud of its astounding accomplishments, which have improved its capabilities to a level undreamed of even a few decades ago. Nevertheless, all the while such progress was occurring, unproved, unorthodox, and fraudulent practices have continued to flourish, ranging from the medically trivial (but economically important) remedies for baldness and obesity to the 'alternative' practices promoted for serious disease. Their impact on traditional practice has been underestimated. These practices should be understood to represent an unalterable opposition to the basic premise of modern medicine, its cornerstone of objective scientific investigation . . . A lack of clear, consistent and active opposition to such approaches by our profession may be perceived as at least tacit support of unorthodoxy . . . When established methods have been ineffective and the patient is unwilling to forgo all treatment, it is our ethical imperative to discourage unorthodox therapies. (Holohan, 1987)

These, by no means untypical, extracts are from a commentary in the *Journal of the American Medical Association*. The titles of some others give the flavour of some of the stronger editorials and commentary 'Cancer Quackery' (Lerner, 1987), 'Paranormal health claims' (Skrabanek, 1988) and 'Alternative medicine a cruel hoax—your money or your life' (Beaven, 1989).

The main themes of these editorials are the lack of scientific evaluation of complementary medicine, the lack of ethical standards and safeguards for patients and, most importantly, the danger of patients being denied orthodox treatment for serious disease. These are all important points, discussed in more detail elsewhere in this book. The major criticism that can be made of these editorials is that all forms of non-orthodox medicine are lumped together and tarred with the same brush: thus the dedicated, skilled and trained osteopath is condemned along with the fraudulent quack knowingly peddling dubious and perhaps dangerous remedies for cancer.

The stimulus for many of these editorials seems often to be an understandable horror of sick and dying patients who, feeling that they have been written off by orthodox medicine, turn to dubious forms of unorthodox medicine. In the United States laetrile, an untested cancer treatment, provoked particular outrage. However, another important theme emerges: the suspicion that patients no longer see doctors as offering care and emotional support. Holohan (1987), while castigating the quacks, also offers a lament for the loss of care, especially in those cases where cure is not possible.

> Written off . . . How sad that patients would perceive themselves as therapeutic failures that are best forgotten. A painting by Sir Luke Fildes, The Doctor, depicts a physician of the last century, sitting by the bedside in the sickroom of a seriously ill child. He simply watches; but he is with his patient, committed to providing care, even in the absence of a possibility of cure. He has not written her off to the nostrums of peddlers of vegetable extracts, laetrile, colonic irrigation, macrobiotic diets and the like. (Holohan, 1987)

This theme is echoed by Baum (1987), a surgeon concerned both with the failings of conventional medicine and the misuse of complementary medicine. Certainly, he considers doctors and others in orthodox medicine often fail as communicators and fail to fulfil the pastoral role that seriously ill patients require, which may be an important and valid reason for a patient turning to complementary medicine. In this sense, doctors need to approach seriously ill patients in a more holistic manner. Both Baum (1987) and Freer (1985) find it hard to understand how complementary medicine has been able to hijack the notion of holism, the implication being that doctors are no longer concerned (or do not have time to be concerned) with the patient as a person. At the root of this is a confusion, discussed in the previous chapter, between holism in the sense of total, alternative views of the way body and mind function and holism as meaning a willingness to tackle psychological, social and even spiritual issues in the care of patients.

Many of the systems of complementary medicine are holistic in the first sense and this has perhaps too easily been equated with the latter. These two aspects of holism are usefully distinguished in the following study by Goldstein and colleagues who compared holistic physicians with their, supposedly non-holistic, colleagues.

HOLISM IN MEDICINE

Goldstein et al (1988) compared physicians who were members of the American Holistic Medical Association (AHMA) with a comparable group of family practitioners on a variety of demographic and attitude measures. The aim of the study was to examine the extent to which there was a real divergence between the groups, with a view to considering how far integration of holistic or alternative medicine with orthodox approaches was possible. Holistic and complementary approaches were seen as one broad movement, although their results indicate that this assumption was probably erroneous.

There was little difference in social, demographic or practice characteristics between the two groups; AHMA members tended to see fewer patients, hospitalize them less often, and be less highly qualified. Holistic physicians' personal experiences of health and illness was no different from family physicians, and both groups were (in California) equally likely to have been in psychotherapy. The characteristic that strongly differentiated the two groups was the importance the AHMA members attached to the religious or spiritual dimension in their lives, and the fact that they felt that spiritual factors had been important in shaping their medical views.

The particular importance of the study from our point of view comes from the estimates of the value of 26 healing techniques (see Table 4.1), derived from 50 preliminary interviews with self-described holistic physicians. Goldstein and colleagues comment that there is considerable variation among both groups in their views. Indeed, 15 of the techniques are not felt to have much value by the AHMA members; the more unusual, and newsworthy, techniques such as polarity therapy have only a small number of advocates even in the holistic group. Techniques which are valued and used (personally or by referral) by AHMA members (e.g. exercise, diet modification, meditation, counselling) are also widely used and valued by the family practitioners, though generally given slightly less prominence. However, as we move down the table to techniques that are less used by AHMA members, the divergence between the groups becomes more apparent. Almost three-quarters of AHMA members have used chiropractic techniques, and over half spiritual or religious healing, massage and

Table 4.1 Evaluation and utilization of techniques by AHMA members ($N = 340$) and FPS ($N = 142$)

Technique	'Much value' for medical practice (%)		'Some or much value' and utilized in practice (%)	
	AHMA	FP	AHMA	FP
Physical exercise	89.4	78.2	87.4	84.5*
Diet modifications	87.9	55.6	88.3	80.3
Self-care instructions	78.5	52.8	83.2	70.4
Meditation/relaxation	77.9	36.6	85.9	69.7
Counselling/psychotherapy	73.5	66.9*	83.5	84.5*
Biofeedback	64.1	28.9	74.7	71.2
Nutritional supplements	61.8	11.3	83.0	52.9
Stress/wellness inventory	56.8	23.2	66.5	46.5
Hypnosis/guided imagery	56.5	19.7	72.6	50.0
Acupuncture	55.9	17.6	68.6	51.4
Autogenic training	46.5	7.7	47.9	14.0
Chiropractic manipulation	45.9	12.7	72.4	50.7
Spiritual or religious healing	45.6	9.2	53.5	20.4
Homeopathy	31.8	1.4	42.1	8.4
Massage/rolfing	30.0	6.3	52.4	21.8
Psychological tests	27.9	21.8*	64.7	71.1*
Acupressure	27.4	8.5	56.4	31.6
Herbal medicine	26.8	2.1	47.3	9.1
Dance or movement therapy	25.0	11.3	37.0	21.8
Laying on of hands	19.7	3.5	30.6	5.6
Psychic diagnosis and healing	18.8	1.4	30.3	3.5
Applied kinesiology	15.9	4.2	34.7	8.4
Polarity healing	9.1	0.7	20.9	1.4
Reflexology	7.4	0.7	22.7	2.1
Iridology	4.4	0.0	13.2	1.4

* Test is not significant at the 0.001 level. Items were measured by a 4-point scale. Scaling for left column: not familiar with technique = 1, familiar but no value for medical practice = 2, some value = 3, much value = 4. Scaling for right column: not familiar with technique or familiar, but no value in medical practice, never used = 1, some or much value, never used = 2, no value but used = 3, some or much value and used = 4.

(From Goldstein et al, 1988. Reproduced by permission of Elsevier Science Inc.)

acupressure. Nevertheless, Goldstein et al write that 'the overall picture that emerges . . . shows most AHMA members to be involved with techniques and approaches that are relatively acceptable to doctors who do not specifically identify themselves as "holistic"'.

The list of healing techniques in fact contains relatively few that we would strictly describe as complementary. Psychological and self-help techniques are prominent and quite highly valued by both groups. Other differences between the two groups tend to indicate that what differentiates a 'holistic' physician may not necessarily have very much to do with complementary medicine, except perhaps a willingness to explore it. More important is the difference in their overall practice styles, which tends to emphasize a more collaborative personal relationship with their patients (Table 4.2). Differences between groups emerge particularly in their views on emotional involvement, a more equal relationship and less reliance on traditional barriers between physicians and their clients. It is interesting that differences emerge not because family physicians think that these things are unimportant, but because a significant proportion of holistic physicians attach very great importance to a particular kind of relationship with their patients.

This study has emphasized again that a holistic approach may be only loosely associated with advocacy of complementary techniques. Holistic physicians do perhaps have a willingness to consider such techniques, and their emphasis on a more equal relationship with their patients probably encourages more discussion of complementary therapies. In the remainder of this chapter we consider studies examining knowledge, interest and attitudes in complementary medicine *per se* among doctors.

KNOWLEDGE AND INTEREST IN COMPLEMENTARY MEDICINE

Although doctors' increasing interest in complementary medicine had been noted in the medical literature, no formal studies were published in the United Kingdom until Reilly (1983) published a survey of young doctors' views.

The survey of 86 general practitioner trainees showed a remarkably high interest in complementary medicine and a surprisingly positive attitude. Over 80% considered acupuncture to be useful, and about 50% considered homeopathy and osteopathy to be useful. More than a third of these trainees had referred patients for some alternative treatment; 13% had received some form of complementary medicine (and a further 13% had undergone hypnotherapy). Whether or not they were users of complementary medicine themselves, a high proportion expressed interest in training; 24% in manipulative therapies, 22% in acupuncture, 12% in homeopathy and one in herbalism.

Reilly stated that a pilot study found that hospital doctors had less interest in complementary medicine, and suggested that complementary techniques

Table 4.2 Practice styles among AHMA members and family practitioners (%)

Trait	Always		Often		Sometimes		Never		Mean*	
	AHMA	FP	AHMA	FP	AHMA	FP	AHMA	FP	AHMA	FP
Emphasize a personal responsibility	37.0	24.6	53.4	54.2	9.6	20.4	0.0	0.7	2.27	2.03+
Connect psychological and physiological	32.6	19.7	47.8	52.1	19.3	26.8	0.3	1.4	2.13	1.90#
Get detailed personal history	46.0	22.5	37.7	43.7	16.0	31.7	0.3	2.1	2.29	1.86+
Share personal feelings and experiences	7.7	2.1	43.6	23.9	48.1	68.3	0.6	5.6	1.58	1.23+
Collaborative relations with patients	20.9	9.5	44.2	43.1	30.0	41.6	4.8	5.8	1.81	1.49+
Touch patients more than most	27.7	9.5	48.0	43.1	21.6	41.6	2.7	5.8	2.01	1.56+
Feel free to express caring	30.7	12.7	51.0	43.7	18.4	42.3	0.6	1.4	2.1	1.68+

* Always = 3, often = 2, sometimes = 1, never = 0.
# $p < 0.01$, two-tailed t-test
+ $p < 0.001$, two-tailed t-test

(From Goldstein et al, 1988. Reproduced by permission of Elsevier Science Inc.)

Table 4.3   Training and use of complementary medicine by general practitioners

Therapy	Training received	Practising	Training intended
Acupuncture	3	3	6
Herbalism	1	1	1
Homeopathy	5	5	6
Hypnosis	12	5	3
Spinal manipulation	26	24	10
Spiritual healing	5	7	1

Figures are percentages of respondents

(Adapted from Wharton and Lewith, 1986. Reproduced by permission of the BMJ Publishing Group)

might have a lesser role in the more specialized and technological environment of the hospital. Reilly commented that holistic care, the need to consider the person and his or her life as well as the illness, is hardly a new idea in general practice. Because primary care doctors might have a greater awareness of the need for holistic care, they might be more willing to consider complementary forms of treatment.

Later studies have substantiated and enlarged on Reilly's findings. Wharton and Lewith (1986) found that although British general practitioners did not claim to know a great deal about most complementary therapies, 59% of them believed that they were useful and many were practising complementary techniques. Over 40% reported referrals to medical practitioners of homeopathy and herbalism, and 28% to medical acupuncturists. Corresponding figures for non-medical practitioners were slightly lower. Table 4.3 shows that almost a quarter were practising spinal manipulation, though this should not necessarily be considered a complementary technique. A small percentage were practising acupuncture, homeopathy and herbalism and more intended to train in these techniques.

In a similar, but larger, study of 222 British general practitioners, Anderson and Anderson (1987) found that 31% of doctors claimed a working knowledge of at least one form of complementary medicine, 12% had received training and 42% wanted further training in at least one area. The proportions receiving and intending training were comparable to the figures reported by Wharton and Lewith (1986). Of the 222 doctors (16%) in the Anderson and Anderson sample, 35% were practising some form of complementary medicine themselves; in the year of the study they had treated over 2000 patients with complementary medicine, about 5% of the total number of patients seen. Manipulation for spinal problems (900 patients) and acupuncture for pain (700) made up the bulk of the treatments.

Referrals to complementary therapists are perhaps a cause for concern, as many doctors have little understanding of the widely varying skills and standards of complementary practitioners. In a comparison of the attitudes of medical students, general practitioners and hospital doctors (to the major systems of complementary medicine), Perkin, Pearcy and Fraser (1994) found that 70% of hospital doctors and 93% of general practitioners had suggested a referral to a complementary practitioner on at least one occasion. They found that 12% of hospital doctors and 20% of general practitioners were practising some form of complementary medicine, most commonly acupuncture. Medical students were the most enthusiastic, and least well-informed, but many doctors had little knowledge of the qualifications of complementary therapists, even though they were making referrals.

General practitioners outside the United Kingdom have shown a similar interest in complementary medicine. Almost all of a sample of 360 doctors in The Netherlands reported referring patients to complementary practitioners (Visser and Peters, 1990). As 600 doctors were originally circulated, this is probably an overestimate; the respondents may well have had a more positive attitude to complementary medicine. Almost half the respondents (47%) gave some form of complementary medicine themselves, generally homeopathy, but the number of patients given such treatments was small. In Germany, Himmel, Schulte and Kochen (1993) found that 95% of the 40 respondents to the questionnaire used some form of complementary medicine, most commonly herbal medicine. As the response rate was low, 95% is almost certainly an overestimate of the true level of use. In New Zealand, 30% of respondents in a survey (11% of total sample) practised one or more forms of complementary medicine and 69% (24% of sample) referred patients for complementary treatment, most commonly to acupuncturists (Marshall and Gee, 1990). Musculo–skeletal problems, pain, headache and back problems, fatigue and psychological problems, smoking and weight loss made up 90% of the referrals. Even with a relatively high level of use, patients' demands for complementary therapies exceeded their practitioners' willingness, or ability, to provide it.

These generally positive views of complementary medicine are also found in preclinical medical students, who are studying basic medical sciences but not yet seeing patients. Furnham (1993) found that the majority (77%) of his sample of over 200 medical students believed that complementary practitioners did have effective forms of treatment. They generally rejected the negative stereotypes sometimes associated both with complementary practitioners and their patients; they did not, for instance, believe that complementary practitioners were unstable or their patients neurotic. They agreed that many patients had found complementary medicine effective and just under half knew someone personally who had been helped by complementary medicine. The students were, however, well aware of the low status of complementary medicine within orthodox medicine and most would try to dissuade a colleague from leaving orthodox medicine to practise complementary medicine.

Furnham examined medical students' perceptions of the efficacy of complementary medicine in more detail, asking them to rate the efficacy of both orthodox and complementary medicine for 27 common complaints and diseases. Orthodox medicine was seen, not surprisingly, and perhaps reassuringly considering the subjects were medical students, as more effective for most serious illnesses. However, complementary medicine (the type of therapy was not specified) was seen as more effective in the treatment of a considerable number of chronic and stress-related conditions: back pain, fatigue, insomnia, stress, obesity, menstrual problems, migraine, rheumatoid arthritis and the common cold.

A criticism that can be made of many of the studies reviewed in this section concerns the precise definition of complementary medicine. Hypnosis is routinely included, as is spinal manipulation, which is used in orthodox medicine (though not osteopathy and chiropractic, which have a wider remit and different underlying theories). Anderson and Anderson (1987) even included relaxation and psychotherapy, certainly standard practice among National Health Service psychologists, although not specifically part of general practice training. The effect of these inconsistencies is to exaggerate the interest in those therapies that would be generally agreed to be complementary; when specific therapies are considered, however, it is clear that there is still substantial interest, and that a sizeable proportion of general practitioners have a positive attitude to complementary medicine.

DOCTORS' VIEWS OF THE VALIDITY OF COMPLEMENTARY MEDICINE

The results of trials of the effectiveness of complementary medicine are considered in Chapters 9 and 10. Here we will simply consider doctors' views of the usefulness and efficacy of complementary therapies. As we shall see, although doctors have much easier access to the medical and scientific literature than the general public, their personal opinions of complementary medicine may have less lofty origins.

Table 4.4   General practitioners' views of the value of complementary therapies

Therapy	Very useful	Useful	No opinion	Not useful	Harmful
Acupuncture	8	59	26	8	–
Herbalism	1	22	48	3	1
Homeopathy	3	44	36	16	1
Hypnosis	8	71	17	3	1
Spinal manipulation	27	62	6	2	2
Spiritual healing	6	40	31	16	6

Figures are percentages of respondents

(Adapted from Wharton and Lewith, 1986. Reproduced by permission of the BMJ Publishing Group)

Several studies have assessed doctors' overall views of the usefulness of different forms of complementary medicine. Table 4.4, taken from Wharton and Lewith (1986), shows that almost 90% of general practitioners consider manipulation useful or very useful, with acupuncture (67%), homeopathy (47%) and spiritual healing (46%) also scoring highly.

In The Netherlands, Knipschild, Kleijnen and ter Riet (1990) examined general practitioners' beliefs in the efficacy of a long list of complementary therapies, with the interesting and sensible addition of specific diseases in some cases. Thus the efficacy of acupuncture was separately rated (on a 10-point scale) for chronic pain, asthma and smoking cessation. Their results for acupuncture, homeopathy, manual therapy, healing, hypnosis and reflexology are shown in Table 4.5. We have included healing and hypnosis as interesting comparisons with the mainstream complementary therapies, and reflexology as an undoubtedly complementary, but rather marginal, technique.

Acupuncture was considered to be effective for chronic pain by over half the doctors replying (74% response rate in study) and homeopathy for respiratory tract infection by 45%. Manual therapy seems not to be perceived as unorthodox any longer in The Netherlands, being seen as equivalent to physiotherapy. Many fewer give credit to faith healing (7%) or healing (17%); massage of various kinds is thought to be beneficial, but reflexology (massage of the feet) is seen as effective by only 14%. The authors commented: 'We are surprised at the high amount of credit that is given to certain (to us) incomprehensible practices such as acupuncture, homeopathy and anthroposophy. It must be realized that even low percentages of positive scores represent a good many doctors.' They go on to suggest that if there is a large gap between the perceived and actual efficacy of these practices, then literature reviews evaluating the efficacy of

Table 4.5 Dutch general practitioners' beliefs in the efficacy of complementary medicine

Therapy/complaint	Mean	Distribution (%)				
		0–1	2–3	4–5	6–7	8–10
Acupuncture Chronic pain	5.0	12	12	26	36	14
Acupuncture Asthma	3.1	35	19	23	17	5
Acupuncture Smoking	3.7	26	22	24	20	8
Homeopathy Pain	2.3	51	15	19	11	4
Homeopathy Upper respiratory tract infection	4.7	20	10	24	32	15
Homeopathy Chronic joint disease	4.5	20	11	25	32	11
Faith healing (general)	1.5	65	17	11	4	3
Healing (general)	2.6	43	18	23	14	3
Hypnosis Smoking	3.6	28	18	24	26	4
Manual therapy Chronic neck/back problems	6.4	4	4	12	47	33
Physiotherapy Chronic neck/back problems	6.3	3	4	21	43	28
Reflexology General	2.4	49	16	21	11	3

Ratings on 10-point scale of efficacy (high = effective)

(From Knipschild, Kleijnen and ter Riet, 1990. Reproduced by permission of Elsevier Science Inc.)

such studies should be published in both the scientific journals and the lay press.

Admittedly, the literature on the evaluation of many complementary therapies is scant, and in some cases non-existent. Nevertheless, there is a fairly substantial literature, albeit of a very variable standard, on some of the major complementary therapies (see Chapters 9 and 10). However, the existing scientific literature may not be a crucial determinant of doctors' views. Wharton and Lewith (1986) found that:

General practitioners views indicated that their views had been influenced in a positive way by: observed benefits to patients (41%), personal or family experience of benefit (38%), the media (14%), post-graduate education (11%) and colleagues who practised (6%). The negative influences were: the lack of observed effects on patients (26%), the lack of scientific evidence (22%), their own inadequate knowledge (22%), the tendency for non-medical therapists to charge large fees and persist with ineffective treatments (14%) and the harmful effects of treatment (11%).

The problem of disseminating scientific literature to practitioners of all kinds is very great. It is perhaps understandable that doctors, like most other people, rely on personal experiences and observation in assessing the value of complementary medicine. In many cases the evidence is not of sufficient quality to permit a definitive judgement. However, some studies indicate that although general practitioners are sceptical of the theories underlying complementary therapies, they may take a pragmatic attitude to their value for individual patients.

Using a slightly different question, which may more closely reflect doctors' views on efficacy and scientific credentials, Anderson and Anderson (1987) asked general practitioners if they considered each therapy to have a valid theoretical basis. Manipulation was considered valid by 32%, acupuncture by 15%, hypnotherapy by 8%, homeopathy by 7% and faith healing, in contrast, by less than 1%. In The Netherlands a majority of doctors conceded that complementary medicine 'included ideas from which official medicine could benefit', but only 19% disagreed with a statement that most effects of complementary medicine were due to the placebo effect (i.e. primarily psychologically mediated) (Visser and Peters, 1990). Verhof and Sutherland (1995) looked at 200 Canadian general practitioners' assessment of and interest in alternative medicine. Whereas three-quarters agreed that general practitioners should have knowledge about the most important alternative treatments, only a quarter believed it important to know the practitioners in their area. Over half (65%) perceived a demand from their patients, especially for musculo–skeletal problems, chronic pain and illness. Interestingly, the general practitioners saw chiropractic, hypnosis and acupuncture (for chronic pain) as most efficacious and homeopathy and reflexology less so. Overall, these doctors seemed more cautious and sceptical than many of their European equivalents, but this could be accounted for by sampling differences. Similarly, Furnham (1993) found that medical students believed that complementary medicine was primarily effective for functional conditions where psychological factors could be said to play a part.

These studies provide evidence that general practitioners believe that complementary medicine is both useful and effective. However, they give little indication of why doctors believe these therapies are effective. Do they think they are effective placebos or do they believe that they have specific therapeutic effects? It would be entirely logical to believe that homeopathy was a useful form of treatment for those patients who found its philosophy sympathetic, to believe that it played some part in assisting recovery and yet also to believe that homeopathic preparations had only a psychological effect.

Visser and Peters (1990) point out that most general practitioners are not scientists, concerned with the developing and testing of theories and techniques, but pragmatists whose main aim is to cure patients, by whatever means. Consequently 'they are willing to give a method the benefit of the doubt, even if its scientific basis has not yet been assessed. They are even more willing to do so at the patient's request and when regular care has not shown sufficient positive results. Once a larger number of practitioners make use of a method, the professional group tends to 'legalize' it in order to prevent the front from cracking' (Visser and Peters, 1990).

While general practitioners are pragmatists, it does seem that they do not all view complementary techniques as simply placebos. Visser and Peters (1990) found that a third of Dutch general practitioners viewed complementary medicine as 'something more than a placebo effect', though interest in complementary medicine was confined to the major therapies. It seems unlikely though that doctors would wish to train in a therapy that they believed was little more than an elaborate placebo; at least those who have trained or intend to train in a complementary therapy probably consider that it is a truly valuable and effective form of therapy.

TRAINING IN COMPLEMENTARY MEDICINE

The interest in complementary medicine shown by general practitioners has led many to consider training in one or more of the complementary therapies. Reilly (1983) found that 82% of his group of general practitioner trainees wished to train in at least one method; 30–40% of general practitioners in Britain had attended classes or lectures on complementary medicine (Wharton and Lewith, 1986; Anderson and Anderson, 1987); over half of Dutch general practitioners actually practised some form of complementary medicine (Visser and Peters, 1990), 30% in new Zealand (Marshall and Gee, 1990), 16% in Britain (Anderson and Anderson, 1987).

With such a high level of interest and acceptance of complementary medicine, some authors (e.g. Anderson and Anderson, 1987) have argued that adequate and recognized training should be provided in complementary techniques. However, critics of this approach have pointed out that many of the techniques sometimes labelled 'complementary' are regularly used in orthodox settings (e.g. manipulation, hypnosis), and that interest in complementary medicine has thus been exaggerated. In Anderson's sample of 222 doctors, only 6 practised acupuncture and 2 homeopathy. Some critics also argue that the evaluation of complementary medicine is the primary concern; until there is firm evidence for its efficacy, over and above a placebo response, there is no argument for including it in medical training, at either student or postgraduate level (Skrabanek and McCormick, 1987). This seems reasonable at first sight, but not much of orthodox medicine would be left if doctors were only allowed to use treatments which had been fully evaluated in controlled trials.

General practitioners, certainly in the United Kingdom, already have many opportunities to learn about complementary medicine. Medical practitioners of acupuncture and homeopathy are comparatively common, and many courses are advertised. The more difficult question is whether complementary medicine should be taught within the already overcrowded medical school curriculum. Training in the techniques might be better left to the post-qualification period. However, an introduction to the methods and the widespread use of complementary medicine would certainly seem to be indicated, if only because many patients, whether their doctor knows it or not, consult complementary practitioners. Several of the studies have pointed out that doctors' interest in complementary medicine exceeds their knowledge of the various techniques. As Reilly points out lay complementary practitioners greatly outnumber medical complementary practitioners and the 'exclusion of these methods from medical training carries certain implications for the future'. In other words, the absence of teaching on complementary medicine in medical school may, paradoxically, foster a stronger body of lay practitioners.

In the United Kingdom there are isolated examples of courses on complementary medicine. George Lewith at Southampton and David Taylor Reilly at Glasgow medical school have both offered introductory courses. However, these initiatives have relied on the presence of particular interested and knowledgeable individuals; the subject has not necessarily been formally incorporated into the teaching. A series of colloquia on the relationship between conventional and complementary therapies at the Royal Society of Medicine has resulted in proposals for a short course in complementary medicine, that is largely self-directed and does not require a faculty member with particular expertise in the area (Box 4.2). The course does not involve any training in complementary techniques, but should enable the student to become familiar with complementary therapies and to consider the arguments and counterarguments for their use and efficacy. It

Box 4.2   A suggested medical curriculum for learning about complementary medicine

Medical students should have an opportunity to consider the scientific (or non-scientific) backgrounds to these alternatives, and the ethics of their practice, since their future patients will ask about and use them, and since an alternative therapy may sometimes be as efficacious as standard treatment. At the end of the curriculum all students should have achieved:

(a) knowledge about complementary medicine and the placebo effect, from both scientific and social points of view
(b) skills in collaborative problem solving, including hypothesis formation and testing; in finding and critically appraising information; and in articulating ideas and arguments
(c) attitudes of open-mindedness about patient autonomy, about coping with uncertainty, and about ethical decision-making when counselling patients about unproven therapies.

The proposed curriculum is described below:

(a) Pairs of students are randomly assigned one of the various types of complementary medicine being practised in the community, and then attached to a practitioner who has volunteered to the project.
(b) The pair search the current literature on their type of complementary medicine, and select and read key articles. They determine what is considered to be the scientific basis for the therapy, and describe ethical problems that they think might be encountered in its practice.
(c) To find out whether their ideas correspond to actuality, the students then interview their practitioner, some of his or her patients who have benefited from treatment, and medical doctors, scientists and unsatisfied patients.
(d) Each pair prepares arguments for and against the use of the complementary medicine as if to convince an educated, intelligent patient.
(e) A half-day is then allocated to debating the issues that have emerged during the students' library and field researches. The debates could be organised in a number of ways. For example, the class could be divided into a number of groups so that each includes pairs of students who have investigated all the types of complementary medicine studied. Students could be randomly assigned to speak for ten minutes for, or against, the therapy they have studied. Randomisation at the time of the debate will have the effect of ensuring that each student is conversant with both sides of the argument. If a mark were required the students within each group could assess the presentations, using a descriptive rating scale, on the debaters' cogency of argument, recognition of ethical issues, and critical appraisal of information. Students would pass or fail according to the majority assessment of their peers. For added interest, students could vote on the winner of each debate.
(f) The role of the faculty is to solicit the volunteer practitioners, to formulate and explain the objectives and organisation of the curriculum to the students and volunteers, and to act as advisors to students in relation to their investigations.

continues

> ┌──── *continued* ──
> This curriculum may also be useful as a model for learning about and debating the desirability of controversial therapies within conventional and surgical practice.
>
> (From Hansen, 1991. Reproduced by permission of *Journal of Royal Society of Medicine*)

is interesting to note that there is specific reference to the placebo effect. This is certainly an important topic as psychological influences may be the predominant ones in many complementary practices. However, the same may apply to many orthodox medical practices (see Chapter 7), and yet little attention is currently given to placebo effects in the current medical curriculum.

THE INTEGRATION OF ORTHODOX AND COMPLEMENTARY CARE

So far we have mainly considered doctors' own use of complementary medicine; there are, however, signs of a growing willingness of many general practitioners to work quite closely with at least some complementary practitioners. Referrals to complementary practitioners are certainly common (incidentally an argument for at least some basic education on the nature and efficacy of complementary medicine, both for medical students and trained doctors). Referrals to medically qualified complementary practitioners are made by between 59 and 76% of general practitioners, and only slightly fewer to lay complementary practitioners (Wharton and Lewith, 1986; Anderson and Anderson, 1987; Marshall and Gee, 1990). In The Netherlands, however, Visser and Peters (1990) found that most doctors preferred to limit their contacts to complementary practitioners who at least had para-medical qualifications (e.g. physiotherapists). They comment that in The Netherlands, accepting complementary medicine means not just tolerating it, but accepting that complementary techniques are increasingly being actually integrated into medical care.

Some general practices in the United Kingdom (and most probably elsewhere) have introduced lay complementary practitioners. Until recently these initiatives have usually been funded as part of a research project, unless the practitioners worked on a voluntary basis. With the advent of fund-holding general practices, the scope for the use of complementary medicine will become greater, especially as it is very much cheaper for patients to see complementary practitioners than doctors (although this is offset by the greater length of complementary consultations). There are also some examples in the United Kingdom of primarily complementary practices bringing in doctors; patients are referred for orthodox or complementary therapy (or a combination) as appropriate.

A report of an experiment in integration is provided by Budd et al (1990), who describe the introduction of an osteopath and an acupuncturist into a London general practice. Each practitioner worked one day a week and 197 patients were referred over a period of 18 months, primarily for musculo–skeletal problems in the case of the osteopath, and for a wide variety of chronic problems in the case of the acupuncturist. The report concentrates on the organization of the service and there are few details of the value of the treatment, except a general comment that patients benefited. However, the introduction of this service led to fewer referrals to hospital physiotherapy departments, fewer referrals to orthopaedic and rheumatology departments and fewer prescriptions for pain-killing drugs. A number of patients successfully treated by the therapists would otherwise have continued to see the general practitioner, probably on a long-term basis. On three occasions serious conditions, which had not been diagnosed by the general practitioner, emerged as a result of the patient talking to the osteopath and revealing symptoms which, perhaps owing to embarrassment or a shorter consultation time, had not been disclosed to the doctor. The doctors and complementary practitioners involved suggest that some complementary therapies might be considered as professions supplementary of medicine, and suggest that their own initiative might serve as a model for similar projects elsewhere.

Burton (1990), in a letter welcoming Budd and colleagues' study, suggested that two fundamental issues needed to be clarified before considering the integration of a complementary form of medicine into general practice, or into any branch of orthodox medicine.

> First, does the complementary therapy consider itself to be offering a therapy, or alternative system of medicine? Secondly, is the approach of the complementary discipline effective, and does it offer something that allopathic (orthodox) management does not?

> If the complementary discipline feels that it is providing an alternative system, which by definition renders competing systems redundant, it is difficult to see how the orthodox and heterodox can peacefully co-exist. However, if the complementary discipline believes it is offering a novel method of treatment (albeit based on peculiar diagnostic and assessment abilities) then open dialogue and assessment of efficacy is facilitated. As far as osteopathy is concerned it has been argued that what is being provided is a therapy which does not require invocation of alternative systems to explain its claimed efficacy. Thus, for this profession at least, there is the possibility of following a conventional scientific route to explore its value for specific and recognizable conditions.

Burton goes on to suggest that general practice is an ideal setting in which to evaluate complementary medicine. There are large numbers of patients and the setting is very similar to many complementary practices—office-based environments situated in the community. Any arrangement that involves clinical collaboration is likely to facilitate research collaboration.

Burton appears to suggest not only that the complementary medicine should not be holding itself up as a complete system of medicine wishing to 'take over' from orthodox medicine, but also that it does not require unorthodox explanations of its efficacy. She allows, however, that the diagnostic practices may be unusual without upsetting the collaboration. Osteopathy, which is apparently quite similar to some aspects of conventional medicine, can fairly easily meet these requirements. Acupuncture, homeopathy and naturopathy, with rather more unusual theories, might find these requirements more difficult to meet (though an acupuncturist was involved in the Budd study). Medical acupuncturists, of course, most of whom have ignored or abandoned traditional acupuncture theory altogether, would generally not have these problems.

Complementary Medicine: a New Dilemma for the Doctor

When complementary practitioners work alongside general practitioners, problems can potentially be resolved by discussion between orthodox and complementary practitioners, much as they are between different professions within the health service. When patients are separately consulting a number of practitioners, both orthodox and complementary, problems may arise because each practitioner may be unaware of the potentially conflicting treatments of the others.

Following the discovery of several 'multiple therapy users' Murray and Shepherd (1988) surveyed the use of complementary medicine in a South London general practice. Over 30% of 35-year-olds had used one of 20 forms of complementary medicine, not rejecting orthodox medicine but often using complementary medicine alongside it. They commented that use of complementary medicine does not necessarily lead to a reduction in the use of general practitioner services if all forms of treatment are used concurrently and without discussion between practitioners. A later study (Murray and Shepherd, 1993) reported that 34% of men and 46% of women patients in a South London general practice had used complementary medicine in the previous 10 years. The study confirmed that use of complementary medicine may not involve a reduction in the use of general practitioner services. Users of complementary medicine had higher than average general practice consultation rates, reflecting their high prevalence of chronic conditions such as asthma, back pain and skin disorders. They also had a relatively high frequency of psychosocial problems and affective disorders, though this may represent the consequences of chronic illness rather than indicating psychological problems *per se*.

Murray and Shepherd (1988) consider that the widespread concurrent use of complementary medicine poses a number of problems for the general practitioner, which are as yet unresolved. Does the general practitioner continue to accept overall clinical responsibility if their patient is receiving a form of complementary treatment that might be harmful? How are patients to avoid a potential conflict of medical management? Even when they are seeing only a complementary therapist, the general practitioner may still be involved as the only person providing 24-hour cover. They also express concern about the absence of information passed between complementary and orthodox practitioners, and the lack of ethical and disciplinary codes governing some branches of complementary medicine.

The most difficult problem for the general practitioner who wishes to refer patients for complementary treatment revolves around the need to assess the qualifications and credentials of the complementary practitioner. The GMC states that:

> A doctor who delegates treatment of other procedures must be satisfied that the person to whom they are delegated is competent to carry them out. It is also important that the doctor should retain ultimate responsibility for the management of his patients because only the doctor has received the necessary training to undertake this responsibility . . . For these reasons a doctor who improperly delegates to a person who is not a registered medical practitioner is liable to disciplinary proceedings. (General Medical Council, 1992)

It seems that the general practitioner may open him- or herself to disciplinary proceedings or allegations of negligence if a patient is harmed by a complementary practitioner he or she refers to, or even 'gives permission to consult', if he or she does not have grounds for considering the complementary practitioner competent (Murray and Shepherd, 1988). As Murray and Shepherd point out, there are a plethora of professional and diploma awarding associations in the complementary sector, and it is difficult to be assured of the qualifications of individual therapists. General practitioners may even be susceptible to attacks for both errors of omission and commission in respect of referral for potentially valuable complementary therapies.

If complementary practitioners and orthodox practitioners are to function as potential therapeutic allies, then the problems of referral will have to be addressed. It is absurd for a doctor to face possible disciplinary proceedings for referring to a practitioner whom he believes may benefit a patient. The problems facing a doctor wishing to refer a patient to a complementary practitioner will, in some cases, be eased as various complementary therapies are seeking statutory registration.

It is important to note the divergence between the views of the GMC and the actual behaviour of the general public. The GMC still adheres to a model of medical practice in which the doctor retains ultimate clinical responsibility in all situations. Many patients, on the other hand, regard the doctor as one specialist among others, to be consulted when appropriate but not necessarily to be regarded as the final arbiter of appropriate and acceptable treatment. This observation brings us back to Helman's (1990) point that most medicine and therapeutic help is either self-administered or derived from the 'folk' sector, which includes complementary medicine. Orthodox, professional medicine, is relatively infrequently used for many minor or chronic conditions, although it, of course, assumes a far greater importance when serious illness is encountered. From this perspective the activities of doctors and other members of the health professions are seen as one part, albeit a vital one, of a much wider effort towards health involving a great variety of lay and professional people.

Chapter 5

Knowledge, Attitudes and Beliefs of Patients of Complementary Practitioners

What do lay people believe or know about health and illness? Are the philosophical tenets and assumptions of each complementary therapy important for patients and part of the explanation for its appeal? Do complementary practitioners offer more autonomy and control to patients? Do complementary practitioners 'educate' their patients more thoroughly than those in orthodox medicine? Alternatively, the relationship between patient and practitioner may be the determining factor. Complementary practitioners may spend more time, listen more carefully, appear more sympathetic and be more likely to touch the patient: the philosophical issues may have little to do with it. The next two chapters are devoted to a discussion of the often sparse empirical research on these questions. As research findings are limited, in fact the whole research area is barely developed as far as complementary therapies are concerned, we will also set out the general conceptual and empirical background to show its potential relevance to complementary medicine and to future research in this field.

LAY BELIEFS ABOUT HEALTH AND ILLNESS

Social scientists from many disciplines (anthropology, education, psychology, sociology) have for some time shown considerable interest in patients' beliefs about health and illness. These beliefs, it is argued, play an important role in determining whether, when, and why patients seek help, to what extent they follow advice and may also influence the outcome of treatment. Experience of complementary and, indeed, orthodox medicine may in turn contribute to these beliefs and theories, enrich and reinforce them.

Nearly all people have theories as to the cause and most effective cure both of minor, frequently occurring ailments (e.g. coughs, colds), and more serious complaints. Various analogies (metaphors, models) are used by people in different cultures or subcultures to describe and 'explain' illnesses and their aetiologies. Chrisman (1977) identified eight ways of conceptualizing the origins of illness: *time running out* or degeneration, where illness is attributed to the wearing out of the body; *mechanical* faults or damage, where illness is attributed to broken or faulty body mechanisms; *imbalance* or lack of harmony, either between various parts of the body or between the individual and his or her environment; *invasion* or penetrations of the body by germs or other foreign bodies causing illness. *Debilitation*: a weakness of the body that results from overworking, being 'run-down', a chronic disease or a weak spot in the body; *stress*: usually from work, relationships, environmental sources; *environmental irritants*: such as allergies, pollens, poisons, food additives, smoke, etc.; *hereditary proneness*: genetic transmission of a particular illness, quality or trait which includes general weakness.

These metaphors or analogies are the natural ways in which lay people think about illness, but they often contrast dramatically with the concepts of Western medical science. Though these lay beliefs are complex they are often inconsistent or unscientific. Indeed, patients may feel self-conscious about the relatively unsophisticated, foolish or even superstitious nature of their beliefs about illness when confronted by an orthodox medical doctor, and may therefore be loath to disclose them. Others, on the other hand, may challenge their doctors' view with their own conceptions and understanding. These beliefs are often highly idiosyncratic, being derived and adapted from a wide variety of sources, yet they are also flexible and changeable in particular circumstances. Such beliefs form a 'system', in the sense that they are related to other non-illness related beliefs and also to the beliefs of other people in the community (Furnham, 1988).

Helman (1990) described a set of commonly held beliefs about 'colds', 'chills' and 'fevers' in a London suburb. Colds and chills are seen to be caused by the penetration of the natural environment (particularly areas of cold or damp) across the boundary of the skin and into the human body. In general, damp or rain (cold–wet environments) cause cold–wet conditions in the body, such as a 'runny nose' or a 'cold in the head', while cold winds or draughts (cold–dry environments) cause cold–dry conditions such as a feeling of cold, shivering and muscular aches. This belief system suggests that once they enter the body, these cold forces can move from place to place—from a 'head cold', for example, down to a 'chest cold'. Chills occur mainly below the belt ('a bladder chill', 'a chill on the kidneys', 'a stomach chill'), and colds above it ('a head cold', 'a cold in the sinuses', 'a cold in the chest'). These conditions are caused by careless behaviour, by putting oneself in a position of risk *vis-à-vis* the natural environment; for example, by 'walking barefoot on a cold floor', 'washing your hair when you don't feel well', or 'sitting in a draught after a hot bath'. Temperatures intermediate between hot and cold, where the former gives way to the latter, such as going outdoors after a hot bath, or else in autumn, where 'hot' summer gives way to 'cold' autumn, are specially conducive to 'catching cold'. Many of these images and metaphors, although of modern, Western origin, are very reminiscent of the explanatory concepts of traditional Chinese medicine. The apparently exotic concepts of Chinese medicine (wind, damp, heat, etc.) may in fact seem comfortingly familiar to some Western patients, as they echo their own natural way of describing and reflecting on illness.

These lay theories about health are sometimes difficult to change because they are based on extensive personal experience and many socially accepted ideas. People can be highly motivated to retain them, either because they support various social behaviours, or because they are firmly embedded in other beliefs about the physical and social world. However, there is evidence that concepts of illness do change in response to changing circumstances. For instance, Hunt, Jordan and Irwin (1989) studied a group of women over time and found that they 'continually tried out, adjusted and reworked the construction of their illness to adapt them to the exigencies of everyday life'. Illness explanations are dynamic, and their change is partly due to their usefulness within the extra-medical social environment.

Lay Aetiologies of Illness

People may site the cause of illness either in the individual patient (behaviour, diet, vulnerability) or the natural, social or even supernatural world (Helman, 1990). Blaxter (1983) interviewed a sample of working-class, middle-aged women in Scotland about their ideas of health and illness, and who discussed 587 examples of episodes of disease. The issue of cause was mentioned in 74% of examples, classified by Blaxter as follows. Infection was by far the most common category of cause invoked. Next most frequent was heredity, followed by environmental hazards, secondary effects of other diseases, stress, childbearing and the menopause, and trauma and surgery. Less common as a category of cause was the notion of a self-inflicted disorder through neglect or behavioural choice. Blaxter observed that the search for causal patterns in their health histories was extremely important to the women and she refers to a 'positive strain towards accounting for their present bodily state ... by connecting together the relevant health events' (Blaxter, 1983).

More recently, Stanton-Rogers (1991) conducted a thorough investigation of lay beliefs and explanations about health and illness using social constructionist research methods. (Extensive in-depth interviews and subsequent sorting and rating of attitude statements by a large group of subjects.) Explanations for good health divided into two categories (those which arise *inside* and those *outside* the individual) which were further subdivided. Four types of explanations related to those that were internal: *behaviour* (looking after yourself, adopting a healthy lifestyle, using preventative services like inoculations); *mind* (positive attitudes, not worrying, taking responsibility for yourself); *heredity* (health constitution); and *the body's defences* (fighting off disease). External explanations divided into three categories: *chance, social policy* (public health measures, good living standards) and *medical advances* (inoculations, contraception). Asked the question: 'What makes people ill?' a similar categorization occurred at least for internal factors (unhealthy behaviour, mind and heredity) but there were rather more external factors: *chance, other people* (upsetting one or exposing one to germs), *disease* organisms (infection), *products of social forces* (inequality, pollution, advertising) and *medical intervention*. Stanton-Rogers (1991) was also able to identify seven quite different 'theories' or 'accounts' which represented the way different people thought about medical and health-related matters.

> The 'cultural critique', 'inequality of access', 'willpower' and 'robust individualism' accounts all assumed that lifestyle and social circumstances are crucial determinants of health status, and hence all couched their explanations within the interplay between the individual and society. They were, however, informed by opposing models of society. The 'willpower' and 'robust individualism' accounts took a 'structural functionalist' or 'pluralist' view of society. They assumed that various social or cultural groups (i.e. different social classes, different genders, different ethnic groups) co-exist in a functional manner and that individuals have a choice about their lifestyles and living conditions. Consequently health status in this view is a product of individual decision making and circumstances. By contrast, the 'cultural critique' and 'inequality of access' accounts operated within a 'dominance' or 'conflict' world view, in which individuals' choices and life chances—and consequently health status—are largely constrained and defined by their social position. Indeed, individual freedom to choose was at the very heart of the 'robust individualism' account's view of the world, whereas the lack of choice for the most vulnerable and oppressed groups was focal for the 'inequality of access' account. (Stanton-Rogers, 1991)

Predictions about the role these lay aetiologies might play in complementary medicine are difficult. It could be that prospective and actual patients of complementary medicine, as opposed to orthodox medicine, are more prone to offering some explanations (e.g. imbalance, environmental irritants) than others. As complementary therapists stress personal responsibility we might also expect a preponderance of 'robust individualism' and 'will-power' accounts from complementary patients in Stanton-Rogers's framework.

THE THERAPEUTIC SIGNIFICANCE OF LAY BELIEFS

Fitzpatrick (1984) has identified five issues of therapeutic significance regarding lay beliefs:

1. *Identifying the problem* Because patients present problems rather than diseases and select which aspects, particularly physical, they report, the way they personally define, categorize and link factors concerning the illness are crucially important in diagnosis.
2. *Monitoring the impact of diagnostic information* Patients assign meaning to the diagnosis that they receive, some of which is highly inappropriate. That is, because of their incorrect understanding of the disease label they have been given, lay people react and even medicate inappropriately. Hence, it becomes important to address the meanings that patients assign to professional diagnoses.
3. *Reassurance in relation to 'non-disease'* Many patients need careful and sensitive assurance that apparent symptoms are normal and not worth worrying about. Patients feel more reassured if they are convinced that doctors have understood their perspectives on the illness.
4. *Obtaining co-operation with long-term treatment* Patients appear to be more compliant with their prescribed long-term treatment of chronic illness when their health beliefs have been elicited and, where appropriate, modified.
5. *Supporting the patient* Patients perceive their doctor to be more supportive if his or her behaviour expresses their concerns in their own terms. Studies have shown that patients who were more satisfied that their specialist consultations had been appropriate to their personal concerns showed less severe negative symptoms a year later than those who found the consultation superficial or inappropriate.

After a thorough review of the area Fitzpatrick (1984) concluded that: 'The evidence . . . suggests that the patients' interpretations of their symptoms are governed by concepts and ideas of considerable complexity and variety . . . There are firm grounds for arguing that attention to patients' interpretations of their health problems has been shown to be clinically fruitful and can be successfully incorporated into the practice of health care.'

Complementary medicine practitioners may have learnt, more effectively than general practitioners, to take lay theories into account, though there is little research aimed directly at answering this question. It may also be that some branches of complementary medicine offer both explanations and remedies that are part of folk 'wisdom' and ordinary language, and hence more approachable for lay people.

The Health Belief Model

Social and medical psychologists, as well as medical sociologists, have developed a model of mainly Western lay people's health beliefs, to account for patients' response to illness. These health beliefs might be better called 'health understanding', as they in fact concern knowledge, attitudes, values as well as beliefs (Pendleton and Hasler, 1983). The health belief model was developed and tested exclusively in the 1970s. According to King (1983) the model has five major points, all of which stress that it is the person's subjective perceptions of health and illness rather than actual or objective medical facts that really determine health behaviour.

King (1983) argues that the model contains the following main elements:

1. *Health motivation*   An individual's degree of interest in, and concern about, health matters.
2. *Perceived susceptibility*   Perceived vulnerability or susceptibility to the particular illnesses, including acceptance of the diagnosis of others.
3. *Perceived severity*   Perceptions concerning the probable seriousness of the consequences (organic and social) of contracting the illness or leaving it untreated.
4. *Benefits and costs*   The individual's estimate of the therapeutic benefits of taking recommended, possibly unpleasant, health action, weighted against the costs involved. Costs might include financial expense, physical and emotional discomfort, or possibly side-effects.
5. *Cue to actions*   Something must occur to 'trigger' these perceptions and lead to the appropriate health behaviour. These stimuli may be either internal (such as symptoms), or external (such as magazine articles, a reminder from the doctor, or illness in the family).

The health belief model has inspired a considerable amount of research in all areas of health. The model has proved to be a good predictor for participation in programmes for the early detection of breast cancer, initial drug therapy defaulting, compliance with alcoholism treatment, though not all studies have found health beliefs to be significant predictors of health behaviour and, even when significant, are not always strong predictors in relation to other factors. No studies, alas, have looked at the model and beliefs about, attitudes towards or use of complementary medicine.

As one might expect, the health belief model has been criticized, adapted and even abandoned by some. For instance, various *omissions* in the model have been noted that include: the patient's social environment, which therefore omits lay referral (e.g. by friends and relations), and social support networks, which may help or hinder health and health-related behaviour; the doctor–patient interaction, which does not operate in a vacuum, but in specific settings and perceptions of symptoms and lay constructions of illness and the sick role. Many other factors—social class, geographic location, cultural reasons—may also be powerful predictors of health behaviour.

King (1983) has pointed to various limitations of the model. She argues that for the health belief model to be useful, all its factors need to be considered simultaneously, as it is often only the *interaction* between these that can predict health behaviour. She also laments the fact that there has been no research on the *stability* of the model's major variables over the individual's life span or on the conditions under which the health beliefs were *acquired*: 'What are the determinants of these patient health beliefs? Why does one patient see himself as more vulnerable than another, to a particular illness? How does the patient come to see himself or herself as susceptible in the first place? How does a person come to believe a specific action is preventive? What governs the desire for a particular level of health?' (King, 1983, p. 120).

Social class has an important influence on health beliefs, which may be important with respect to complementary medicine. In an in-depth study of 60 British adults, Calnan (1987) sought to understand lay concepts of health, health threats, disease causation and health management. He found three major factors appear to shape these beliefs about health maintenance:

1. Experience and knowledge derived from folk culture.
2. Socio–political values about health and its control.
3. The perspectives and values of powerful groups (i.e. the medical profession) which are legitimized experts.

In Calnan's (1987) study, middle-class women tended to integrate ideas about mental and physical health, while working-class women tended to keep them more separate. Working-class women tended to be very sceptical about official and professional ideas about disease prevention, inequalities in health and so on. They appear to draw heavily on personal experience rather than abstract models of disease causality in their lay theory models. Middle-class people were better informed, more critical and had higher expectations of help. Middle-class patients tended to adopt a consumerist approach to patient need, emphasizing the need to be pro-active and critical. It is this group, middle class, better educated and more willing to be critical, who may be most likely to turn to complementary medicine.

The way in which perceived susceptibility and perceived seriousness influence the health-related actions people take was summarized by Bishop (1987). He found that adults used four basic dimensions in conceptualizing symptoms: virally caused; psychological versus physical causation; upper versus lower part of the body; and the extent to which symptoms are disruptive to a person's activities. Perceived cause of the symptoms was a critical determinant of action.

> Thus it appears that when deciding what to do about specific symptoms, people pay particular attention to the perceived source of the symptoms and use this perception to guide their actions. Specifically, the perception of a symptom as being physically caused appears to trigger help seeking from a professional, but the perception of the symptom as being viral tends to lead to self-care. In the former case it appears that people are differentiating between symptoms that are perceived as 'real' and those thought to be psychogenic, and only wish to consult doctors for those that are 'real'. In the latter cases, viral symptoms (including, among others, symptoms of the common cold and 'flu) may be ones that people believe will pass with time and palliative care and for which physicians have no real cure anyway. Thus over-the-counter medicines or home remedies are seen as the most useful response. (Bishop, 1987, pp. 142–143)

Thus various factors are involved in the health assessment of one's health. First, there is the *perceived seriousness* of the health problem. People first consider how severe the organic and social consequences are likely to be if they develop the problem or leave it untreated; the more serious they believe the effects will be, the more likely they are to take preventative action. Second, there is the *perceived susceptibility* to the health problem. People evaluate the likelihood of their developing the problem; the more vulnerable they perceive themselves to be, the more likely they are to take preventative action. Third, *cues to action* in that people who are reminded or alerted about a potential health problem are more likely to take preventative action than are those who are not. Finally, in weighing the pros and cons of taking preventative action, lay people consider whether the *perceived benefits*—such as being healthier or reducing health risks—of the action exceed its *perceived barriers* or costs.

Studies on patients' perceived susceptibility and vulnerability have shown that these perceptions are strongly related to the patients' compliance with medical advice, be it as serious as cancer or as common as dental problems. Studies on the effects of the patients' perceptions of severity of the illness have not demonstrated such conclusive results, in that not all studies have shown a positive association between perceived severity and compliance, probably because both high and low levels of perceived threat are associated with a low likelihood of taking preventative action (Furnham, 1988).

THE HEALTH BELIEFS OF PATIENTS RECEIVING COMPLEMENTARY MEDICINE

Very little work has been carried out on the health beliefs of complementary medicine patients. Only in the past decade have researchers begun to look at the attitudes, beliefs and values of patients of complementary practitioners and contrasted them with patients of orthodox practitioners. The authors carried out a series of preliminary studies which have begun to explore this complex area. In these studies, various specific hypotheses were tested, each of which attempted to address the question about the difference between orthodox and complementary medicine patients. The various themes are explored in turn in the remaining sections of the chapter.

Biological Knowledge

Furnham and Forey (1994) predicted that those consulting a complementary practitioner would have a greater biological knowledge. Subjects were shown a picture of the human body and a list of human anatomical parts and functions: patients were asked to match items on the list to the picture. A strongly significant finding indicated that those who consulted homeopaths had a higher biological and physiological knowledge of the body and its functions. Of course, showing difference in biological knowledge does not necessarily imply that increased knowledge in part or total 'caused' them to choose (or avoid) complementary medicine. It could well be that many complementary medicine practitioners see it as their specific duty to educate their clients in relevant biological knowledge, so that biological knowledge is a consequence not a cause of this choice. Only longitudinal studies can tease out this difference. A further possibility, discussed later in the book, is that the difference is simply due to higher educational levels of complementary patients.

The Determinants of Illness: Physiological or Psychological

A large proportion of patients' illnesses are designated as psychosomatic in that they are thought to be partly, or even wholly, psychological rather than physical in origin. Indeed, some general practitioners feel that the majority of their patients present with psychological as opposed to physical symptoms. Lay people also have ideas about whether illness is caused primarily by psychological factors like stress (family, work/mental states) or personality, or by physical factors like biological changes, genetic dispositions or physical abnormality. Beliefs about the origins of illness may be important in the way people make sense of symptoms and in the treatment they seek. If people are partly attracted to complementary medicine because its practitioners attach greater importance to psychological factors, this may reflect an underlying belief in the importance of psychological factors in the onset and maintenance of disease.

However, Furnham and Forey (1994) found few dramatic differences when comparing the responses of patients of general practitioners and homeopathic patients. Subjects were presented with 23 illnesses (e.g. cancer, diabetes, obesity) and asked to indicate whether they thought the cause was primarily in the mind (psychological) or the body (physiology). The results indicated that there was no real difference in the way the two groups view the origins of illness. Both groups believed that illnesses were made up of physiological and psychological elements to some degree. It is unlikely then that this factor distinguished those people who chose to receive complementary medicine.

Attitudes to Medicine and Science

Furnham, Vincent and Wood (1995) examined attitudes to science and medicine among 250 patients attending an osteopath, homeopath, acupuncturist or an orthodox general practitioner. The first group of attitudes examined were concerned with belief in medical science, covering such matters as following a doctor's advice and belief in the efficacy of modern medical techniques. Significant differences were found between the four groups, with the general practice groups showing most faith in orthodox medicine, while the acupuncture group showed the least, significantly less than any of the other three groups. A similar pattern emerged as regards positive attitudes to scientific methodology. A third group of attitudes concerned the psychological factors in physical illness. Items concerned the importance of positive emotional states, the influence of the 'will to live' and the use of psychological treatments in medicine in achieving good physical health. The acupuncture patients placed the most importance on a healthy state of mind, significantly more so than either homeopath patients or general practice patients, who placed the least importance on state of mind. The report concluded:

> It appears that to talk of patients of complementary practitioners as a homogeneous group is fundamentally wrong. Patients consulting different types of complementary practitioners hold different beliefs about their own health, and hold differing levels of scepticism about orthodox medicine. Rather than talking about general practice patients and complementary patients, it would seem more appropriate to talk about a continuum ranging from orthodox medicine, through various types of complementary medicine, to those types of treatment that have least in common with orthodox medicine. Patients differ by degrees in their health beliefs, and scepticism of orthodox medicine, and do not fall neatly into two distinct groups. (Furnham, Vincent and Wood, 1995)

Box 5.1   Attitudes to science, health and medicine

Positive attitude to science

1. Medicine is a science and should be based upon rigorous scientific principles.
2. Treatments which are not based upon modern scientific discoveries are worthless.
3. Every treatment should be thoroughly tested by doctors and scientists before people are allowed to try it.
4. Complementary (alternative) therapies should be scientifically evaluated.

Importance of psychological factors

1. Psychological treatment (e.g. relaxation, counselling) should be used much more widely.
2. Being fit and well depends as much on your state of mind as on the functioning of your body.
3. The 'will to live' can be a significant factor in whether people recover from a serious illness or injury.
4. State of mind is a crucial part of achieving better health; positive thinking can enhance physical health.

Harmful effects of modern medicine

1. The side effects of modern drugs are often severe and sometimes dangerous.
2. People sometimes feel worse rather than better after orthodox medical treatment.
3. Many forms of medical treatment do more harm than good.
4. Patients are sometimes operated on when they do not need it.

(From Vincent, Furnham and Willsmore, 1995. Reproduced by permission.)

Vincent et al (1997), in a further similar study, gave 82 acupuncture patients a simple attitudes to medicine questionnaire which had three themes, and also covered the ratings of efficacy of complementary therapies that are described later in this chapter. The purpose of the study was to see which, if any, of the attitudinal variables was associated with a belief in the efficacy of complementary therapies. A positive attitude to science was associated with a strong belief in the efficacy of orthodox medicine. Further, a belief in the importance of psychological factors was associated with a belief in the efficacy of acupuncture and homeopathy though, once demographic or other attitudinal variables were taken into account, these results did not quite reach significance. Significant associations were found, however, between attitudes to psychological factors and a belief in the efficacy of herbalism. Associations between perceived efficacy and the importance of psychological factors in illness do not necessarily mean that patients view complementary therapies as placebos. Patients may be drawn to complementary medicine because it is seen as more able to take a psychological perspective into account. Some complementary therapies (e.g. homeopathy, some forms of acupuncture) explicitly take emotional factors into account in the diagnoses and underlying theory, though it is not clear how far this matters to (or is indeed noticed by) most patients. It may be that complementary practitioners simply have more time, or that they are seen to be more receptive to discussing emotional aspects of illness.

The results of this study differ from the previous one in one important respect. The earlier study showed that a stronger relative belief in orthodox medicine among patients of different complementary therapies was associated with attaching less importance to psychological factors in illness. Here, in contrast, in a group of people attending a highly traditionally oriented acupuncture centre, the distinguishing factors were scientific attitudes and beliefs about harm. There may be a general lesson to be drawn from this, concerning variations in philosophy and styles of treatment within complementary therapies. These studies are interesting in that they demonstrate that differences between groups are present, but we should not assume that the same patterns will necessarily be seen when different complementary centres, which may have their own individual characteristics, are sampled.

Health Consciousness

Does health consciousness have anything to do with the type of medical treatment sought? Are complementary medicine patients particularly sensitive to health and health issues? Work in this field is again limited, but three studies have attempted to compare and contrast health consciousness in patients of orthodox and complementary medicine.

Furnham and Forey (1994) asked matched groups of homeopathic and general practice patients 14 questions about health consciousness and awareness of health issues. Questions covered such topics as awareness of health issues in the media, knowledge of nutrition and food additives and general environmental issues. There were consistent differences between the two groups, with homeopathic patients generally showing greater health consciousness and awareness and greater concern for the environment. Furnham and Kirkcaldy (1996) asked exactly the same questions of 200 German patients of either general practitioners or complementary practitioners and found a similar pattern of results.

In a further, similar study Furnham, Vincent and Wood (1995) gave over 250 patients a health beliefs and lifestyle questionnaire. Six questions, which concerned nutrition, diet and environmental issues, attracted a similar pattern of response. They found acupuncture patients believed in the importance of these issues more strongly than general practice patients, with homeopathic and osteopathic patients falling between the two. The results of all these studies tend to indicate that homeopathic patients, at least, are more health conscious than orthodox medical patients and complementary patients in general may be more concerned with a healthy lifestyle and environmental issues. These factors may encourage people to choose complementary medicine, or be the *result* of visiting a complementary practitioner. The most likely scenario is perhaps that these beliefs are both cause and consequence, that is their initial health interests are reinforced.

Beliefs about the Prevention of Illness

Beliefs about how to prevent illness may also discriminate between complementary and orthodox patients. Furnham and Smith (1988) asked general practice patients to rate the efficacy of eight preventative measures to stay healthy which, it should be pointed out, were measures of intended, not actual, behaviour. Only two yielded significant differences between the groups. General practice patients thought regular exercise was less effective, but taking pharmaceutical medication more effective, than patients attending a homeopath.

In a similar study, Furnham and Bhagrath (1993) found many more differences between a matched homeopathic and general practice group in their

Table 5.1 Beliefs about the prevention of illness

	GP	Homeopathic	F ratio
Regular exercise	3.40	3.38	0.01
Taking medicines	2.28	2.28	0.00
Good diet	3.50	3.73	5.20*
Cutting down on smoking	3.57	3.81	4.05*
Cutting down on drinking	3.32	3.72	9.47**
Reducing stress at work	3.31	3.76	14.71***
Having time to relax	3.38	3.78	13.99***
Good sleeping pattern	3.33	3.72	9.91**
Meditation	2.61	3.18	12.9***

* $p < 0.005$
** $p < 0.01$
*** $p < 0.001$

(From Furnham and Bhagrath, 1993. Reproduced by permission of The British Psychological Society)

study (Table 5.1). The nine questions concerning illness prevention showed seven significant differences. Homeopathic patients believed more than orthodox medicine patients that a good diet, cutting down on drinking and smoking, reducing stress at work, increasing relaxation time, having a good sleep pattern and meditation helped prevent illness. Homeopathic patients believed in treating the whole person, not just the symptoms, and also believed more strongly than the patients of a general practitioner that the body could heal itself, so endorsing some of the central tenets of homeopathy. Again, there seem to be important systematic differences in the belief of the two groups, which may have an influence on the choice of an orthodox or complementary medical specialty.

Perceived Susceptibility to Illness and Health Risk

Are patients of complementary medicine particularly sensitive to health risks? Do complementary medicine clients believe that they are more susceptible to illness than orthodox medicine patients? And could this differential perception be responsible for them choosing complementary medicine? Two studies done in this area suggest there is little or no difference between patients of orthodox and different types of complementary practitioners on these factors.

Furnham and Smith (1988) gave matched groups of general practice and homeopathic patients a list of 21 'medical problems' including infections, cardiovascular problems, neurological and psychosomatic illnesses, and asked them to rate how likely they were personally to develop each condition. Various analyses were performed comparing the general practice with the homeopathic group, yet no findings of significance emerged. In other words, there was no difference between the groups in their perceived susceptibility to illness and disease. Furnham and Bhagrath (1993) also found fewer than may be expected by chance differences. Patients were asked about their chances of getting one of the 21 illnesses or complaints. Of these, only two (less than one would expect by chance) showed differences. The homeopathic group thought that they were significantly more likely to get asthma and suffer from sleeplessness. The fact that there were no more than chance significant differences suggests that complementary medicine (or at least homeopathic) patients do not hold different beliefs about their susceptibility to illness compared to general practice patients.

Locus of Control

A number of commentators have suggested that patients of complementary practitioners may have a stronger belief that they can influence their state of health, possibly linked to their emphasis on both psychological and lifestyle factors in the cause of serious illness, such as heart disease and cancer. Locus of control is a concept underlying beliefs about internal versus external control of outcomes of various kinds. It assumes that individuals develop a general expectancy regarding their ability to control their lives. People who believe that the events that occur in their lives are the results of their own behaviour and/or ability, personality and effort are said to have the expectancy of internal control, while people who believe events in their lives to be a function of luck, chance, fate, God(s), powerful others, or powers beyond their control or manipulation are said to have an expectancy of external control. People with high internal locus of control tend to have higher aspirations, to be more persistent and respond more to challenge, and to see themselves as the source of their success. It is without doubt one of the most extensively measured individual differences dimensions measured in the whole of psychology (Furnham and Steele, 1993). Locus of control has been significantly, consistently and predictably related to many beliefs and behaviours, with psychologically adaptive features nearly always being associated with inner locus of control.

If the tendency to seek information about one's surroundings and the desire to maintain personal control characterize internals, we would expect them to differ in important ways from externals in the area of health maintenance. As Strickland (1978) has said: 'One would expect that internals, in contrast to externals, would be more sensitive to health messages, would have increased knowledge about health conditions, would attempt to improve physical functioning, and might even, through their own efforts, be less susceptible to physical and psychological dysfunction.' In fact, research has shown that internals are more likely to show enhanced efforts to maximize their health and well-being and minimize illness. From the review by Strickland (1978), the following are some of the health-related behaviour or characteristics in which internals have been found to surpass externals (although the evidence is not always completely clear-cut):

- information seeking about health maintenance
- precautionary health practices
- greater knowledge of their own illness when stricken
- more positive attitudes to physical activity
- greater participation in physical activities
- greater likelihood of refraining from smoking or of having given it up
- lessened susceptibility to essential hypertension and heart attacks
- better prognosis once a heart attack occurs.

Lau and Ware (1981) have developed a specific health locus of control inventory. The 28-item questionnaire, scored on a 7-point agree–disagree scale, attempts to measure subjects' beliefs as to how much they have control over their own health. It has four subscales: self-control over health (e.g. 'People's ill health results from their own carelessness'); provider control over health (e.g. 'Doctors can rarely do very much for people who are sick'); chance health outcomes (e.g. 'Recovery from illness has nothing to do with luck'); and general health threat (e.g. 'The seriousness of many diseases is overstated'). A series of studies have brought some conflicting findings, but clearly indicated that complementary patients differ from general practice patients on some aspects of health locus of control.

Furnham and Smith (1988) used the health locus of control scale in a study comparing patients attending either a general practitioner or a homeopath. They found only one of the four scales, provider control, yielded a significant result. An analysis of the subscale showed that seven of the eight items showed a significant difference in the predicted direction. Homeopathic patients were by and large more critical and sceptical about the efficacy of traditional doctors in curing illness. This is very clearly illustrated in the item-by-item analysis of the subscales presented in Table 5.2. However, the difference between the groups on the provider-control scale must be very carefully interpreted in view of the wording of the items which refer to 'doctor' and 'medical' as the provider. If the subjects perceived the homeopath not to be a doctor (in the conventional sense), the

Table 5.2 Locus of control scores for general practice and homeopathy patients

Subscales	GP ($N=44$)	Homeopath ($N=43$)	F ratio
1. Chance health outcomes	5.01	4.70	1.03
2. Provider control over health	5.44	4.36	16.93***
3. Self-control over health	5.14	5.12	0.07
4. General health threat	3.88	3.67	0.46
Item by item analysis of provider-control scale			
1. Seeing the doctor for regular check-ups	4.45	3.32	7.93**
2. Doctors can rarely do much for sick people	2.36	3.22	4.98*
3. Doctors relieve or cure only a few problems that their patients have	3.05	4.62	20.33***
4. Doctors can almost always help their patients feel better	5.29	4.24	10.72**
5. Recovery from illness requires good medical care more than anything else	5.02	4.34	4.49*
6. Most people are helped a great deal when they go to the doctor	5.71	4.22	24.13***
7. Doctors can do very little to prevent illness	3.33	3.46	0.10
8. Many times doctors don't help their patients get well	2.90	3.88	6.69*

Scale: 1 = strongly disagree—7 = strongly agree
*** $p<0.001$; ** $p<0.01$; * $p<0.05$.

(From Furnham and Smith, 1988. Reproduced by permission of Elsevier Science Inc.)

results would reflect a scepticism about orthodox medicine, rather than a lack of belief in medical intervention generally in the homeopathic group.

In a similar study, Furnham and Forey (1994) found two of the four subscales yielded a significant result. As before, the complementary medicine patients had a significantly lower score on the provider control over health, but, in this study, also on the general threat to health subscales, though this was due to differences on a single item. However, Furnham and Bhagrath (1993) found no significant difference on the total subscale score for provider control, though the self-control over health score was significantly different for a homeopathic group. Four of the seven items revealed a significant difference. The general health threat score also showed no sign of any significance. Furnham and Kirkcaldy (1996) used the same scale translated for 200 German patients. As in two of the previous studies, it was the 'provider control over health' items that showed the most consistent, statistically significant findings. Thus, compared to general practice patients, the complementary medicine patients agreed less that 'Seeing a doctor for regular check-ups is a key factor in health', 'Doctors can almost always help their patients feel better' and 'Most people are helped a great deal when they go to a doctor'.

Overall, the results show some consistent findings. Complementary patients, unlike equivalent groups visiting a general practitioner, tend to have more internal beliefs about the control of their health. They have some tendency to believe that they, rather than, say, doctors or bad luck, are responsible for their health or illness. The most consistent finding, on the provider subscale, may reflect a particular scepticism about orthodox medicine rather than provider control as usually conceived, which would indicate a lack of faith in medical intervention generally.

Perceived Efficacy of Orthodox and Complementary Medicine

Some studies have considered how people generally, as opposed to patients of complementary practitioners, perceive the efficacy of complementary medicine. Vincent and Furnham (1994) gave a questionnaire to 135 British adults, of whom 12% had experience of complementary medicine. The study examined the perceived efficacy of four different types of complementary medicine (acupuncture, herbalism, homeopathy and osteopathy) and orthodox medicine in treating 25 common complaints, ranging from cancer to the common cold. Subjects completed a questionnaire measuring the state of their health; experience of complementary medicine; sources of information about complementary medicine; and perceived efficacy of orthodox and complementary therapies in the treatment of each condition. Personal accounts of treatment appeared to be particularly important sources of information on complementary medicine and also highly valued in assessing its efficacy.

Ratings of efficacy were calculated for four groups of conditions:

1. Major medical conditions—appendicitis, bronchitis, cancer, diabetes, heart attack and pneumonia.
2. Minor conditions—common cold, hay fever, insomnia, menstrual problems and migraine.
3. Chronic conditions—allergies, arthritis, asthma, back pain, blood pressure and skin problems.

Table 5.3 Perceived efficacy by illness type

Type	Acupuncture	Herbalism	Homeopathy	Osteopathy	Orthodox
Major	1.41	1.70	1.67	1.24	3.98
Minor	2.02	2.52	2.23	1.41	3.05
Chronic	2.26	2.37	2.38	1.92	3.45
Psychological	2.15	2.02	1.80	1.50	2.48

(From Vincent and Furnham, 1994. Reproduced by permission of Longman Group UK Ltd)

4. Psychological problems—depression, drinking problems, fatigue, nerves, obesity, stopping smoking, stress and weight loss.

Ratings on these various complaints were averaged to form four scores per subject. Table 5.3 shows the mean efficacy for each therapy, in each of these four groups of conditions.

The results showed that orthodox medicine was clearly seen by the great majority of subjects as being more effective in the treatment of most complaints, especially in the treatment of major, life-threatening conditions. Complementary medicine was seen as more effective in the treatment of minor and chronic conditions, though generally not superior to orthodox medicine. For psychological problems orthodox and complementary medicine were seen as very much equivalent. For some specific conditions, complementary medicine was seen as the most effective treatment: osteopathy and acupuncture were both perceived as valuable in the treatment of back pain and herbalism was perceived as a valid treatment for fatigue and stress. The fact that people are able to specify which complementary therapies are likely to be effective in which conditions suggests that people are not necessarily for or against complementary medicine, but see specific therapies as useful in the treatment of specific problems.

Do patients of individual complementary therapies believe them to be particularly efficacious? On a five-part (5 = very effective) scale Vincent, Furnham and Willsmore (1995) asked an acupuncture, homeopathy, osteopathy and a general practice group to rate the efficacy of various specialties (see Table 5.4). The acupuncture group gave significantly higher efficacy ratings than the general practice group for acupuncture, homeopathy and osteopathy. For acupuncture the mean scores are significantly higher than all the other groups, indicating a degree of loyalty to their specific therapy. The comparatively low ratings for osteopathy for a wide variety of complaints disguise its high ratings for chronic pain and musculo–skeletal problems.

Table 5.4   Mean scores for perceived efficacy of complementary therapies

	Patient groups				
Therapy	Acupuncture	Homeopathy	Osteopathy	GP	F ratio
Acupuncture	3.54	2.52	2.20	2.21	7.28***
Herbalism	3.31	2.81	2.57	2.36	1.48
Homeopathy	3.07	3.16	2.68	2.05	1.46
Osteopathy	1.81	1.59	1.89	1.60	1.23
Orthodox medicine	2.46	2.89	2.86	2.81	0.952

*** $p < 0.001$

(From Vincent, Furnham and Willsmore, 1995. Reproduced by permission.)

This study has in fact been replicated, with a simplified and refined questionnaire, this time looking at the perceptions of 82 patients attending a British acupuncture clinic. Vincent and Furnham (1997) asked them to complete a brief questionnaire which covered: (a) demographic information and experience of complementary medicine; and (b) ratings of the perceived efficacy of acupuncture, osteopathy, homeopathy, herbalism and orthodox medicine for 16 illnesses, divided into four categories: major, minor, chronic and psychological. Osteopathy and acupuncture were seen as particularly useful for back pain, with acupuncture being seen as beneficial for other chronic conditions and for psychological problems by these acupuncture patients. Orthodox medicine was seen as least effective in curing chronic and psychological conditions. Acupuncture patients perceived their own chosen therapy as more effective than other complementary therapies and, for many complaints, as more effective than orthodox medicine. Orthodox medicine was clearly seen, even by complementary patients, as more effective for major, life-threatening conditions, but acupuncture patients still rated acupuncture as highly effective even for these complaints. However, they may have been considering acupuncture as a preventative measure or as an adjunct to conventional treatment, for instance to promote recovery after surgery, rather than as a replacement for orthodox medicine.

We have seen that people have complex beliefs about health and illness shaped by their personal and social circumstances, their medical history and encounters with professionals. Demographic and psychological factors also play a part in shaping, maintaining and changing health beliefs. There is rich, multidisciplinary literature on the nature and function of health beliefs and how they operate. These beliefs play a part in many health-care decisions and would appear to be important in the decision to consult and receive treatment from complementary practitioners.

Research on the beliefs of patients of complementary practitioners is still in its infancy. The literature is sparse and the findings necessarily preliminary. Patients of complementary practitioners tend, as might be expected, to perceive complementary therapies as more effective, relatively speaking, than general practice patients, though orthodox medicine is still preferred for serious illness. They appear on the whole, compared to general practice patients, to have better biological knowledge, to be more health conscious and to believe more strongly that people can influence their own state of health, both by physical means and through maintaining a psychological equilibrium. The work on locus of control has provided mixed findings, but complementary patients do appear to have less faith in 'provider control', that is in the ability of medicine to resolve problems of ill health. They do not appear, on the limited evidence available, to have different ideas about the determinants of illness or their own perceived susceptibility to illness.

Many of these 'explanations' are overlapping and there may be other valid explanations which have not been considered. Although the results from various studies were examined, the current research has two major drawbacks. The first is that it is cross-sectional, which means it is not possible always to look at longitudinal causal patterns. Indeed, it is frequently difficult to separate cause and consequence. Second, most studies have been restricted to patients/clients of a few specific branches of complementary medicine. It is quite possible that quite different patterns exist for clients of the different complementary practices, particularly those from the more well-established specialties versus those from the more fringe areas.

Chapter 6

Consultations with Orthodox and Complementary Practitioners

What do patients value about consultations with either an orthodox practitioner or complementary practitioner? How does the consultation style of complementary practitioners differ from that of general practitioners? Can the frequently reported satisfaction with complementary practitioners be accounted for by features of their consultation style such as having a simpler more user-friendly language, taking more time with each patient, touching the patient more often or giving the patient more autonomy and control? Are complementary practitioners more in tune with the consequences of the consumerist movement and more willing and able to provide 'the service' the modern, middle-class patient wants? There is, alas, a paucity of research on this topic though it is possible to speculate on some of the major differences and their consequences.

The British Medical Association (BMA, 1986) has suggested that the growth in complementary medicine implies a criticism of orthodox medicine, although the evidence that this is the case is equivocal. However, the growth in consumerism within health care has led to concern about patient satisfaction because 'while doctors may be required to become more concerned with meeting consumers' demands, the actual relationship between themselves and their patients may become more formal and bureaucratic and consequently neglect the crucial aspects of patient satisfaction . . .' (Williams and Calnan, 1991). The crucial aspects of patient satisfaction, identified from Williams and Calnan's (1991) large-scale UK study, are professional competence, together with the nature and quality of the practitioner–patient relationship.

Taylor (1985) has discussed the doctor–patient encounter and the nature of the relationship between complementary practitioner and patient in some detail. She recognizes the differences between the various complementary therapies and the fact that they share no common epistemological basis. Yet she argues that they are distinguished and distinguishable from orthodox medicine in their emphasis on the subjective experience of the patient and their insistence that all therapists should focus on the whole person, not just the disease. In contrast, Taylor suggests that scientific medicine sees the human body as a machine like any other which needs servicing; patients, who are cases, should not distract the doctor with their unique feelings and experiences. Too many people have become accustomed to the sort of medicine which 'relies on magic bullets administered by harassed physicians who cannot distinguish us one from another as we flow from waiting room to examination room to billing office' (Taylor, 1985). Many doctors and their patients would feel that this is too strongly stated, and Taylor recognizes that complementary medicine is not necessarily very different. Complementary practitioners may characterize orthodox medical practices as technological and aggressive and their own as natural and non-invasive, yet as Taylor notes:

> There seems to be little that is 'natural' or noninvasive about the acupuncturist's technique of sticking needles into various parts of the anatomy. Some kinds of alternative specialists train in schools which do not look very different from medical schools, go into private practice and, when their services are recognized as competitive with mainstream medicine, their prices become competitive too. (Taylor, 1985)

Taylor examines the various, by now familiar, reasons for the growing popularity of the complementary therapies, but argues that the failures, cost and uneven distribution of modern medicine cannot alone account for the rise in alternative medicine. For Taylor the one factor above all which explains the rise and fall of different healing systems is the changing nature of the medical encounter. The next section summarizes her position.

THE CHANGING NATURE OF THE MEDICAL ENCOUNTER

The consumer movement, the women's movement and the more general demands for professional reform and accountability have brought pressures for change in the medical encounter, but traditional medical schools and practising doctors have resisted populist demands and the pressure for democratization and customer service. Not only has medicine resisted change, but for many there has been a perceptible deterioration of the medical encounter. Malpractice law suits have made doctors more cautious; there are fewer generalists and more specialists, so a long-term relationship is less likely; patients have neither a 'voice option' in the medical encounter nor an 'exit option' to leave. Changing doctors, getting second opinions, paying for insurance is very difficult for most, and patients have to confront many problematic aspects of the relationship with an orthodox medical doctor. On the one hand, medicine has acquired great power, prestige and influence, and demand for medical services has never been greater. On the other hand, increasing costs and the rationing of some services has led to a perception of the withdrawal of services. Taylor (1985) notes that:

> Medicine has acquired enormous political and cultural significance as its jurisdiction over social life has been extended . . . Doctors are the gatekeepers to many benefits such as sickness compensation and abortion, and major protagonists in a host of complicated social decisions required to resolve controversies about who has the right to die, who is dangerous to themselves and their community, who may conceive children and who can obtain a new lease on life through an organ transplant. Visions of unlimited technical advances in medical care are now tempered by concerns about the growing 'medicalization' of social life and personal troubles. Paradoxically, the sense of entitlement which the 1960s are supposed to have brought about, particularly with regard to consumers and their services, has probably led to a situation where patients want and expect *more* from their doctors just as, for different reasons, both the managers of services and social critics are instructing them to ask for less.

Just when the complex and fragile relationship between the orthodox healer and healed is in most jeopardy and pressure on health care is intense, complementary medical practitioners have appeared in large numbers. However, the stress of self-care and the popular desire to reduce doctor dependence may also work in favour of orthodox medicine.

> A movement which promises to deliver a new generation of compliant, intelligent patients and to provide relief from both onerous responsibilities and trivial medical tasks obviously holds many attractions for a beleaguered profession. More important, it does not undermine professional authority since it neither denies the efficacy of modern medicine nor criticizes its practitioners. (Taylor, 1985, p. 223)

The changing relationship, however, is not always satisfactory for the patients. While they expect more, less is offered for a host of economic, political and demographic reasons. Patients complain of still being met by an insistence on clinical autonomy and a refusal to share information, not being able to participate in clinical decisions about their own care. Not being respected, crowded waiting rooms, being patronized, and being processed are common complaints. Thus, for Taylor, medicine is a relationship. The appeal of complementary medicine is determined less by the proven efficacy of its methods than by the willingness and ability of complementary practitioners to deliver what patients want from the medical encounter. When medicine cannot offer cure or even relief, as with much chronic illness, then the quality of the patient–practitioner relationship becomes paramount.

THE CONSULTATION AND ITS PROBLEMS

Kleinman (1980) has noted that the consultation is a transaction between lay and professional explanatory models—though it is also a transaction between two parties separated by differences in power (both social and symbolic) and knowledge. The main functions of the consultation are:

1. Presentation of 'illness' by the patient, both verbally and non-verbally.
2. Translation of these diffuse symptoms or signs into the named pathological entities of medicine, that is, converting 'illness' into 'disease'.
3. Prescribing a treatment regime which is acceptable both to doctor and to patient.

For the consultation to be a success, there must be a *consensus* between the two parties about the aetiology, diagnostic label, physiological processes involved, prognosis and optimal treatment for the condition. The search for a consensus or understanding is in a sense a negotiation. Thus each party attempts to influence the other regarding the outcome of the consultation, the diagnosis given and the treatment prescribed. Patients may try to reduce the seriousness of a diagnosis or the severity of a treatment regime, or more usually strive for diagnoses and treatments that make sense to them in terms of their lay view of ill health. The patient is thus a much more active participant than is generally appreciated, or at least can be active if they choose and circumstances allow.

Within the consultation, one can isolate a number of recurring problems that interfere with the development of consensus or understanding. These in turn can provide hypotheses about the characteristics of the complementary consultation and the appeal of complementary therapy. Kleinman (1980) lists a number of problems that can arise, but five are of particular relevance in that they highlight areas in which a complementary consultation might prove attractive.

1. *Differences in the definition of 'the patient'*   Orthodox medicine generally focuses increasingly on the individual patient and his or her problems, but it may be the *family* who are the cause of the problem, and not the individual. A greater willingness to focus on social issues may be a factor in the appeal of some complementary practitioners.
2. *Problems of terminology and language*   Clinical consultations are usually conducted in a mixture of everyday language and medical jargon. The language of medicine itself has become more and more technical and esoteric over the past century, and increasingly incomprehensible to the lay public and non-specialist. The same term, for example, may have entirely different meanings for doctor and patient. We have already seen in the previous chapter how lay theories about illness have parallels

with the metaphors used in traditional Chinese medicine. There could in some circumstances be a better fit between complementary medical explanations and patients' views.

3. *Incompatibility of explanatory models*   The disease perspective of modern medicine, with its emphasis on quantifiable physical data, may ignore the many dimensions of meaning—psychological, moral or social—that characterize the illness perspective of the patient. Emotional states, such as guilt, shame, remorse or fear on the patient's part, may not be taken into account by the doctor, who concentrates primarily on the diagnosis and treatment of physical dysfunction. Again, it may be that the explanatory models and concepts of complementary medical practitioners can sometimes be more attuned to these aspects of a patient's illness.

4. *Disease without illness*   This is a common phenomenon in modern medicine, with its emphasis on the use of sophisticated diagnostic technology. Physical abnormalities of the body are found, often on the cellular or chemical level, but the patient does not feel ill. Examples include hypertension and raised blood cholesterol, which are detected in routine health screening programmes. The fact that 'ill' patients do not 'feel unwell' may also partly explain much of the reported non-compliance with prescribed medication. Complementary medical practitioners may also perceive subtle imbalances or non-optimum functioning, in fact may be more apt to do this than the orthodox practitioner. However, they may be able to offer less drastic forms of treatment.

5. *Illness without pathology*   Patients feel that 'something is wrong' and may have various physical symptoms, but despite their subjective state they are told, after a physical examination, that there is nothing wrong with them. However, in many cases, they continue to feel unwell or unhappy, perhaps even more so. Cynics would argue that it is particularly this group of patients that are attracted to complementary practitioners who take them (more) seriously. More plausibly, however, the appeal may be the willingness of complementary practitioners to diagnose and treat such conditions, and provide an explanation, perhaps in terms of energy imbalance, for their occurrence.

THE CHARACTERISTICS OF EFFECTIVE COMMUNICATION

In a comprehensive and scholarly review on doctor–patient communication, Pendleton and Hasler (1983) have shown how the doctor's skills and consultative style can have considerable effects on the immediate, intermediate and long-term outcomes of patient health. A considerable number of studies in the burgeoning doctor–patient communication literature have attempted to identify which precise, independent features of that relationship predict a range of outcomes. Ong, de Haes and Lammes (1995), in a very comprehensive review, identified three relationship or communication variables of importance: creating a good interpersonal (trusting, warm, open) relationship; the clear and comprehensible exchange of information; and skill in making treatment-related decisions. These factors have direct consequences for four major medical outcomes: overall satisfaction; compliance and adherence to the treatment programme; the recall and understanding of exchanged information; and final health status and psychiatric morbidity.

Research has identified a long list of factors which have been found to be positively related to patients' reports of satisfaction. These include: the practitioners' 'contract' with the patient, empathy, expression of positive affect, the amount and type of information given, and the degree to which patients perceived their expectations to be met. Patients' perception of the practitioners' overall competence is naturally a powerful factor in satisfaction. To some extent, these many factors can be reduced to two: warmth and information. Interpersonal skills which are linked to the communication of warmth, friendliness, empathy, respect for and interest in the patients make a significant difference, as more complementary than orthodox practitioners have realized.

How do the patients' expectations about doctors relate to their utilization and evaluation of health care? Ditto et al (1995) suggest simply that some patients expect doctors to adopt one of two styles:

- *Authoritarian* Assume role of expert and primary decision maker; have clear-cut answers and have exceptional abilities.
- *Egalitarian* Assumes the doctor will make recommendations for treatment, discuss options and allow patients to participate in decision making.

They found authoritarian role expectations were associated with more visits to medical professionals, more overall health care utilization, greater satisfaction and more compliance than those with egalitarian role expectations. One would perhaps anticipate that patients with egalitarian role expectations and associated health behaviours might be more drawn to complementary medicine.

There is some evidence to suggest that, with time, general practitioners become more directive. Robinson and Whitfield (1987) compared the way patients behaved with trainees and with experienced doctors. The patients talked more to the trainees who, in turn, asked patients more about their suggested treatment. There could be many explanations for this finding: patients may, for instance, be more at ease with trainees, more trainees might be women, or trainees might give less clear instructions. The authors believed it was the trainees' willingness to engage patients in discussion about treatment that encouraged patients to think of queries which otherwise might not have occurred to them. This might also explain why complementary practitioners take longer and seem to engage their patients more. However, there may be equally simple practical explanations for these findings. Experienced general practitioners may simply be under more time constraints than either trainees or alternative practitioners. Equally, general practitioners may be better at giving clear instructions or closing interactions than the other two groups.

Communication Skills Training

Until recently, little or no attempt was made to train doctors to communicate more effectively with their patients. It was, and for some still is, assumed that this skill or set of skills is no more than common sense, which, anyway, will be acquired or improved on the job with increasing experience. However, over the past 20 years there has been considerable interest in social-skills training and research (Argyle, 1981). The underlying message of this approach is that the ability to communicate efficiently and effectively is a skill that can (and must) be taught and learnt.

Maguire (1981) reviewed numerous studies on junior and experienced hospital doctors and general practitioners, and showed that there was a consistent lack of certain key, history-taking skills that were not compensated for, or acquired with, greater experience or postgraduate training. He also argued that doctors lacked skills of exposition in the giving of information and advice to patients. The reasons these important skills were not acquired were as follows:

1. The time-honoured apprenticeship method was inappropriate, both because the role models can be poor, and also because social and psychological aspects are ignored.
2. Doctors were assumed to possess these skills despite the considerable evidence that they do not.
3. Doctors could not acquire these skills, believing that they could not be learnt—either one has them or not.
4. The use of these skills would only create problems, in that practising them would lead to patients disclosing difficult-to-handle problems.
5. The skills were assumed to have no important effect on care despite the considerable evidence to the contrary.

Maguire (1981) argued that these five objections were misplaced, and that more effective communication skills training methods should be developed to identify deficiencies, measure performance and provide feedback. Maguire et al (1986) and Maguire (1990) documented the sort of key communication skills that all doctors need: those of eliciting patients' problems (information gathering), establishing patients' responses (exploring how patients have responded to diagnoses, explanations and treatments), correcting misconceptions that patients may hold about their illnesses, and monitoring the impact of treatments. A decade later these ideas have taken root and communication skills training, though still very limited, is finally on the agenda in most British medical schools (e.g. McManus et al, 1993). However, despite the importance, relevance and efficacy of communication skills training, it appears that the medical profession has generally not laid down any formal requirements for the training or assessment of communicative competence in doctors. The same is, of course, true of complementary medicine training organizations. We should not assume that complementary practitioners necessarily have superior communication skills.

Efforts have also been made to improve communication from the patients' side. King et al (1985) encouraged patients who were about to see their doctor to make lists of: what had been happening to them and how it had affected their daily routine; what they thought might be wrong with them; what they were most afraid of; what they would like the doctor to do; what they wanted to know about their problem; what they had already tried to do about the problem. Studies on the participation of patients during general practice consultations have shown that following these steps is useful for both doctor and patient. Robinson and Whitfield (1987) noted that patients' passivity presented problems for doctors and that participative patients also improved treatment and satisfaction from the doctors' side.

DIFFERENCES IN ORTHODOX MEDICINE AND COMPLEMENTARY MEDICINE CONSULTATION STYLE

The preceding sections of this chapter have shown that communication skills have not been to the fore in medical education, and a considerable number of studies have demonstrated deficiencies in basic clinical skills, such as history taking, giving information and attending to psychological and social issues. It seems at least plausible that the consultation style of complementary practitioners may sometimes be preferred, and this may be part of the appeal of complementary medicine. There has, however, been little research on this question.

Hewer (1983) reviewed 10 studies all addressing the encounter between complementary practitioners and their patients in some measure. The studies were carried out between 1954 and 1980 in America, Australia, Germany and The Netherlands, with a variety of complementary medical practitioners, and identified a number of common themes. The duration of the contract was much longer with the complementary practitioner compared to the general practitioner (7 versus 20 minutes on average). The average consultation with a general practitioner lasted less than 10 minutes; a consultation with a complementary practitioner could last ten times that long. Though the quality of the diagnosis and recommended therapy need not suffer from the time constraints, patients of orthodox medicine tended to feel rushed, stressed and as if they were neither able to fully give, or receive, a full explanation of their problems. As Tate (1983) points out, a longer, less structured, more time-consuming approach does not necessarily lead to a better clinical outcome, though it is likely to be more satisfying for the patient, and hence lead to better compliance with treatment. The complementary medical practitioner relationship tends to be more patient-oriented, with better explanations for the nature of illness, an egalitarian relationship between patient and practitioner, and the patient experiencing a high level of acceptance from the complementary therapist. But Hewer is also careful to note that, whereas patients of complementary practitioners believe they are given a better diagnosis and have their worries and opinions taken more into consideration, well over 90% of patients are also happy with their general practitioner.

The studies reviewed by Hewer were of variable quality and did not necessarily address all the key themes. Orthodox medicine practitioners are more formal in their dress, style and behaviour than many complementary medicine practitioners and may be perceived as more authoritarian than complementary medicine practitioners (King et al, 1985). Many patients are surprised if the doctor does not undertake some sort of physical examination, however cursory; in some branches of complementary medicine (osteopathy, chiropractic, massage therapy), patients will always be examined and treated physically. There are two reasons why this is important: because patients expect it and because of the power of touch. In many Protestant cultures touch is infrequent, and for this reason it can be very powerful. Touching, through physical examination, reassures, calms, and establishes intimacy (Argyle, 1972). The counselling skills and holistic attitude of complementary practitioners may also be responsible for their popularity. They may, for this reason, be seen as more caring and compassionate. The fact that patients have to pay complementary practitioners, whereas they may often have to consult a general practitioner for free, should not be overlooked. It might encourage attentiveness on the part of complementary practitioners and it could lead the patient to value the treatment more highly.

Perceptions of Complementary Practitioners and General Practitioners

A small number of studies have directly examined patients' perceptions of their practitioners. Furnham, Vincent and Wood (1995) asked three groups of complementary patients and an orthodox medicine group to compare the consultation styles and willingness to deal with emotional issues of general practitioners and complementary practitioners. Complementary practitioners were generally perceived as being more sympathetic, and having more time to listen, by all the groups to some extent. Significant differences were apparent between all groups, with the general practitioner group agreeing least with such statements, while the acupuncture group agreed more than any of the other three groups. As before this may reflect the characteristics of a particular centre rather than acupuncture patients *per se*. All groups also tended to agree that complementary practitioners were better at explaining treatments and, perhaps more surprisingly, some also agreed that complementary practitioners were better at explaining why a patient was ill (see Table 6.1).

In a study of German patients, Furnham and Kirkcaldy (1996) found strong evidence that complementary medicine patients were less impressed by their general practitioner than patients of general practitioners only. Complementary patients believed that their general practitioners were less interested in patients' well-being and listened less than complementary practitioners. All this could be a function of consultation time, rather than of communication skills, but the effect on the patient is the same (see Table 6.2). Of course, these small-scale studies need to be replicated. Nevertheless, the results do appear to indicate that for the reasons set out above, complementary medicine practitioners may be providing a more satisfying consultation.

Perceptions of Competence and Satisfaction

The perceived competence of complementary practitioners, rather than the actual experience of the consultation, may be another important reason

Table 6.1 Patients' perceptions of the consultation

Items	GP	Ost	Hom	Acu	F ratio
Compared to GPs, complementary practitioners:					
are more sympathetic	4.41	5.38	5.04	6.31	14.79***
have more time to listen	4.88	5.54	5.09	6.71	17.50***
have less knowledge of disease	3.67	3.37	2.83	3.09	2.23
are more sensitive to emotional issues	4.44	5.32	5.07	6.55	19.28***
are better at explaining the treatment	4.26	5.49	4.87	5.98	11.47***
are better at explaining why you are ill	4.26	5.44	4.67	6.15	14.99***

1 = strongly disagree; 4 = neutral; 7 = strongly agree).
*** $p < 0.001$

(From Furnham, Vincent and Wood, 1995. Reproduced by permission of Liebert Inc.)

Table 6.2 Satisfaction: with GPs and their competence

Question	GP Mean (SD)	CM Mean (SD)	F ratio
At your last visit to your general practitioner, how satisfied were you with your treatment?	3.65	3.22	6.02*
Do you think your general practitioner is concerned with your well-being?	3.35	2.91	4.37*
Do you feel your general practitioner treatment is effective?	3.79	3.31	5.00*
Do you think your general practitioner listens to what you have to say?	3.90	3.50	4.55*
Do you believe that general practitioners can help their patients feel better generally?	3.91	3.30	4.54*

Coding: 1–5: 1 = not at all, 5 = very much
* $p < 0.05$

(*Source*: Furnham and Kirkcaldy, 1996. Reproduced by permission of The British Psychological Society)

for their appeal. Although prospective patients may remain sceptical on their first visit, presumably perceived competence passes some threshold which encourages further visits. Subsequently it is likely to be a function both of the actual efficacy of the treatment and the clinical manner of the practitioner.

Furnham and Forey (1994) examined complementary and general practitioner patients' perceptions of their practitioners' competence. They found the difference between the two groups concerned the higher perceived competence of complementary practitioners from their patients, rather than higher satisfaction. They also presented the subjects with 30 common illnesses and asked whether they would consult a general practitioner or complementary practitioner first. All but one illness showed significant differences. For minor illnesses, patients of complementary practitioners might consult them, rather than their general practitioner. However, for some specific illnesses even those consulting complementary practitioners would consult a general practitioner first. These were angina, high blood pressure, bronchitis, cancer, kidney problems, leukaemia and pneumonia.

Practitioners' Views of the Consultation

In spite of a wealth of research into the practitioner–patient relationship and patient satisfaction with orthodox medical treatment (Fitzpatrick, 1984; Ong, de Haes and Lammes, 1995), few studies have investigated what practitioners themselves view as important. Choi and Tweed (1996, unpublished data—private communication) surveyed 231 general practitioners and 110 complementary therapists in a postal survey. Given the greater emphasis in complementary medicine on the holistic approach, they hypothesized that complementary therapists would place greater importance on the practitioner–patient relationship than general practitioners would. Their questionnaire measured the importance of practitioner–consultation variables (e.g. have time to talk, patient being able to relax, practitioner's personality) and patient variables (e.g. patient's fear of treatment, patient's state of mind, duration of condition).

As they predicted, Choi and Tweed found in their survey that the patient–practitioner relationship was more important to complementary therapists than to general practitioners, this being particularly accounted for by the complementary group's stress on practitioner consultation variables. In contrast, patient variables were more important to general practitioners than to complementary therapists reflecting, they suggest, the different approaches of orthodox and complementary medicine. However, Choi and Tweed point out that differences in the characteristics of the specific study groups could account for these results. Complementary practitioners' consultation times were considerably longer (a mean of 51.03 minutes compared to the general practitioners' mean of 9.40 minutes), indicating that the formers' approach to health care is necessarily very different to that of general practitioners. The general practitioners were significantly older and had been practising for twice as long as the complementary therapists and were thus more experienced. Moreover, the sample of complementary therapists contained practitioners of at least 13 different kinds of complementary treatments, all with different origins, philosophies and training requirements. They were not therefore a homogeneous group.

In the same survey, Choi and Tweed also found that although general practitioners did not rate practitioner and consultation variables as highly as complementary therapists did, they did consider them more important than patient variables. This indicates that general practitioners are indeed concerned with factors that yield the highest degree of patient satisfaction, that is the practitioner–patient interaction. The findings highlight the conflict for the general practitioner, whose average consultation time, within the UK National Health Service, is 10 minutes. Future research needs to ask the question whether the general practitioner can facilitate a satisfactory practitioner–patient relationship in such a short time, and, if so, how?

The experience of the consultation and medical treatment as a whole may be one of the most powerful forces determining whether people go or stay with either orthodox or complementary practitioners. The sparse empirical research in this area, as well as a great deal of speculation, suggest that at least a proportion of patients are more positive about the consultation styles of complementary practitioners. They take much more time—as much as ten times that of general practitioners; they express more compassion and sympathy; they are probably more likely to touch the patient and they attach particular importance to their own behaviour in the consultation. While there are good reasons for these differences—the pressure on practitioners in the two sectors is quite different—it does seem that orthodox medical practitioners find it harder to meet the changing needs and demands of their patients.

Chapter 7

The Placebo Effect in Orthodox and Complementary Medicine

*Phil Richardson**

In the preceding chapters we have reviewed research which sought to explain the appeal of complementary medicine. A person's knowledge, attitudes and beliefs may lead them towards complementary medicine, and a number of different facets of the treatment, of which the consultation style is one, may persuade them that the treatment is worth while and should be continued. These factors, along with a variety of other psychological and social influences, have another importance, however, in that they may also affect the outcome of both orthodox and complementary treatment.

There is now a wealth of evidence that psychological factors play a substantial role in determining patients' responses to orthodox medical treatments. Recovery from surgical operations can be accelerated if patients receive appropriate psychological preparation (Weinman and Johnston, 1988). Survival following life-threatening diseases, such as cancer, appears to be influenced by the patient's emotional reaction to the original diagnosis as well as to their state of mind during the period of treatment and follow-up (Levy and Wise, 1987). The patient's faith in the treatments they receive, and their associated expectations of benefit (or otherwise), undoubtedly contribute in some measure to the curative power of modern medicine (Brannon and Feist, 1992).

These influences are rather unhelpfully described by the term 'the placebo effect', a phrase which embraces a wide variety of ill-understood effects. The placebo is a portmanteau concept, in that a single term is used to describe a set of quite disparate phenomena. This effect has been variously described as the therapeutic impact of 'non-specific' or 'incidental' treatment ingredients to distinguish it from those aspects of a patient's response

* Senior Lecturer in Psychology, UMDS (London University) and Consultant Psychologist, Lewisham and Guy's Mental Health Trust

to treatment which can be unequivocally attributed to some characteristic aspect of the treatment and its presumed 'specific action' on the disorder being treated (Shapiro and Morris, 1978). In the case of a drug the specific action would refer to its particular pharmacological effect, while the placebo component would refer to any other aspect of the treatment that might exert a therapeutic effect. This might include the expectations of the patient (and the doctor), the power and prestige of the physician, the credibility of the treatment and so on.

THE PLACEBO IN COMPLEMENTARY MEDICINE

For critics of complementary medical techniques who can find no scientific basis for the specific action of homeopathy, say, or traditional Chinese acupuncture, it is tempting to attribute all improvements in patients treated by these techniques to the placebo effect. To them the practices of many complementary medical practitioners appear to have much in common with the largely psychotherapeutic aspects of placebo treatments. For this reason it is important to ascertain what is known about placebos and placebo effects if we are adequately to evaluate the effectiveness of complementary medicine.

A complementary practitioner who has no interest in dismissing his or her remedies as 'mere' placebos might find little of interest in the findings of research on placebos administered in conventional medical settings. These attitudes could, however, be based on a misconception about the action of treatments—a misconception which is implicit in the way in which orthodox treatment trials (e.g. drug trials) are commonly described in the conventional scientific literature. The simplistic view, which appears to underlie this misconception, is that treatments are either active (or 'specific') or are placebos (with a 'non-specific' action). If active, they 'work' as a result of their physically active ingredients; if placebos, their impact is psychological. This view fails to acknowledge that all treatments, physically active or otherwise, have some psychological impact when administered to a conscious patient. The interest of placebo studies is that they isolate the relevant psychological processes by eliminating the possibility of a direct physical effect of treatment. Placebo research is therefore relevant to our understanding of the psychological impact of all treatments whatever their nature, for the simple reason that all treatments are in this sense capable of generating 'placebo' effects.

A recent contribution to the language of placebo effects helps us to see how this is so. Grünbaum's approach distinguishes so-called *characteristic* treatment ingredients, which are specified by a theory of therapy to be remedial for a particular disorder, from *incidental* ones, which are not so specified. Placebo effects are those effects on a disorder which are brought about specifically by incidental treatment ingredients, *regardless of whether the treatment itself is a non-placebo or a placebo* (when none of its characteristic ingredients is in fact remedial for the disorder) (Grünbaum, 1981). For many physical treatments, orthodox or complementary, the psychological processes accompanying treatment administration would qualify as incidental ingredients and hence be the prime contributors to the placebo effect of the treatment.

From this perspective the placebo effect ceases to be a nuisance variable which merely hinders the evaluation of drug treatments. Instead it can be seen as an essential element of any approach to therapy which claims to be holistic. Many of the most positive and valuable aspects of the therapeutic encounter contribute to the placebo effect. The rapport between patient and practitioner, the belief of the patient, the enthusiasm of the doctor, although of great importance are all in a sense incidental to the specific action of a drug, needle or homeopathic remedy. The placebo can thus be seen as a simple form of psychotherapy.

The History of Medicine is the History of the Placebo

It has seldom been disputed that the history of orthodox Western medicine is largely the history of the placebo. Indeed, the majority of medicines and medical practices prior to the turn of the twentieth century have since been recognized to be inert or, in some instances, positively toxic (Shapiro, 1960). Historical precursors to the inert *medicines* dispensed to patients in modern-day placebo-controlled trials were often more elaborate, exotic and at times repellent than their bland contemporary counterparts. In previous centuries therapeutic properties were ascribed to a bizarre assortment of substances, including *usnea* (the moss scraped from the skull of a victim of a hanging), the Bezoar stone (a common gallstone masquerading as the crystallized teardrop of a deer bitten by a snake), and the circulio antiodontaligiosus (a crushed worm applied locally for toothache) (Shapiro, 1960; Volgyesi, 1954).

In recent years coloured water—in the guise of a tonic, an injection of sterile water offered as a painkiller, empty capsules, and pills made of chalk or sugar have established themselves as elements in the orthodox physician's armoury (Richardson, 1995). In fact, anonymous surveys have found that placebo use is far from rare among hospital doctors. In one study more than 80% of US hospital clinicians admitted to their occasional use in routine clinical practice (Gray and Flynn, 1981). Sadly, however, the reasons commonly offered to justify their use, e.g. fobbing-off the demanding patient, *proving* that the symptom thereby reduced was psychogenic, betray a limited knowledge of relevant empirical research findings and poor psychological sophistication among users (Goodwin, Goodwin and Vogel, 1979).

STUDIES OF THE PLACEBO EFFECT

Since the 1950s, when the placebo-controlled trial came into its own as a method for evaluating new treatments, evidence has been accruing for the therapeutic power of the placebo treatments themselves. Early placebo studies commonly inferred that a placebo effect had occurred simply on the basis of a reduction in symptoms after the administration of a placebo (Richardson, 1994). The placebo was often administered as the only comparison condition in the evaluation of a drug. However, basic studies of this kind, not directly aimed at monitoring placebo effects, do not offer strong evidence for the occurrence of placebo effects. The observed changes could simply be spontaneous symptom fluctuation, including spontaneous long-term improvement, which might then be erroneously attributed to the placebo. More recent studies, however, have incorporated a no-treatment control condition, and these provide more compelling evidence that the symptom relief which is seen to follow placebo administration can in reality be attributed to the placebo itself—and thus be considered a true placebo effect.

Examination of the available evidence suggests that placebos administered in an orthodox medical context may induce relief from symptoms in an impressively wide array of illnesses, including allergies, angina pectoris, asthma, cancer, cerebral infarction, depression, diabetes, enuresis, epilepsy, insomnia, Meunière's disease, migraine, multiple sclerosis, neurosis, ocular pathology, Parkinsonism, prostatic hyperplasia, schizophrenia, skin diseases, ulcers and warts (see for example White, Tursky and Schwartz, 1985).

Placebo response rates vary enormously from study to study and may range from 0 to 100% of patients showing improvement, even for the same condition (Ross and Olson, 1982). This variability is not altogether surprising if one considers that the apparent benefits of treatment for any complex condition will depend on both the symptoms being targeted and the way the symptoms are measured. Each of these may vary from study to study, as may the overall context in which the study is carried out.

Pain is the commonest symptom giving rise to a medical consultation and has also been the commonest outcome measure in studies of the placebo effect (Richardson, 1995). Experimental pain, induced in laboratory volunteers, generally shows a poor placebo response rate—commonly 16% of subjects will show a 50% or greater reduction on whichever pain measure is in use. In studies of clinical pain, an average response rate of 35% has been reported by a number of reviewers (Beecher 1955; Evans, 1974). Specialized placebo studies, where the primary focus of interest is the placebo effect itself, have often yielded much higher response rates still (up to 85%), as have those in which the main target symptom is itself psychological (e.g. anxiety, depression) (Richardson, 1995).

As well as the impact of placebos on symptoms, placebo effects have also been demonstrated on objective measures of certain bodily processes, including blood pressure, lung function, postoperative swelling, and gastric motility (Richardson, 1989, 1994). For example, dental patients undergoing wisdom tooth extractions showed significantly greater reductions in postoperative swelling when treated with placebo ultrasound than those who were simply monitored over the same period without treatment (Hashish, Feinman and Harvey, 1988). This sort of evidence reduces the likelihood that placebo effects can be attributed simply to a wish on the patient's part to please the doctor or therapist by reporting symptom relief. In addition adverse effects of placebo administration have been noted in many studies. These include dependence, symptom worsening (the *nocebo* effect) and a multitude of side-effects, both subjective (headache, concentration difficulties, nausea, etc.) and objectively visible (skin rashes, sweating, vomiting, etc). In drug trials the action of placebos has proved hard to differentiate from that of the drugs with which they have been compared: several studies have found parallel time–effect curves and dose–response relationships, along with closely comparable performance on various other pharmacokinetic parameters (Ross and Olson, 1982).

The idea that placebo effects can be understood as the direct or indirect result of psychological influences on the patient's physical state has not gone unchallenged. One proposal has been that data distortion, through some form of measurement error on the part of the investigator or patient, might account for placebo effects, particularly in view of the extensive evidence for the influence of experimenter bias and therapist expectancy effects on patient outcome (Feldman, 1956; Evans, 1985). According to this view the placebo effect would be largely epiphenomenal. The effect of systematic biases in the measurement of symptoms may, of course, be reduced in controlled studies by the use of assessors who are blind to the patient's treatment. A problem remains, however: it is usually impossible to blind the patient to the simple fact of having received treatment.

Systematic overreporting of symptoms by patients during pretreatment assessment (e.g. to 'earn' treatment) and under-reporting of symptoms after treatment (e.g. to 'thank' the doctor) would create the impression of a positive treatment effect. Patients in a waiting-list control group who overreported on the first pretreatment assessment have no reason to alter their report at the second assessment, if still awaiting treatment, and will therefore show less change than those in the placebo group. This source of potential bias is seldom acknowledged by researchers and yet is clearly not eliminated by the usual expedient of a no-treatment control group. Nevertheless, though it may account for some placebo effects, it is hard to see how simple misreporting could explain objectively measured change in physiological processes, including those of which the patient would normally have no awareness (e.g. blood pressure, lung function) (Richardson, 1994).

Taken together, the above findings strongly suggest that the psychological impact of any treatment is potentially great. While these findings are based on studies carried out more or less exclusively in conventional medical settings, it would be truly remarkable if such processes were not also at work in the domain of the complementary therapies, especially as complementary therapists rightly attach great importance to the psychological aspects of treatment. It is worth stating again that the fact that placebo effects occur in no way implies that the associated treatment is a placebo. In fact a maximally effective treatment can be expected to maximize the placebo effect. Recognizing that a treatment has a powerful placebo effect does not imply that it is entirely psychologically mediated and should not therefore be taken as a criticism.

Understanding the Placebo Effect

The simple recognition that placebo effects occur in orthodox medicine, and most probably also within the complementary therapies, does little to advance our understanding of the psychological power of these differing forms of treatment. The therapeutic exploitation of placebo power requires an understanding of the determinants and correlates of placebo effects. Once again our knowledge of the relevant variables and processes has been largely restricted to research in an orthodox medical context.

Attempts to further our understanding of placebo effects have typically involved one of two kinds of strategy: firstly to identify which variables make a placebo response more or less likely, and secondly to test hypotheses about presumed mechanisms of the effect. The first kind of study has typically looked at patient variables, treatment characteristics, or aspects of the therapist and therapist–patient interaction.

Differences between placebo responders and non-responders have long been a focus of interest. Attempts to spot such differences on sociodemographic characteristics (age, gender, ethnicity, educational level) have generally yielded weak and inconclusive findings (Shapiro and Morris, 1978; Richardson, 1994). Other studies have looked at possible individual differences in intelligence and personality. Locus of control, field dependence, emotional dependence, extraversion, introversion, neuroticism, suggestibility, autonomic awareness, acquiescence, tolerance of ambiguity, affiliation, autonomy and impulsivity have all been contenders in this domain (Richardson, 1995). Once again, however, conflicting and equivocal findings (e.g. both extraversion and introversion have emerged as predictors of placebo responsiveness) suggest that the placebo responder cannot be characterized by this kind of personality variable.

It seems more likely that the archetypal placebo responder is a mythical beast. The evidence suggests that placebo responders on one occasion may no longer be so on the next (Shapiro and Morris, 1978). Conversely, conditioning studies have shown that previous non-responders can be turned into responders (see below). Thus placebo responsiveness may not be an enduring trait. Any patient may benefit from the placebo effect, not just a gullible minority. An awareness of this fact may do much to destigmatize the placebo effect and counter the suggestion that any psychologically induced improvement in health status must be a sign of neuroticism on the part of the patient or quackery on the part of the clinician.

Research has also been conducted on the simple physical characteristics of the placebo in whatever form it is administered. The colour and size of capsules and pills have been repeatedly subject to experimental manipulation, but with little reliable impact (Buckalew and Ross, 1981). Despite this, there is a popular myth among orthodox clinicians that pill colour may in itself be influential and, despite evidence to the contrary, one frequently encounters bizarre claims in this regard. For example, one reviewer has reported that for a placebo to be maximally effective it should be very large and either brown or purple or very small and either bright red or yellow! (Evans, 1974). More serious, 'major' or invasive procedures do appear to have stronger placebo effects. Injections *per se* would appear to have a greater impact than pills (Carne, 1961; Grenfell, Briggs and Holland, 1961) and placebo surgery has yielded unusually high positive response rates. In the work of Cobb, Thomas and Dillard, for example, 85% of patients with angina showed improvements on various measures, including ECG and exercise tolerance test performance, following placebo 'surgery' in which they received only an operation scar (Cobb, Thomas and Dillard, 1959; Dimond, Kittle and Cockett, 1960). Treatments that employ sophisticated technical equipment also have enhanced placebo power. For example, Langley and colleagues obtained a higher than usual 55% response rate to placebo transcutaneous nerve stimulation when the machinery was given additional technological trappings such as an oscilloscope, flashing lights, dials (Langley et al, 1984).

Why certain treatments provoke stronger placebo responses than others is unclear. There is some evidence that technically sophisticated treatments have greater credibility for the patient, and may thus generate a stronger expectation of successful outcome (Petrie and Hazleman, 1985). Electro-acupuncture might be expected to benefit from this effect. The use of high technology is though, with rare exceptions, an infrequent feature of comple-mentary approaches, and complementary therapies are generally minimally invasive. From this point of view complementary therapies should have limited value as placebos. On the other hand, patients receiving comple-mentary therapies perceive them as highly credible and effective, which would tend to enhance their placebo effect, as might a positive relationship with the practitioner concerned (see Chapters 5 and 6). This may therefore be an important way in which complementary treatments can justifiably be viewed as *alternative*—for those whose weak faith in orthodox methods might actually diminish their potential therapeutic impact—by weakening the placebo effect.

The style of treatment administration and other qualities of the therapist appear to contribute substantially to the impact of the treatment itself. Recognition of the potential impact of a therapist's expectations on the patient's response to treatment has long been embodied in the double-blind procedures used in treatment evaluation studies (see Chapter 8). Therapist variables have also been extensively explored in the placebo literature, with the majority of studies pointing to their importance (Richardson, 1994). Those therapists who exhibit greater interest in their patients, greater confidence in their treatments, and higher professional status, all appear to promote stronger placebo effects in their patients (Shapiro and Morris, 1978). How this occurs remains a subject of speculation.

Studies of doctor–patient communication have demonstrated the influence of certain therapist behaviours on patient satisfaction and adherence to medical advice, and there is reason to believe that adherence may have an important impact in its own right. In one study, for example, the risk of death during the year following myocardial infarction was significantly (and substantially) greater in patients who took less than 75% of their prescribed medication, *regardless of whether the medication was a beta blocker or a placebo* (Horwitz et al, 1990). The reasons for this effect are unclear, however, and there has been insufficient cross-fertilization between research on therapist influences on the placebo effect and other related fields of psychological enquiry (e.g. psychotherapy process research and studies of doctor–patient communication). In view of the holistic philosophy adopted by most complementary practitioners, it would seem highly likely that the therapist–patient relationship would have an equally important role in the complementary therapies as in orthodox medicine.

MODE OF ACTION OF PLACEBOS

Hypotheses concerning the way in which placebos exert their effects are numerous and have drawn upon diverse theoretical concepts, including operant conditioning, classical conditioning, guilt reduction, transference, suggestion, persuasion, role demands, faith, hope, labelling, selective symptom monitoring, misattribution, cognitive dissonance reduction, control theory, anxiety reduction, expectancy effects and endorphin release (Richardson, 1994). Investigations driven by such theories are sadly small in number and often entirely absent. Explanations of placebogenesis that have received greatest attention from researchers are the anxiety-reduction, expectancy, classical conditioning and cognitive dissonance accounts.

As noted above, the relief of pain has been a prime focus for placebo research. Anxiety is thought to increase the experience of pain, and it is therefore not surprising that the reduction of anxiety has been proposed as an explanation of placebo effects (Evans, 1974). The lower placebo response rates with experimental, as opposed to clinical, pain could be accounted for by the fact that healthy experimental volunteers are initially less anxious than patients who may be ill or injured; unlike medical patients, volunteers have less chance to experience anxiety reduction when offered treatment, whereas the relief at being offered treatment may alone alleviate to some extent the symptoms of the patient group. In similar vein, the pain relief associated with swallowing an aspirin, yet which occurs well in advance of any possible pharmacological effect, might be explained by the immediate relief of anxiety which accompanies the knowledge of having received treatment. Scientific evidence for this interpretation of placebo effects is sparse and despite one or two positive findings (c.f. Evans, 1974) most investigators have found no clear association between changes in state anxiety and placebo-induced symptom change (Richardson, 1994). The role of anxiety reduction as a mediator of placebo-induced symptom change therefore remains unclear. Its likely role as a source of symptom reduction in the complementary therapies is also reduced by the consideration that many recipients of complementary medicine experience chronic health problems of the kind that are less likely to be associated with the high anxiety and uncertainty of an acute illness. In cases where anxiety is absent, placebo-induced symptom relief can hardly be attributed to its reduction.

Patients' expectations of treatment being beneficial have been advanced as a possible explanation for placebo effects. The role (if any) of therapeutic expectancies is probably as great in complementary medicine as in orthodox medicine and possibly more so, in that patients must usually actively seek out a complementary practitioner. Actively seeking a consultation surely implies at least some hope or expectation of benefit on the part of the patient. Patient expectations have been shown to predict the outcome of psychotherapy and of drug treatments and there is some evidence that expectancy manipulations may influence responses to a placebo. Other investigators have found that therapeutic instructions may influence analgesic responses both to placebos and to standard painkillers (see Richardson, 1994). In contrast, a review of the research literature on cognitive coping strategies has concluded that verbal expectancy manipulations alone are not effective in reducing pain (Fernandez and Turk, 1989). Other aspects of treatment administration are therefore likely to interact with expectancy if it does play some role in determining outcome. Furthermore, in comparative studies testing alternative accounts of the placebo effect, expectancy-based explanations have typically fared worse. Although they appeal to common sense, such accounts have limited explanatory force unless they can also specify the precise mechanism(s) by which a particular expectancy translates itself into a particular form of symptom relief. To aver that change occurs 'because the patient expected it' begs many questions about what really happens between expectation and outcome.

According to the classical conditioning view, many of the standard accompaniments of effective non-placebo treatments (e.g. doctors, syringes, stethoscopes) have the potential to become conditioned stimuli by dint of their repeated association with symptom relief (Wickramasekera, 1985). Thus, if a drug routinely provides relief from pain, after a while the syringe which contains the drug becomes associated with the relief of pain and comes to have pain-relieving properties itself. Conditioned drug responses have been demonstrated both in animals and in humans, though their direct relevance to placebo phenomena has only recently emerged through a series of studies conducted by Voudouris and colleagues (Voudouris,

Peck and Coleman, 1990). In experimentally induced pain, the pairing of reduced shock intensity with the application of a placebo 'analgesic' cream subsequently led to significantly lower pain ratings to a given level of painful stimulation than when no prior pairing had occurred. A verbal expectancy manipulation (simply telling the patient that this was a power-fully effective analgesic) obtained a smaller degree of placebo-induced pain relief than the conditioning procedure. Conditioning accounts of the placebo effect therefore look promising, but do not yet appear to have been tested directly on clinical populations. Their relevance in complementary medicine may be reduced, however, by the probable unfamiliarity and/or inexperience of most patients with most complementary techniques; conditioning effects require repeated prior exposure to the conditioned (therapeutic) stimuli.

The holding of two or more psychologically inconsistent beliefs is thought by some to create a state of tension which will motivate the individual to reduce the inconsistency (Festinger, 1957). This tension is described as *cognitive dissonance*. Undergoing treatment on the one hand, and deriving no benefit on the other, would for many patients be inconsistent, and the resultant dissonance might motivate the patient to alter the symptom or its perception—to reduce the inconsistency. Laboratory studies suggest that dissonance arousal is a powerful force capable of producing physiological as well as psychological change (Zimbardo, 1969). There have also been many demonstrations of the relevance of dissonance theory to clinical phenomena in general, and its relevance to the placebo effect is supported by a small series of experiments reported by Totman (1987). Through various conventional dissonance-inducing experimental paradigms he was able to demonstrate that patients in whom greatest dissonance was aroused during placebo administration were those who showed greatest subsequent symptom relief. His dissonance-based interpretation of these findings has not gone unchallenged, however, and alternative accounts of his findings have been proposed (Richardson, 1994).

Unlike the previous accounts of placebo effects, whose immediate relevance to complementary medicine is less clear, cognitive dissonance accounts may have much to offer in understanding the placebo component of complementary treatments, and indeed of any novel or unusual treat-ment a patient elects to have. From this standpoint, factors which enhance dissonance should increase the potential for a therapeutic effect brought about by consequent dissonance reduction. Effort expended on a treatment and displeasure associated with its application are both likely to increase dissonance, along with any element which increases the patient's commitment to the treatment. A distinctive feature of the complementary therapies is that in most cases the patient will have actively sought them out, thus increasing—or at least reflecting—their self-perceived commitment. Moreover, many complementary techniques require special efforts on the part of the patient and may entail unpleasant or distasteful consequences. For example, in Chinese herbal medicine it is common place for patients to be expected to prepare infusions and/or decoctions themselves. This can involve elaborate and time-consuming rituals. Moreover, the taste of the finished product typically takes it to the limits of what most people would regard as drinkable! Dissonance-induced placebo effects may of course be equally, probably more, important in unpleasant or distressing orthodox treatments.

IMPLICATIONS OF RESEARCH ON PLACEBO EFFECTS

The above overview of the psychological processes through which a treatment, which in physical terms should be ineffective, can none the less produce impressive levels of symptom relief in patients with a wide variety of physical health problems, should be food for thought for all clinicians who are seeking an explanation for the therapeutic power of a treatment whose efficacy is established but whose mechanisms of action remain opaque. It remains to be established which of the differing accounts of placebo genesis can best elucidate the psychological processes which commonly mediate patients' responses to their medical treatments. In any case, it seems unlikely that a single approach will successfully account for all placebo phenomena with respect to all symptoms and all response modalities. Where complementary medicine is concerned the dissonance-reduction hypothesis would appear to offer one of the more promising explanatory accounts.

Whatever the reasons for placebo-induced symptom change, it has become axiomatic that the use of a placebo-control condition is essential to the proper evaluation of the specific effectiveness of any form of medical treatment. As noted earlier in this chapter, however, it will often be overly simplistic, in the evaluation of physical treatment methods, to ask whether this or that treatment is a placebo or not. The more pertinent question may be: In what proportion may the effects of this treatment be accounted for by psychologically-mediated as opposed to direct physically-mediated changes? Nevertheless, where the evidence is unclear and the presumed physical mechanisms of a given treatment are poorly defined and understood, it may be more parsimonious to assume that any given treatment works through any one of a variety of known psychological mechanisms rather than through unknown physical ones. This position would imply that in the absence of direct evidence from placebo-controlled double-blind trials it is right and proper to regard any new or unusual form of treatment, be it orthodox or complementary, as potentially a form of psychotherapy. This is an extreme, though logically defensible, view which starkly illustrates why the controlled trial, the principal subject of the next chapter, has assumed such importance in medicine.

Chapter 8

Research Methods and Research Problems in Complementary Medicine

In order to evaluate the efficacy of ginseng, find two people and let one eat ginseng and run, and the other run without eating ginseng. The one that did not eat ginseng will develop shortness of breath sooner.

Bencao Tujing, *Atlas of Materia Medica*, 1061 AD

This Song dynasty text, cited by Tsutani (1993), shows that controlled trials in complementary medicine are not a completely new innovation. Nevertheless, most branches of complementary medicine, and indeed many aspects of orthodox medicine, have not benefited from this early methodological rigour until comparatively recently.

Before reviewing the evidence on the efficacy of complementary medicine in the next two chapters, we will consider some of the difficulties that have arisen in defining an appropriate methodology for its evaluation. Some complementary practitioners, and others who value the more individual approach of complementary therapies, have suggested that the classic experimental methodology of the randomized controlled trial may not do justice to complementary medicine and perhaps should be avoided. A new methodology may be needed which reflects the unique characteristics of complementary medicine (Heron, 1986).

Critics of complementary medicine have responded, sometimes with irritation, that complementary practitioners are simply seeking to avoid empirical scrutiny, accusing both its patients and practitioners of a 'flight from science' (Smith, 1983) and a wish to leave medicine in the age of superstition. These extreme positions were more common a decade ago. The colleges of most of the major complementary therapies have now realized that they need to take research seriously if they are to maintain respect and withstand scrutiny from government and orthodox medicine, whether or not their patients mind if they are engaged in research.

WHO WANTS RESEARCH INTO COMPLEMENTARY MEDICINE?

Given the remarks of the critics of complementary medicine seen in previous chapters, it may seem unnecessary to ask why research into complementary medicine should be carried out. Complementary practitioners have been challenged to submit their therapies to experimental test and, if they are aiming for statutory registration, there is a pressure to develop a programme of research. From the complementary practitioners' point of view, this outside pressure can lead to mixed feelings about research. Are they doing research to pacify their critics or to develop a discipline that they believe in? This depends partly on the questions addressed and the people to whom the research is oriented. Mills (1993a) has usefully addressed the question of audiences for research into herbal medicine, but his comments apply equally to other forms of complementary medicine. He considers that there are three broad groups who might be thought to have an interest in the results of such scientific enquiries.

1. *The public (patients and consumers)* Consultation with complementary practitioners usually occurs because of word-of-mouth recommendation or information in the media, not because of the reading of scientific journals. However, the public is indirectly influenced by research through reports in the media, and is certainly concerned with the safety of medicines of all kinds.

2. *Those speaking for the public* Although various government departments are involved in monitoring the safety of medicines, they rely on expert medical evidence. The group who must be convinced of the value of a complementary therapy, particularly where legislation is concerned, are therefore the medical advisors. They are presumably influenced, to some degree at least, by the research literature and in particular by the evidence from controlled trials.

3. *Practitioners of complementary medicine* Complementary practitioners may engage in research, willingly or unwillingly, because of a need to justify and protect their therapy from critics and those who might legislate against their practice. However, this is only one aspect of research. Practitioners may also wish to audit their own work or carry out more formal studies aimed at improving the quality of their practice and their understanding of its action. The audience for this research is primarily other practitioners.

4. *Sympathetic orthodox practitioners* We have added a fourth group to Mills's list: doctors and other health professionals with an interest in complementary medicine, who may both value research in the area and

also conduct it. Their interest is probably mainly in outcome studies. Their question is, essentially, will this therapy aid me in the treatment of patients?

THE SCIENTIST–PRACTITIONER MODEL

For many practitioners, both orthodox and complementary, their primary work is treating patients; any interest in research is secondary. This sentiment, as applied to herbal medicine, is nicely expressed by Mills (1993a):

> Knowledge within traditional medicine has generally been in the form of received wisdom moulded to the individual needs and prowess of each practitioner. Such means of acquiring healing skills seem temperamentally suited to most practitioners, herbal and conventional, even today. Their interest in inquiry for its own sake, with secure truths up for constant possible refutation, is understandably secondary to their concern to survive in practice.

In medicine there are various external pressures to carry out research and, in some posts at least, research is regarded as an essential part of the work. For practitioners in private practice, as most complementary therapists are, the situation is rather different. Why should he or she concern themselves with the time-consuming process of research, which has little or no immediate reward? In an ideal world, practitioners might also be scientists, evaluating and developing their practice through a constant programme of applied research. Many doctors, psychologists and others would endorse this model. Are complementary practitioners just being feeble or are they refusing to face up to empirical scrutiny? It is salutary to consider the conclusions of a study of psychotherapy, though we suspect that similar remarks could be made about medicine and other disciplines with equal justification. 'The typical practising psychotherapist does not do research, publishes little or nothing, is unwilling to participate in research, and has a more generally negative attitude to research than have academic colleagues in clinical psychology' (Morrow-Bradley and Elliott, 1986).

Another study found that psychotherapists spend little time reading about research and only about half of them find research to be of any clinical use (Cohen, Sargent and Sechrest, 1986). There may only be a minority of complementary practitioners interested in research, but the reluctance of some of the complementary professions to engage in research is certainly not a phenomenon confined to complementary medicine.

ATTITUDES OF COMPLEMENTARY PRACTITIONERS TO RESEARCH

There are, as far as we know, no studies of the reasons complementary practitioners have for entering training. The motives no doubt vary according to the particular type of therapy and the extent to which the practitioner is interested in the underlying theory or philosophical background. Some acupuncturists, for instance, have an interest in Taoist or Buddhist philosophy and in related physical/meditational practices such as T'ai Chi, Qi Gong or martial arts. However, the basic motives are probably more pragmatic—a wish to make a living in a way that it is useful and helpful to others and interesting to the practitioner.

An interest in science or clinical research is not a requirement for training as a complementary practitioner, though courses on research and a research project have been introduced in some schools (e.g. British School of Osteopathy). This is a pattern that is likely to continue as more of the professions seek statutory registration. Doctors who practise some form of complementary medicine will also have received some introduction to research, although even in medical school teaching in research methodology is fairly rudimentary.

We know of only two studies examining the attitudes of complementary practitioners to research, both carried out with acupuncturists. Vincent and Mole (1989) surveyed 100 senior practitioners to discover why acupuncturists had failed to take advantage of funding opportunities that existed for research into complementary medicine. Almost all (93%) of the 58 respondents thought that research was important and that acupuncture would benefit from formal evaluation. Over half were interested in taking part in a research project. A proportion of acupuncturists were prepared to consider the value of a placebo-controlled trial and there was little evidence of any entrenched opposition to conventional methodology.

A similar, but more substantial, survey was carried out by Fitter and Blackwell (1993) of 1158 acupuncturists. Of the 423 respondents, 32% were already committing at least half a day a week to research and development, and over 80% were willing to commit that time if properly supported. The most important reasons given for engaging in research were to promote the wider acceptance of acupuncture (96% agreement) and to aid personal learning and development (90%). About a quarter of respondents were very interested both in reviewing literature and carrying out studies. With a 36% response rate the study no doubt overestimates the interest in research. However, it is clear that there is a substantial number of

acupuncturists willing to put time and effort into research and, in particular, to acquiring the necessary skills for research. Very few had any
knowledge and experience of research, though a small group had gained
some experience. Vincent and Mole (1989) comment that as acupuncturists
have almost no experience of research of any kind, it is hardly surprising
that they do not submit applications for funding or initiate research.

FUNDAMENTAL QUESTIONS AND RESEARCH STRATEGIES

A number of different questions can be asked about any form of treatment,
and these will vary according to the existing state of knowledge and the
novelty and stage of development of the treatment. Questions about
mechanism or the optimum method of giving the therapy may predomi-
nate in a well-established treatment, whereas questions about efficacy and
safety may be primary in relatively untested treatments, such as those of
complementary medicine. They may have stood the test of time and been
accepted by many patients, but there is still considerable scientific debate
about effectiveness. Once there is evidence that a complementary treatment
works, research on its mode of action and the treatment process may come
to the fore.

In our view the fundamental questions for research into complementary
therapies are:

1. Does the therapy have a beneficial effect on any individual disease or
   disorder?
2. Does the treatment have any advantage over existing treatments in
   terms of efficacy, safety, patient preference, cost and availability. If it is
   not at least equally effective, the therapy might be scientifically or
   philosophically interesting, but it will be of little practical value.
3. Is this effect primarily, or even partly, due to the specific and intended
   action of the treatment (needles, herbs, manipulation, etc.), or is it due to
   psychological processes? To put it another way, is the therapy just a
   placebo, or is there some specific treatment effect?
4. What mechanism might underlie the therapy's action?
5. There is also a range of 'process' questions, primarily of concern to
   practitioners. These might concern the reliability and validity of diagnosis, the value of individual techniques and approaches in the overall
   treatment package, the role of the practitioner in the treatment process
   and perhaps the attitude of the patient.

The first two questions are essentially questions about outcome and they might be of less interest to practising complementary therapists already convinced of the value of their therapy. However, they are certainly the questions that mostly concern the wider medical and scientific community, whether critics or sympathizers. The question of the extent to which psychological factors are responsible for observed changes could also be seen as the most basic question about mode of action. Is there any specific action at all? Questions of the mechanism of action of complementary therapies are more likely to follow research into outcome, though a certain amount of work has been carried out in the major therapies.

TYPES OF STUDY

Studies of any therapy fall into various categories. The following categorization is very straightforward, and only meant to offer a broad indication of the range of studies that can be carried out. The classical test of the effectiveness of a therapy is the randomized controlled trial, and we will concentrate on this type of study when evaluating complementary therapies. But other types of study can offer valuable information and we will briefly introduce them. *Evidence-based medicine*, that is, clinical practice based as far as possible on the results of controlled trials, is currently being advanced as the gold standard for orthodox medicine, but it should be noted that a number of authors (e.g. Black, 1996) have pointed out that randomized controlled trials are neither feasible nor desirable in all circumstances.

Case Studies and Case Series

Case reports provide a detailed account of the effect of a treatment on a single patient, with a case series simply being the description of a group of patients having the same treatment. Case reports have always been used as the guides to the study of rare clinical situations, for the reporting of new information about side-effects of treatment or for introducing views which challenge existing theories of disease (Aldridge, 1993). The clinical account of single cases was once the primary form of medical knowledge. Now their primary use is to provide hypotheses that may then be tested in formal studies. The use of case studies (as opposed to single case designs) is probably limited at this stage in the development of complementary medicine as there is already a wealth of clinical description in the complementary medical journals, and a wealth of hypotheses that now need testing.

Single Case Designs

Single case designs are an attempt to formalize case studies, the design implying a prior hypothesis, measurement and formal statistical analysis. At its most elaborate, different treatments, perhaps including a placebo, may be given in sequence and the effects of each observed and compared with a baseline no-treatment stage. Where multiple observations are collected (from diaries or repeated clinical measures), extremely sophisticated statistical analyses can be used to disentangle the effects of the treatment from trends and both regular and random variations in the data (Chatfield, 1985). Aldridge (1993), after reviewing the use of single case designs in a wide range of disorders, has suggested that these methods are well suited to the study of complementary medicine. They are cheap, flexible in approach, offer different levels of formality and rigour, and can incorporate an emphasis on providing the best, individually tailored, care of the patient. There are various problems if the treatment has long-term or irreversible effects, and they are not suitable for the broad questions about the applicability of treatments across a range of individuals (such as whether homeopathy is generally more effective than conventional medicine in the treatment of hayfever). The methodological rigour can, however, equal that of controlled trials (Barlow and Hersen, 1984; Kazdin, 1984).

Clinical Audits

Audit in medicine has been developing strongly in the last few years, but is only just starting in the complementary sphere. The aim is to monitor the quality of care, evaluate its effectiveness and, where necessary, make changes to clinical procedures (Moss, 1992). The progress of patients under treatment is carefully monitored, and any adverse effects of therapy noted, but there is not usually any comparison group of patients receiving some other form of treatment or placebo. Audits may be carried out on any aspect of treatment, the quality of diagnostic information recorded, the frequency with which a particular technique is used by different practitioners, or the outcome of a particular procedure. Similar formal studies may be made of the process of treatment: practitioners might, for instance, study the reliability of their diagnoses or the relation between a particular intervention and the patient's therapeutic progress; in the latter case the study of process and outcome take place simultaneously. Audit is now required in all areas of health care and will probably be expected in complementary medicine, at least in any complementary profession that is seeking statutory registration.

Studies on Mechanism of Action

Studies on the mechanism of action of a complementary therapy do not necessarily require different designs, but they are likely to differ in several ways from clinical studies of the treatment. They are more likely to be laboratory based, to concentrate on short-term effects, to focus on one single aspect of the treatment and they will certainly try to relate the findings to existing scientific knowledge. In complementary medicine this might concern the role of trigger points or endorphins in mediating the effects of acupuncture, the precise pharmacological properties of different herbal remedies or a possible mechanism for the action of the extremely dilute remedies of homeopathy. Studies of mechanism might also attempt to validate the theories underlying a complementary therapy, for example, examining the evidence for the existence of acupuncture points and meridians.

Understanding the mechanisms that might underlie the action of complementary therapies is an enormously complex area, which we will not attempt to review. However, we will comment on this research when it affects the evaluation of the results of outcome studies. Homeopathy, for instance, uses very high dilutions of materials in some of its preparations, so high that few if any molecules of the original substance remain. It seems, in pharmacological terms, highly unlikely that such preparations could have any therapeutic action and positive results for trials of homeopaths are therefore often viewed with some suspicion. Other complementary therapies do not suffer from the problem of an implausible mechanism to the same extent. Acupuncture, herbalism, manipulative therapies and even naturopathy may or may not be effective, but could certainly act on principles that are known and accepted, even if their practitioners choose to conceptualize their action in other terms. Complementary therapies that require the existence of a subtle energy body or some other occult phenomena are clearly less likely to be accepted by orthodox medicine and science, even if studies of their validity and effectiveness should provide positive findings.

Controlled Trials

An uncontrolled trial is essentially an extended case series in which a large group of patients is treated and their improvement monitored. The main disadvantage with this method, especially when dealing with complaints that will eventually resolve naturally, is that there is no way of knowing whether the improvement is due to the passage of time, the attention of the therapist, or other factors unconnected with the treatment (Pocock, 1985; see also Chapter 7). The randomized controlled trial, discussed below, attempts to overcome these problems by evaluating the treatment in an experimental paradigm, albeit in a clinical setting. Most of the important studies of complementary therapies are formal trials, though they vary greatly in overall methodological rigour and the extent to which they are randomized and controlled.

The remainder of the chapter will concentrate on the methodology of randomized controlled trials and the problems that arise when this method is applied to complementary medicine. The randomized controlled trial is generally regarded as the most potent scientific tool for evaluating medical treatments. This is not to say that other approaches and methodologies are not important; single case designs, for instance, would seem to have great potential within complementary medicine. However, for the wider medical and scientific community, controlled trials remain the final arbiter of a therapy's efficacy and, for that reason if for no other, controlled trials must be a central component of research into complementary medicine. Before addressing the methodological issues we will briefly review the history of the randomized controlled trial, which is a comparatively recent innovation in medicine, to review the reasons both for its development and its preeminence in the evaluation of clinical treatments.

THE DEVELOPMENT OF THE RANDOMIZED CONTROLLED TRIAL

Randomized trials were established in agricultural tests in the early part of the twentieth century, following the pioneering work of the statistician Ronald Fisher (1923, 1926). There were isolated examples of clinicians following the same logic in tests of medical treatment, but no formal adoption of similar methods until the 1930s. In 1931 the British Medical Research Council set up a Therapeutic Trials Committee, and in the late 1930s the committee's statistician, Professor Austin Bradford Hill, laid the foundations of the randomized controlled trial with a series of articles in the *Lancet* (Pollock, 1989).

The turning point in the history of randomized controlled trials came in 1946 with the trial of streptomycin for the treatment of pulmonary tuber-culosis. The trial had several important innovative features (Pollock, 1989). The most important was that patients were randomized to a treated or control group, by consulting sealed envelopes held at a central location. Bias in allocation was therefore avoided. The second feature was that the entry criteria were strict and determined prior to the allocation to treatment. Thirdly, great care was taken to avoid bias from any source. There was no placebo control though, as it would have meant giving four painful intramuscular injections every day for four months; treated patients were simply compared with untreated patients. However, the clinical assessment was carried out by independent observers who had no knowledge of the patient's allocation. The trial also marked the first attempt to grapple with the ethical issues involved in controlled trials, in that the committee considered it would be unethical not to attempt a speedy, formal evaluation of a potentially fatal disease, presumably as opposed to waiting for an accumulation of clinical experience. However, there was at that time no question of informing patients, in either group, that they were taking part in a special study.

This study heralded a new approach to the evaluation of medical treatments, although it was not until 1960 that the first controlled trial of surgery was carried out and many standard treatments have still not been formally evaluated (Smith, 1991). Its appeal stems from its similarity to a laboratory experimental setting and the basic method is still the same: the random allocation of patients to one or more treatment conditions. As it is recognized that psychological factors may affect the response to treatment, the patient may be kept 'blind' to the nature of the treatment. Psychological factors may also affect the clinician giving the treatment; he or she may unknowingly communicate their beliefs to the patient, so biasing the result of the trial. Where both patient and clinician are unaware of the nature of the treatment (drug versus placebo, for instance) the trial is referred to as *double blind*. Where the clinician is aware, but the patient is not, the trial is *single blind*. A further important refinement, crucial where blinding of patient or clinician is not feasible, is that the assessment is carried out by an independent observer who is unaware of the treatment allocation.

The control condition varies according to the nature of the question that the trial addresses. If the question is simply the overall efficacy of a treatment, the comparison (the control) will be simply with an untreated group of patients. As disease has a natural ebb and flow, often improving steadily over time, a comparison with untreated patients is essential if one is to be convinced that the treatment is offering an additional benefit over and above the 'tincture of time'. For this reason alone uncontrolled studies cannot provide definitive answers to questions of efficacy (Pocock, 1993). More common now is the comparison between a novel treatment and an existing standard treatment, to see if the new treatment confers any advantage in respect of efficacy, safety, cost or other benefits. Where the fundamental question, especially important with novel or unusual treatments, is whether the treatment has its effect through psychological means then the comparison is with a group receiving placebo treatment. In the case of drugs, it is relatively straightforward to produce sugar pills, identical in appearance to the true tablets. With treatments requiring a physical intervention (such as surgery, physiotherapy or acupuncture) the definition of an appropriate placebo is extremely problematic, as well as raising additional ethical problems.

METHODOLOGICAL ISSUES IN THE RANDOMIZED CONTROLLED TRIAL

Complementary practitioners are often concerned that subjecting their therapy to the scrutiny of a randomized controlled trial will distort the true purpose of what they are doing and disguise or negate the efficacy of their therapy. These concerns are not confined to complementary medicine. In recent years, especially with the extension of the methodology of the randomized controlled trial to assessments of non-drug treatments and interventions, such as health education, psychotherapy and health-care provision, a considerable number of problems have emerged. Clinical investigators have become increasingly aware of certain difficulties in the interpretation, feasibility and ethics of controlled trials (Kramer and Shapiro, 1984). Complementary practitioners in particular may be unaware that many of their doubts and concerns have already been encountered, especially in trials of physical therapies or those that require an individual approach to the patient. We will therefore summarize some of the main methodological problems before considering those that are especially important in the evaluation of complementary therapies in more detail. Kramer and Shapiro (1984) focus on six major issues, with other authors raising a number of others (Pocock, 1985; Heron, 1986; Pollock, 1989; Canter and Nanke, 1993; Lewith and Aldridge, 1993):

1. Problems may arise because subjects randomized to different treatment groups may meet and discuss their treatment. Assignment to natural groups (e.g. comparison of two schools or two geographical regions) may be preferable to randomization.
2. Blinding may not be feasible for some treatments. While neither doctor nor patient may be able to distinguish a real tablet from a dummy, placebo tablet, there are no clear equivalents to placebo drugs for some treatments.
3. Participation in a study may affect the behaviour of people taking part. Simply being monitored and assessed regularly may have a beneficial effect. For instance, Blanchard and Andrasik (1982) found in their review of treatment for headache that migraine patients improved when just keeping diaries before being treated.

4. Subjects agreeing to take part in a trial may not be typical of the general population of patients with that particular problem. Entry criteria to a trial are strict to ensure comparability between groups and give the best chance of showing a treatment benefit. Patients with atypical symptoms, multiple problems or a poor prognosis may be excluded (Grisso, 1993).

5. Reduced compliance with treatment because of the possibility of receiving placebo treatment. If patients are informed that they might be taking a placebo they may be more inclined to give up the treatment if there are no immediate effects.

6. Using standard treatments in the trial may be artificial and have little relevance to clinical practice. Treatment within the context of a controlled trial may have to be closely specified at the outset, which inhibits a more flexible patient-centred approach. The trial may therefore not be a true test of the therapy as used in clinical practice and the needs of the patient may conflict with the requirements of research.

7. Individual variations in response are often ignored in an analysis that only considers average group responses. Patients who are made worse by the treatment may not be given enough attention in the reports, unless they suffered particularly obvious side-effects.

8. Ethical problems may arise in a variety of contexts, particularly where placebo treatments are involved or the patient or clinician has a marked preference for one treatment option over another. These concerns increase when the disease is potentially disabling or life-threatening.

9. The main outcome measure, based on clinical assessment and objective tests, may not reflect the patients' perspective of what constitutes an important and beneficial change. Patients may be more concerned with the quality of their lives, which may not be closely linked with changes in biochemical parameters or other disease indicators. However, quality of life measures are now much more widely used (see Fallowfield, 1990).

10. The concern with *eliminating* the placebo effect when assessing a treatment in relation to a comparable placebo may mean that important psychological variables are neglected. Therapist characteristics and the attitude of the patient to treatment are seldom examined in a medical context, and yet may be important determinants of the patient's compliance with treatment and attitude towards illness.

These methodological issues have all been discussed in the context of trials of conventional treatments. Many of the concerns expressed about the evaluation of complementary medicine apply equally to the evaluation of more conventional treatments. Complementary medicine is not necessarily therefore a special case requiring radically new methodologies. Criticisms of randomized controlled trials apply in many other contexts than complementary medicine, especially those treatments which are individually based and do not have clear and easily measurable outcomes. There are, however, a number of areas, some already mentioned, which do pose particular problems in complementary medicine. Some are simply major areas of concern to complementary practitioners, and therefore merit special attention; in other cases the problems may be familiar, but the solutions required are not easily transferred from other areas of research and evaluation.

When considering the evaluation of complementary medicine, particularly in relation to randomized controlled trials, we frequently refer to the comparable problems that exist in the evaluation of psychotherapy. This reflects our conviction that the difficulties encountered in evaluating the effectiveness of psychotherapy foreshadow many of those encountered in evaluating complementary medicine. Psychotherapy was similarly embattled 40 years ago when Eysenck (1952) suggested that spontaneous remission accounted for the improvements observed in psychotherapy and threw down the gauntlet to psychotherapists to provide evidence that their treatment was effective. A more important parallel is the obvious need in psychotherapy to tailor the treatment to the individual patient, and yet maintain sufficient standardization to meet the demands of the trial. We are not implying that complementary therapies are necessarily effective because of their psychological effects; it is simply that many of the methodological problems encountered in the evaluation of psychotherapy are particularly relevant to complementary medicine.

The remainder of the chapter reviews the issues which we feel to be of especial concern or especially problematic in the evaluation of complementary medicine: alternative theoretical frameworks, different diagnostic systems, individual differences in treatment and in response to treatment, outcome measures, the contribution of the patient and practitioner and finally, practical difficulties.

Alternative Theoretical Framework

Clearly the issue of an alternative theoretical framework only arises when two different disciplines are juxtaposed in some way. We are mainly concerned with a potential clash between the scientific base of orthodox medicine and the theories underlying complementary medicine. The degree of incompatibility will vary with the therapy in question. Some, such as osteopathy, chiropractic and herbalism, may have modes of action that are entirely conceivable in scientific terms. Homeopathy, on the other hand, differs in both clinical approach and underlying theory. Acupuncture meridians and energy flow are unsubstantiated concepts in scientific terms, but there are other more orthodox explanations for acupuncture's action (e.g. endorphin release, Clement-Jones et al, 1980). There are also some studies purporting to demonstrate the existence of meridians and the energy system (see Bensoussan, 1991 for further discussion).

Where mechanisms are concerned, therefore, there may be great differences of view and opinion between orthodox and complementary therapists. However, this need not matter unduly in clinical trials as long as the complementary therapists are allowed to practise in the way they see fit and the researchers (if they are not also complementary practitioners) are tolerant of this different approach and attempt to understand it. Essentially, both sides must take a black box view of the therapy, which is to evaluate the package and examine the specific ingredients of the package later. A similar approach has been adopted in psychotherapy research, where studies of the therapeutic process have followed on from outcome studies evaluating the particular treatment (Kazdin, 1984).

Curiously, some problems arise because researchers unthinkingly accept some aspect of the complementary therapy and incorporate it into the design of a trial. For instance, acupuncturists hold that needles need to be inserted at particular classical locations; most researchers have taken this to imply that needles inserted in non-classical locations are inactive and can therefore constitute a placebo treatment. Depth of insertion and stimulation are the same; only location differs. This procedure is referred to as *sham acupuncture*, and has been used in a great many studies as a placebo (see Richardson and Vincent, 1986; Vincent, 1993). Where there is no difference between true and sham acupuncture, the conclusion has been that acupuncture is a placebo. This issue is discussed in more detail in the next chapter, but an outline of the argument is given here to illustrate the difficulties that arise.

There are various problems associated with this control condition. To begin with, there is some doubt about whether acupuncture points and non-points can be reliably distinguished (Macdonald, 1989). Even if they can, there is evidence that acupuncture at non-classical points may have analgesic effects. Controlled trials have also shown significant benefits from treatment at both classical and non-classical locations. Studies of the acupuncture treatment of back pain, for instance, show no difference between sham (non-classical) acupuncture and true acupuncture, but acupuncture has shown an advantage over a true placebo control. Acupuncture at non-classical sites cannot be assumed to be a placebo. A sham acupuncture control condition really only offers information about the most effective sites of needling, not about the specific effects of acupuncture. This fundamental error has bedeviled the majority of controlled trials of acupuncture, and set research back by a decade (see Vincent, 1993 for a full discussion). So, while researchers need to understand the ideas underlying a complementary therapy, there can be dangers in importing them into the research design.

Different Diagnostic Systems

Groups of patients in controlled trials need to be homogeneous with respect to their basic disease or complaint. Usually in orthodox medicine, their diagnosis is specified rather than simply their main symptom. Trials will be carried out on asthma or bronchitis or emphysema, not simply on breathing difficulties. Where complementary therapy is concerned, the issue becomes: homogeneous with respect to whose diagnosis—orthodox or complementary? Acupuncturists may diagnose in terms of meridian imbalance, yin–yang or hot–cold, homeopaths by the character of their remedy and so on. The diagnoses are arrived at by taking into account a wide range of information which overlaps with, but does not coincide with, the information used by a doctor in arriving at an orthodox diagnosis. The essential underlying point is that the orthodox and complementary diagnoses are not isomorphic—they do not correspond to each other. This problem has been usefully and comprehensively explored by Wiegant, Kramers and van Wijk (1993) in relation to chronic obstructive pulmonary disease (see Figure 8.1).

Wiegant, Kramers and van Wijk (1993) distinguish three basic kinds of trial (see Figure 8.2). Firstly, those that simply rely on orthodox diagnoses and give a standard complementary treatment with no individual variation. In acupuncture, for instance, Vincent and Richardson (1986) referred to this as 'formula' acupuncture in contrast to the traditional variety based on individual assessment and traditional theory. This approach can be criticized as not doing full justice to the therapy.

In the second type of trial an orthodox diagnosis is used, but the complementary practitioners give the treatment as they would wish. A similar situation arises in psychotherapy research. Psychotherapists may assess a depressed patient in a quite different way from a psychiatrist, but trials of psychotherapy can still employ specific symptom-based entry criteria which are meaningful to both psychotherapist and psychiatrist. Wiegant,

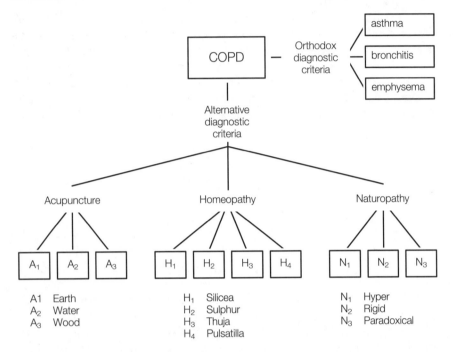

Figure 8.1 Homogeneity of patients from the point of view of orthodox as well as of complementary medicine. Out of a group of patients with COPD, three more or less homogeneous subgroups of patients can be formed, based on orthodox criteria. However, from the point of view of the complementary therapist (either acupuncture, homeopathy or naturopathy) these subgroups are far from homogeneous. Based on their specific diagnostic criteria a different categorization of subgroups takes place (*Source*: Wiegant, Kramers and van Wijk, 1993. Reproduced by permission.)

Kramers and van Wijk (1993) suggest that, in the complementary arena, three problems arise from this approach.

1. Complementary practitioners may, in the absence of specific complementary diagnostic criteria, question the adequacy of the treatment.
2. As the complementary treatment will vary for different patients with different complementary diagnoses, some remedies or therapeutic approaches may be effective and some not.
3. No understanding is reached of the complementary treatment process and the internal logic of the complementary approach.

Wiegant and colleagues point out that some of these difficulties can be overcome at the end of the trial, provided the complementary diagnoses are recorded. The outcome of treatment can be looked at in relation to the complementary diagnosis after the trial is completed. However, this tends

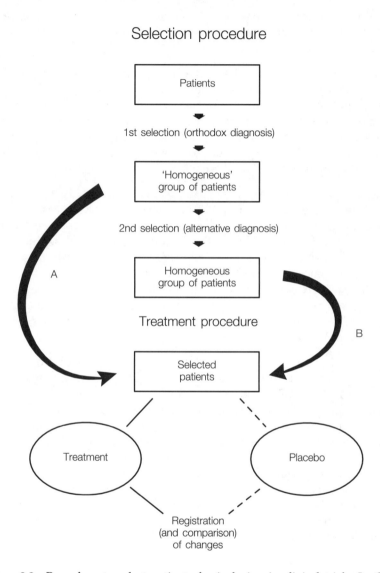

Figure 8.2 Procedure to select patients for inclusion in clinical trials. In the first selection step, a 'homogeneous' group of patients is formed using orthodox diagnostic criteria. This group meets the criteria for a uniform orthodox treatment to be studied in a clinical trial (arrow A). However, to participate in a clinical trial studying the effect of a complementary therapy, a second step should be performed. This twice selected group of patients now meets the criteria for a uniform complementary treatment (arrow B) (*Source*: Wiegant, Kramers and van Wijk, 1993. Reproduced by permission.)

to mean that only small subgroups of patients are involved and there may be a tendency, in the absence of a clear prior hypothesis, to overemphasize any significant findings (Pocock, 1985).

The third approach is to build the complementary diagnosis in from the beginning, and try to achieve homogeneous groups with respect to both orthodox and complementary criteria. The major problem with this approach is that massive patient numbers are needed to identify a small, select subgroup of patients (possibly somewhat untypical) who are homogeneous with respect to both diagnostic systems. A final fourth possibility is to use only complementary diagnoses.

Conventional diagnoses must be used if the research is to be taken seriously in the medical community (Vincent and Richardson, 1986). Complementary practitioners involved in such research may feel that if they are allowed to practise freely, this is quite acceptable, though they are unlikely to learn much about their own therapy. The third strategy, using both sets of diagnostic criteria, in an ideal world might be the strategy of choice. In practice, while it is important to discuss this as a way of clarifying these issues, it is likely to be impractical simply because of the huge numbers of patients required to select a group which is homogeneous on two sets of criteria.

Trials employing complementary diagnoses alone, and suitable outcome measures, might well be of considerable interest to complementary practitioners interested in refining and developing their practice. However, we would argue that there are other prior concerns. Wiegant, Kramers and van Wijk (1993) suggest in any case that clear typologies of patient signs and symptoms need to be developed first, so that complementary diagnoses can be clearly specified. Thereafter the reliability, and perhaps the validity, of such diagnoses should be checked. Only then is it worth bringing them into the much more elaborate and expensive option of a controlled trial. Understanding the treatment process in a complementary therapy and disentangling the various therapeutic components might in any case be more effectively done in an experimental context or in a series of single case designs.

Single-blind or Double-blind Trials?

The *double-blind controlled trial* is a catchphrase taken, as we have discussed, to indicate the gold standard and final arbiter of efficacy of a treatment. Should anyone, and especially a complementary practitioner, protest that a treatment is not a suitable candidate for a double-blind trial, they may be suspected of backing down from a serious test of that treatment's efficacy. Yet some treatments cannot be tested in a double-blind format, or at least only in a highly artificial and suspect way. The reasons for this concern the nature of the treatment, in particular whether it is a physical intervention and requires a skilled practitioner; whether the treatment is complementary or not is really a side issue. We will examine this a little more closely taking acupuncture as an example of a treatment which presents formidable difficulties for evaluation in a double-blind format.

The expectations of both patients and clinicians may affect the outcome of a trial. There is therefore a need to 'blind' both patients and clinicians to the allocation of the treatments under test. In a single-blind trial patients do not know whether they are receiving a true or a control treatment, and in a double-blind trial the clinicians do not know either (Vincent and Richardson, 1986). Reports have appeared of so-called double-blind trials in which patient progress has been assessed by an independent clinician who was unaware of treatment allocation (Gaw, Chang and Shaw, 1975; Henry et al, 1985). This independent assessment is a valuable addition to any trial, but does not make it double blind. In both these trials, the clinician giving the treatment inevitably knew whether he was giving true acupuncture or a sham, control treatment. Such trials are therefore single blind, with independent assessment.

It is difficult to see how a trial of acupuncture could be double blind. It would mean that the person giving the treatment would not know whether he was giving true or sham treatment, and he would therefore have to have little or no experience as an acupuncturist! It is possible that the sites to be needled could be marked on the patient by an experienced acupuncturist and then treated by a technician who had been merely trained in needling technique (Godfrey and Morgan, 1978), but it is questionable whether a technician would produce the same quality of treatment as an experienced acupuncturist. Similarly, it would be impossible to carry out a double-blind trial comparing two surgical techniques. In a single-blind trial, the patient is unaware of which technique is being used—which is quite possible for surgery. A double-blind trial, however, would require that the surgeon would also have to be unaware of the choice of technique—which is hardly feasible when the surgeon is providing the treatment. The same logic applies to trials of acupuncture or any other skilled treatment.

In complementary medicine, herbalism and homeopathy can be tested double blind, in that the person giving the treatment could be left unaware of whether active preparations were given. This admittedly becomes quite complex if the treatment is adjusted during the trial, especially if the substances concerned cannot be disguised in a casing. For treatments requiring the active participation of a practitioner, such as acupuncture, osteopathy, chiropractic, physiotherapy and surgery, no such manoeuvres are possible. The clinician cannot be blind to the treatment, though the patient can be.

Any treatment requiring active, skilled interventions poses formidable problems if a placebo-controlled trial is planned. The definition of a suitable acupuncture placebo comparison group has posed considerable problems (Vincent, 1993), and it is not clear what form a placebo manipulative therapy might take. The crucial point here is the same as that discussed in relation to the blinding of patient and clinician; it is not the fact that a therapy is complementary that poses the problems, but that its nature is such that there is no easy equivalent to the inert tablets routinely used in drug trials.

Individual or Standardized Treatment

It is axiomatic in some branches of complementary medicine that patients should be treated as individuals and that there are no prepacked treatments that are suitable for all patients with a particular complaint. Any good doctor, therapist or practitioner recognizes and responds to the differences between people, their different reactions to their complaint, their individual ways of dealing with pain and suffering, and so on. This is not what divides complementary and orthodox medicine, although part of the appeal of complementary medicine may be that some of its practitioners are more willing, or have more time, to discuss emotional issues. As regards evaluation, the key point is that complementary therapists insist that a treatment strategy must take account of the individual as well as the disease, condition or symptoms. They usually plan therapy individually for each patient and, to some of them, the testing of a standard therapy for a standard disease would fall so far short of optimal therapy that the results would be irrelevant (Anthony, 1987, 1993).

Similar concerns have been expressed in other contexts. The wide gap between the clinical setting and the research context has been noted in complementary medicine (McGourty, 1993), psychotherapy (Kazdin, 1984) and medicine (Kramer and Shapiro, 1984). Controlled trials of drugs can specify a dose, even though it may not be optimum for each patient; in practice a clinician would adjust the dose according to the patient's response and the presence or absence of side-effects. In trials of surgery, however, much greater variability is inevitable; certainly the same operation is performed, but the intervention must always depend on the extent of the pathology revealed during the operation, and so is necessarily tailored to the patient. In psychotherapy it is obvious that, although a general approach may be specified, the treatment must be geared to the patient's particular perspective and needs. Comparative clinical trials of psychotherapy have nevertheless been successfully carried out, even though therapists have been able to treat the patients very much as they would in clinical practice. The less standardized the treatment, however, the more other problems are likely to arise. For instance, if two treatments are being compared, an imbalance or great variability in the time spent with patients or the degree of intervention will make the results more difficult to interpret. None of this is to say that the fears of complementary practitioners are groundless, only that they may not be aware that others have had similar concerns in other contexts.

In some situations, when trying to identify the effective components of a treatment, for instance, it may be useful to closely specify the intervention and carry it out under experimental conditions with volunteers. This strategy is referred to as analogue research, often using students or healthy volunteers as subjects. Research in the clinical setting and analogue research each have their own advantages and drawbacks; it is not a question of one being the right way and the other wrong. Rather it is a case of using the methodology appropriate to the question one is asking.

Whatever strategy one chooses it is crucial that one is able to specify, at least to another experienced practitioner, exactly what was done in the therapy. One of the intriguing findings from psychotherapy is that when therapy sessions are videotaped and analysed, there is sometimes less difference in the behaviour of therapists of different theoretical persuasions than might have been predicted from their strongly divergent theoretical orientations (e.g. Sloane, 1975). If a complementary therapy is so intuitive as not to permit of meaningful description, it does become very difficult to research it, if only because the study can never be replicated. However, as long as the therapy can be specified to another practitioner, replication becomes possible. If an orthodox audience is to be convinced, however, it is preferable that it be specified in a way that can be understood by a general audience. A compromise is to specify guidelines for treatment which allow the practitioner some room for responding to individual patients, but nevertheless prescribe a basic pattern and style of treatment. For instance, Vincent (1989a) specified a range of acupuncture points in a controlled trial of the treatment of migraine, which were allowed to vary according to the patient's presenting complaint and current symptomatology. The control treatment followed similar guidelines.

Individual Response to Treatment

Just as complementary practitioners consider that treatment should be adapted to each individual patient, so they also consider the outcome of treatment to result from a unique constellation of factors that are particular to each individual patient. In this sense, the controlled trial can be anathema to them in that it obscures individual differences in favour of making general statements about a group of patients, statements which should ideally be generalizable to similar groups in other contexts. These difficulties are compounded if the complementary diagnosis does not correspond with the orthodox diagnosis, and the complementary prac-titioners in a trial are using several different treatment strategies for one orthodoxly defined disease.

Many controlled trials pay little, if any, attention to individual differences in treatment response (Kramer and Shapiro, 1984). There will be some reference to complications of treatment and the side-effects of drugs may be carefully documented. The presence of complications may be related to the patient's particular condition, or other concurrent disease, but there will not usually be any attempt at a systematic analysis of individual differ-ences. In psychology, too, where one might hope for a greater appreciation of the individual, some have bemoaned the lack of attention to individual differences in favour of experiments centred around group averages (see, for example, Eysenck, 1983). Larger and more sophisticated trials (both clinically and statistically) do now pay attention to a wide variety of potential confounding variables. For instance, studies of social support for a Type A personality in relation to the onset and recovery from coronary heart disease need to take diet, smoking habits, alcohol intake, physical exercise and cholesterol levels into account when considering the impact of social and psychological variables (e.g. Friedman et al, 1986). No doubt much more attention could be paid in treatment trials to the predictors of good response, whether these be in terms of clinical state, social and psychological variables or clinician–patient relationship. Examination of such variables after a trial has ended opens one to the possibility of spurious findings, especially if a number of subgroup analyses are carried out (Pocock, 1985).

The worry that the individual is being lost in the research may not be simply that not enough relevant factors are taken into account. It may be more a question of how an individual's response to health, disease and treatment can be reduced to an average group response on one or two measures. The answer is firstly that trials are a simplification of the clinical situation, and there should be no pretence that research can ever encompass all the relevant factors in an individual's progress to health. In addition, the fundamental questions addressed in a controlled trial concern *groups* of patients rather than individuals. This is not only a matter of a group design and group-based statistics, but the nature of the questions addressed. Essentially, one is concerned with broad policy decisions, whether made by government or clinicians. Is this treatment *generally* beneficial for this condition? The actual question is often very simple, although the process of answering it with adequate methodological rigour may be horrendously difficult. The results of controlled trials provide general guidelines as to the best overall treatment strategy. Trials are not generally designed to provide information about the treatment process, or about the multitude of potential influences on a patient's condition. These other influences are screened out or controlled not because they are not important, but in order to answer more general questions.

Another fear sometimes expressed by complementary practitioners (and other clinicians and therapists) is that an interest in research is dehumanizing and that it will detract from one's clinical practice. Certainly different types of people may be attracted to clinical work and to research, and the best clinicians may not be good researchers and vice versa. However, there is no inherent contradiction between a concern for the nuances and subtlety of clinical practice and the methodological rigour required for research. It is entirely possible to take research results as a guiding strategy, yet be completely attuned to the moment by moment ebb and flow of the clinical relationship.

Outcome Measures in Complementary Medicine

Clinicians have always enquired about the impact of a disease on a patient's life. Only in the last ten to fifteen years, however, have these concerns been taken into account in trials of the evaluation of treatment (Fallowfield, 1990). Increasingly the impact of the condition on the patient's life, as perceived by the patient, is assessed alongside more conventional measures of disease progress. Measures of disability and handicap, looking at the impact of a disease on essential daily activities, date from the 1960s, but more recent measures take a wider range of social and psychological factors into account. The Nottingham Health Profile, for instance (Hunt et al, 1981; Hunt, McEwen and McKenna, 1985), examines pain, physical mobility, sleep, energy, emotional reactions and social isolation and the effects of the illness on seven areas of daily life: work, looking after the home, social life, home life, sex, interests and hobbies. Scales such as the Sickness Impact Profile (Bergner et al, 1981) and the Psychosocial

Adjustment to Illness Scale (Derogatis, 1986) cover similar ground, each with varying emphasis on different themes. There is also a wide variety of psychological measures of anxiety, depression and other mood states, both temporary and more enduring (e.g. Derogatis and Melisaratos, 1983).

Such developments should be reassuring to complementary practitioners concerned to make as broad an assessment as possible of the various changes that treatment may bring about. Whether or not they regard the patient's perception as the primary source of information about the disease process, it is clear that taking the patient's perspective into account and considering the context of the disease is now seen as both desirable and scientifically respectable. An additional question is whether complementary medicine needs measures that are not encompassed by existing approaches. Clearly the existing measures may be imperfect from a complementary perspective, and perhaps justly criticized, but should different underlying concepts be measured? There seem to be two broad areas where specifically 'complementary measures' may be required, not necessarily for orthodox researchers but possibly for those working within a complementary framework. The first is the assessment of mood and subjective state, the second refers to signs of improvement that derive specifically from the complementary therapy itself. These will be considered in turn.

Homeopaths take a person's character traits and emotional life into account when choosing a remedy (Ullman, 1991). Some acupuncturists consider that the first sign of improvement is that the patient reports feeling 'better in themselves' (Worsley, 1973), implying a change in mood and well-being prior to physical changes. Successful treatment may, presumably, affect psychological reactions as well as the physical condition. Emotional states are important both for diagnosis and for monitoring treatment progress in some branches of complementary medicine. There are now a considerable number of measures of mood which are better able to monitor short-term fluctuations in emotional state, which may be a prelude to more sustained improvements in a patient's physical condition (see, for example, Howarth and Schokman-Gates, 1981). Problems may arise, however, if the emotional reactions in question are highly individual. In a research study it may be difficult to find a measure that is applicable to all the subjects involved; in single case analyses, however, it may be possible to develop measures that are specifically applicable to that particular person.

The second area concerns measures that are peculiar to the complementary therapy under investigation. The assessment of a patient may involve specifically complementary diagnostic techniques; progress in the treatment may be assessed using these techniques. Acupuncturists, for instance, may use the pulse diagnosis as an indicator of the treatment's progress and efficacy; naturopaths may use iris diagnosis; cranial osteopaths detect changes in the energy flow and so on. There is no reason why these kind of measures, however subjective they may be, should not be recorded and correlated with changes in other measures or indices of clinical change. We would suggest that they should not be considered as outcome measures, unless their reliability and validity can first be established. However, monitoring these complementary indicators could be valuable as part of a process of investigating their value, which should be seen as conceptually separate from the evaluation of their associated treatments. It is perfectly possible that acupuncture might be a valuable treatment, even if the pulse diagnosis should prove unreliable (see Cole, 1975). The naturopathic approach might prove extremely beneficial, even if iris diagnosis should prove to be worthless (Knipschild, 1988).

Critics may object that the measures described above are subjective and hence unreliable. Objective measures are rightly valued in clinical trials as being able to provide solid evidence of the effectiveness or ineffectiveness of a treatment. Changes in cholesterol levels, blood pressure, the movement in a joint, changes seen on X-rays, CAT or PET scans are seen as indicators which can be relied upon, in contrast to the more subjective judgements of both clinicians and patients. In reality, the reliability and validity of any measure can be questioned, particularly where an element of human judgement is involved. The fact that a result emerges from a laboratory is not an absolute guarantee of its reliability, as concerns about cervical smear reports demonstrate. However, this is not to deny the importance of such measures, only to suggest that there may not be such a gulf between objective and subjective measures as is sometimes thought. Considerable efforts are devoted to ensuring the reliability and validity of subjective measures.

One particular note of caution should be sounded. It is tempting to record every conceivable item of information about a patient and to have multiple measures of outcome. Multiple endpoints, however, open up the possibility of a Type I error—essentially a chance finding of change on a measure, even though there is in reality no real improvement. The greater the number of measures, the greater the possibility of this kind of error (Pocock, 1985). However, the solution to this problem is not to abandon multiple measures, but to designate one as the primary endpoint and arbiter of improvement. Should the treatment show a change on this measure, then changes in other measures are seen as welcome confirming evidence and as showing that the treatment has widespread effects.

The Contribution of Patient and Practitioner

In the evaluation of orthodox medical treatments the impact of psychological factors is taken very seriously, but usually only in the sense that great care is taken to exclude them. A central purpose of placebo-controlled trials is to separate the specific effects of a drug or other treatment from the psychological effects of taking a tablet, seeing a doctor, taking part in a study and so forth. However, while drug research is a massive industry, little attention is paid to psychological factors, although their power and influence is implicitly acknowledged in virtue of the care that is taken to control for such effects. Research on the psychological influences in a medical context is comparatively rare (Richardson, 1989), although there is a considerable amount of research on patient satisfaction and compliance with treatment (Ley, 1989).

It is certainly regrettable that so little attention is paid, in research terms at any rate, to the role of the relationship between doctor and patient and the various other psychological and healing influences. A suspicion of soft science probably plays a part, as does the fact that it is difficult to patent or market a psychological finding, however robust. Complementary practitioners might reasonably complain, without invalidating their own therapies, that most medical research leaves out many important therapeutic factors. Although a holistic approach is by no means the province of complementary practitioners, most do pay particular attention to their patient's emotional life and social situation (see Sharma, 1992). Some may go further and believe, for instance, that the attitude and state of mind of both practitioner and patient is all important in the healing process. Ideally perhaps these beliefs should be reflected in research into complementary medicine, though it may not be necessary to include them for meaningful research to be carried out. It would seem reasonable to investigate the efficacy of a specific treatment, while still allowing that many other important factors also contributed to the overall therapeutic effect.

Research into patient and practitioner variables is extremely difficult and costly. After some hundreds of studies of psychotherapy, many conclusions are still tentative. Many criticisms have been made of studies that have been carried out (Bergin and Garfield, 1994), although psychotherapy research is characterized by a great concern for methodological rigour. There are some consistent findings. Patient variables such as social class, age and sex do not appear to be predictive of outcome, and definitive statements about the necessary personal qualities of the patient have been difficult to formulate (Bergin and Garfield, 1994). As regards therapists, gender, age, ethnicity, general personality and verbal activity levels all exert definite, although weak, effects (Beutler, Machado and Neufeldt,

1994). These authors also note that the previous decade of research has produced little in the way of substantive findings, although there have been marked improvements in the sophistication of the methodologies employed.

The precise findings in regard to psychotherapy research do not matter for this argument. Complementary practitioners may, in any case, have different concerns and a different conception of which factors are important. The key points are firstly that such research is possible, and secondly that it is extremely difficult. Compared with research into complementary medicine, psychotherapy research has a much longer history and immeasurably greater funding and expertise. If psychotherapy researchers, with these resources, have been painfully struggling with these issues over decades, it suggests that this area, however important, should not be a first priority for research into complementary medicine.

PRACTICAL DIFFICULTIES OF RESEARCH

The last few sections have dealt with some major methodological issues confronting researchers into complementary medicine. All researchers will be aware of the multitude of practical problems that also arise, but there are some practical problems which are particularly acute in complementary medicine.

The first, and in some ways most important, is the lack of research expertise among complementary practitioners (Tonkin, 1987; Vincent and Mole, 1987; Fitter and Blackwell, 1993). Most of them entered complementary medicine because of a desire to practise; an interest in science or research does not, as yet, form any part of either the entrance requirements or the syllabus of many complementary training institutions. This is changing, but at the moment there are only a very few people (whether medical or lay practitioners) with experience of both research and complementary medicine. This means that the main advocates of complementary medicine, who are often called upon to justify their claims, do not have the expertise necessary to provide the evidence that is needed. Additionally, they are usually in private practice and not easily able to give up the substantial time needed to mount a serious research project. Tonkin (1987) suggests that the problem stems from an absence of training in research at postgraduate level in complementary medicine:

> The first (problem) is really so obvious that it is surprising that it has not been more widely recognized before. The plain fact is that the majority of complementary practitioners lack the necessary expertise and experience as

well as the time, material facilities and finance to mount research projects of an adequate calibre . . . The deficit is primarily due to the absence in their training establishments of the intermediate echelon equivalent to the Registrar grades that exist in orthodox medical schools, and whose job specification includes the implementation of research projects under the experienced guidance of their professional mentors. In fact, research of an acceptable quality can really only be achieved with the full and active cooperation of the established profession and of sister disciplines in academic institutions.

Crucially this lack of expertise, training and time affects the ability of complementary practitioners to attract funding for research, unless they have collaborators with experience of applying for grants. Even with such assistance, grants are very hard to come by at a time when research funds are limited. Without such assistance it would be, to say the least, an uphill struggle to obtain a serious level of funding when competing with experienced researchers in major institutions. This difficulty has led some to argue that some research money should be earmarked to pump prime research into complementary medicine (Monckton, 1993). With a massive public interest in complementary medicine, it is surely necessary to research the area and to separate the valuable from the useless or fraudulent. In the United States, the Office of Alternative Medicine has been established with just this aim—to attract and fund research into complementary medicine. Critics of this approach say that research funding is an open competition and that complementary practitioners must compete with everyone else. However, there are undoubtedly cases in which a particular need has been identified and money set aside for development. Clinical audit is a case in point, which has been specifically funded in Britain in an effort to drastically improve the monitoring of quality of care. Once established as a routine activity, specific funding is withdrawn. No one would argue that complementary medicine should receive indefinite special funding. However, there certainly seems to be a case for initial funding to develop research expertise in the complementary community, so that they can later effectively compete for funds.

Chapter 9

The Quality of Medical Information and the Evaluation of Acupuncture, Osteopathy and Chiropractic

We now turn from considering how complementary medicine has been and should be evaluated to examining the evidence for its efficacy. This chapter concerns the physical therapies of acupuncture, osteopathy and chiropractic; the next deals with those involving medicines (homeopathy and herbalism) and supplements and dietary changes (naturopathy). The division is somewhat arbitrary and primarily designed to keep the chapters to a digestible length. Before this, however, we will briefly assess the quality of orthodox medical information.

As we have seen earlier, complementary medicine has often been chastised for the paucity of supportive evidence and the low standard of much of the evaluative work; sometimes these criticisms extend to charges that some complementary therapies are dangerous. These are certainly valid criticisms in some cases, and put practitioners of complementary medicine in a vulnerable and defensive position as they struggle to document their belief in the efficacy of their therapies. They may feel less defensive, however, when they realize that these problems are by no means confined to complementary medicine. While strenuous efforts have been made in many areas of medicine to improve standards of evaluation and methodological rigour, there is, to say the least, room for improvement. The following observations were made not by wild, rebellious critics of orthodox medicine writing in fringe journals, but by writers in the world's leading medical journals.

'WHERE IS THE WISDOM . . .? THE POVERTY OF MEDICAL EVIDENCE'

This title comes from an article by the editor of the *British Medical Journal* (Smith, 1991). The article begins by completing the quote from TS Eliot: 'Where is the wisdom we have lost in knowledge, and where is the knowledge we have lost in information?', the information being the 30 000 biomedical journals in the world. In it Smith summarizes and comments on the work of Professor David Eddy, a leading expert on medical information and decision making (see, for example, Eddy, 1994). Professor Eddy began his medical life as a cardiothoracic surgeon in Stanford in California, but became progressively concerned about the lack of evidence underpinning what he and other doctors were doing. He decided to select an example of a common condition with well established treatments and assess in detail the evidence supporting those treatments. Beginning with glaucoma, he searched published medical reports back to 1906 and could not find one randomized controlled trial of the standard treatment. Later he traced back the confident statements in textbooks and medical journals on treating glaucoma and found that they had simply been handed down from generation to generation. The same analysis was done for other treatments, such as the treatment of blockages of the femoral and popliteal arteries, and the findings were similar. That experience 'changed his life' and after taking a degree in mathematics at Stanford University he became Professor of Health Policy and Management at Duke University. Professor Eddy estimates that only about 15% of medical interventions are supported by solid scientific evidence, partly because only about 1% of articles in medical journals are scientifically sound and partly because many treatments have never been assessed at all: 'If it is true, as the management gurus tell us, that "every error is a treasure" then we are sitting on King Solomon's mine'.

Assessment of the Literature

Doctors are faced with a massive literature, even in a single specialty, and to make sense of it is a formidable task for any clinician. A frequent approach to this problem is for groups of experts to try to achieve a consensus statement about the best treatment for a certain condition, and the circumstances under which it should be varied. When Eddy assists at these consensus conferences he asks the members to list the outcomes they are seeking and to rank the scientific evidence for each outcome from excellent to none and then describe the best evidence available. For 21 problems tackled so far the best evidence has been judged—by the experts—to be between poor and none for 17, and usually the best available evidence was something less than a randomized controlled trial. Often the evidence that was available contradicted current practice: thus of 17 randomized trials on giving lidocaine prophylactically in patients with chest pain, 16 showed no effect and one showed a positive result, yet practice in the United States was to give lidocaine (Smith, 1991).

Further evidence on the quality of medical information is provided by a grand overall assessment of the literature between 1950 and 1980 (Williamson, Goldschmidt and Colton, 1986). Medical statisticians screened 28 articles which themselves assessed the adequacy of study design, data, statistical inferences and documentation. The 28 assessment articles, which were published in major medical journals, are in turn an overview of over 4200 medical reports relating to the evaluation of treatments. These research reports were mainly on drug trials, but they included some studies of surgical, psychotherapeutic and diagnostic procedures. The original 28 articles were written either specifically to improve the quality of clinical medical research, or to provide definitive evidence of the efficacy of medical interventions.

Williamson, Goldschmidt and Colton (1986) summarize their findings as follows:

> The 16 assessment studies reported before 1970 described a median of 23 per cent of 2006 research reports as meeting the assessors' criteria for validity; the 12 published during 1970 or after reported that a median of 6 per cent of 2172 publications met the assessors' criteria. This decrease may reflect rising assessment standards more than falling research quality. Eight assessment articles correlated the frequency of positive findings with the adequacy of the methods used to obtain these results; this rate was 80 per cent in 449 inadequately designed studies and 25 per cent in 305 adequately designed studies. Serious, widespread problems exist in the published clinical literature.

Most of these reports date back to the 1970s or before. Since then standards of reported research have improved, but problems remain. Pocock, a medical statistician writing in the *British Medical Journal* in 1985 stated that, 'though there have been considerable improvements in the use of statistical methods for clinical trials in recent years, there remain major practical difficulties in the design and interpretation of many trials'. His paper concentrated on problems relating to randomization, the overemphasis on significance testing and the inadequate size of many trials and provided many examples of fallacious or misleading conclusions arising from such errors. Williamson, Goldschmidt and Colton (1986) found a strong tendency for sound research to be less likely to report significant findings, suggesting that the evidence for the efficacy of many interventions is much poorer than generally supposed.

Publication Bias

A further problem, often suspected but now demonstrated in one major study, is publication bias. This is the tendency for studies with significant results to be more likely to appear in print than those which turn out to have non-significant findings. The upshot of this, where it occurs, is an overly optimistic view of the efficacy of medical interventions. Easterbrook, Berlin and Gopalan (1991) examined 487 research protocols approved by a research ethics committee between 1984 and 1987. As of May 1990, 285 studies had been analysed and 52% of these published. Studies with significant results were more likely to be published, led to a greater number of publications and presentations and were more likely to be published in journals with a high citation impact factor. The tendency towards publication bias was, however, greater with observational and laboratory-based studies than with randomized controlled trials (Easterbrook, Berlin and Gopalan, 1991).

Further problems arise in attempts to analyse and combine the results from trials of therapies. These procedures, which are known as *meta-analyses*, have their origins in psychotherapy research. They are not simply reviews of evidence, but actually combine the results of a number of studies to produce a composite, and hopefully more reliable, result. However, Sacks et al (1987) summarize their findings as follows:

> We found 86 meta-analyses of reports of randomized controlled trials in the English-language literature. We evaluated the quality of these meta-analyses, using a scoring system that considered 23 items in six major areas—study design, combinability, control of bias, statistical analysis, sensitivity analysis and application of results. Only 24 meta-analyses (28 percent) addressed all six areas, 31 (36 per cent) addressed five, 25 addressed four, 5 addressed three and one addressed two. Of the 23 individual items, between 1 and 14 were addressed satisfactorily. We conclude that an urgent need exists for improved methods in literature searching, quality evaluation of trials and synthesizing of the results.

The weakness and inconsistency of the scientific evidence for many clinical interventions is one reason for the wide variations in the use and outcomes of clinical interventions (Chassein et al, 1986; Moss, 1992). In the absence of hard evidence, clinical decisions are often based on clinical preference. 'Despite science based undergraduate teaching and encouragement of the pursuit of scientific research we seem to pay lip service to scientific principles when it comes to clinical practice and decision making' (Moss, 1992). The problem is not just in the original data, but in the failure to apply the findings in a scientific manner in clinical practice.

This brief overview suggests that the quality of medical information generally, and in particular the evidence for many clinical interventions, is quite poor. This is not to disparage the efforts being made or to detract from the importance of evaluating all forms of medical intervention, whether orthodox or complementary. Our point is only that the difference in the standards of evidence for orthodox and complementary therapies may not be as great as generally assumed. There are certainly, as we shall see, many flaws in studies of complementary medicine. However, in the face of similar problems with the evidence for orthodox medicine it is unreasonable, even hypocritical, for critics of complementary medicine to throw up their hands in horror, dismissing the existing studies out of hand. The paucity of medical evidence, while certainly very serious in complementary medicine, is a general one and not confined to complementary medicine. While complementary practitioners and researchers certainly need to improve the standards of complementary medical research, they should realize that they are not alone in having such problems.

REVIEWING STUDIES OF COMPLEMENTARY MEDICINE

Before reviewing studies evaluating some of the major forms of complementary therapies, we will briefly describe our strategy and the limitations of our review. Our aim is to give the reader, in a series of comparatively short essays on each therapy, an overview of research in each area and a broad indication of the state of the evidence for the efficacy of each therapy or system of therapy. We cannot hope to provide a comprehensive evaluation of all the important studies of each therapy in a book of this length and type, except by reference to other reviews. Where comprehensive reviews exist we have summarized their methods and conclusions and often commented on the review itself. Where the evidence is more scattered, we have presented examples of some of the best available evidence.

Almost insurmountable problems exist in attempting a brief summary of herbal medicine in that there is a massive pharmacopoeia of herbs used worldwide, in addition to numerous drugs derived from herbs. Here we have had to rely, in the absence of more authoritative reviews, on a series of illustrative studies and short reviews of individual herbs. We have tried to give some assessment of the overall standards of research; the major reviews all include such an assessment and it is clear that the quality of evidence available on complementary therapies is generally not of an adequate standard. Although there are some reviews (e.g. Patel et al, 1989) which are described as meta-analyses, there are no real meta-analyses of complementary therapies in the sense of a statistical pooling of data from several similar studies. We consider that there is not a sufficient number of studies of similar disorders of adequate quality in any area to warrant such an approach at the moment.

The central questions addressed in each of the essays concern the efficacy of the therapy:

1. Does the therapy have a beneficial effect on any individual disease of disorder?
2. Is this effect primarily, or even partly, due to the specific properties of that therapy, or is it due to psychological processes or, alternatively, simply to the passage of time?

The second question can, in some instances (homeopathy, herbalism, blind food challenges in naturopathy), be addressed with placebo-controlled trials. Devising a placebo control for physical therapies, such as osteopathy and chiropractic, is not, as we have discussed, always feasible and these therapies are usually compared with alternative treatments. Devising a suitable placebo control for acupuncture has proved a difficult undertaking, but there are a number of acceptable placebo-controlled trials in this area.

We have generally not discussed the validity of the ideas underlying the therapies or the processes which are involved in carrying out the treatment in any detail, unless they bear directly on the evaluation of the treatment. The distinction between studies that use an abbreviated 'formula' version of some complementary therapy and those that allow complementary practitioners to work in the way they wish must be borne in mind, although these two types of studies are not generally distinguished. While this may be a matter of regret and perhaps justified criticism to some complementary practitioners, it is to us secondary to the question of whether any form of the therapy is beneficial. There are, to our knowledge, no studies that directly compare different styles of individual complementary therapies.

The validity of the ideas underlying a complementary therapy is often the source of much criticism and perhaps of the doubt attending its efficacy. For instance, the energy flow and meridians of acupuncture appear absurd to some. We have taken the rather pragmatic view that a therapy may be effective whether or not the theory is valid, or whether all the procedures involved are necessary for its success. There are many elements in most complementary therapies, any or all of which may be important in producing any observed effect. The unpacking of the therapeutic package is for us, at the moment, a secondary question to that of overall efficacy. However, there is little doubt that the plausibility of the underlying mechanism is an important factor in the acceptance of the results of clinical trials.

Acupuncture has been shown to stimulate the release of endorphins and enkephalins and although there is considerable doubt that these short-term effects could explain any long-term clinical effects (Price et al, 1984), such findings have certainly eased the acceptance of acupuncture into the world of orthodox medicine. Similarly, aspects of osteopathic and chiropractic theory might be suspect, but the idea that manipulation or massage might relieve pain would seem acceptable to most people. Herbs clearly contain pharmacologically active ingredients which may have beneficial effects. Homeopathy, on the other hand, appears to defy basic scientific laws and is thus inherently suspect to some people, whatever the results of clinical trials may indicate. We will briefly describe the furore over the results of some experiments that supported the idea that high dilution potions could have specific effects to illustrate this difficulty.

ACUPUNCTURE

Scientific research into acupuncture has a number of different aspects. Experimental studies have sought to demonstrate short-term analgesic effects and examine the biochemical and physiological mechanisms that may underlie such effects (Chung and Dickenson, 1980; Price, Rafii and Watkins, 1984). In this section, however, we are primarily concerned with the therapeutic uses of acupuncture and the evaluation of acupuncture as a treatment for disease. Even when the scope of the review is narrowed to the clinical evaluation of acupuncture, there is still a large literature; certainly many hundreds of papers have been published in English. Many of these, however, are primarily descriptive, of poor quality and little value (Vincent, 1993). While descriptive studies and other approaches (e.g. single case designs) have their value, we will concentrate on controlled trials of acupuncture, commenting particularly on the small group of studies which have used a satisfactory placebo control.

Methodology of Acupuncture Trials

Many studies of acupuncture treatment are seriously flawed by methodological problems. Poor design, inadequate measures and statistical analysis, lack of follow-up data and substandard treatment are all too common. The most important problems are the measurement of outcome, design and choice of control group (Vincent and Richardson, 1986; Vincent and

Chapman, 1989; Vincent, 1993). The various issues are discussed in detail in these papers, but one crucial issue must be raised here: the definition of an appropriate control group. Controlled trials may involve comparisons of acupuncture with a waiting list group, an alternative treatment or a placebo, but the main methodological problems arise with the placebo control (Lewith and Vincent, 1995).

Placebo Control Conditions Used in Acupuncture Trials

A bewildering variety of control procedures have been used in acupuncture trials; sometimes the needles are not even inserted in the control treatment; instead they are rubbed against the skin (Borglum-Jensen, Melsen and Borglum-Jensen, 1979) or glued to it (Gallachi, 1981). It seems unlikely that patients would accept these procedures as credible forms of treatment. In the most commonly used control treatment, needles are actually inserted but at incorrect, theoretically irrelevant sites. Usually this has simply meant carrying out a procedure similar to the true treatment at nearby, non-classical locations. Depth of insertion and stimulation are the same; only location differs. This procedure, which is termed *sham* or *mock* acupuncture, has been used as a placebo in a great many studies (e.g. Gaw, Chang and Shaw, 1975; Godfrey and Morgan, 1978; Mendelson et al, 1983; Henry et al, 1985).

The reasons for sham acupuncture being used as a placebo treatment derive from traditional theory. For acupuncture to be effective, according to the theory, needles must be inserted at designated classical points (O'Connor and Bensky, 1981). Acupuncture at non-classical sites (sham acupuncture) was consequently assumed by most investigators to be ineffective and, therefore, ideal as a placebo. Unfortunately, there are several lines of evidence to suggest that sham acupuncture is an unsuitable and misleading control condition. Even if acupuncture and non-acupuncture points can be reliably distinguished, evidence from laboratory studies and controlled trials suggests that analgesic effects may result from needling at non-classical locations, rendering sham acupuncture useless as a placebo (Lewith and Machin, 1983; Vincent and Richardson, 1986; Vincent, 1993). A sham acupuncture control condition really only offers information about the most effective sites of needling, not about the specific effects of acupuncture. This fundamental error has bedeviled almost all experimental and clinical controlled trials of the acupuncture treatment of pain. It is therefore vital to find a control condition that does not suffer from these defects, which in practice means one with small or non-existent specific physiological effects.

There have been two plausible solutions to the problem of a suitable placebo control. The first was the introduction of mock transcutaneous nerve stimulation (TENS) as a control condition in acupuncture trials. In this procedure, transcutaneous electrical nerve stimulators are used in the usual way, except that no current actually passes between the electrodes. Patients are sometimes told that they are receiving subliminal pulse therapy and they will therefore not feel the current. This control was first used in a trial of acupuncture in the treatment of back pain (Macdonald et al, 1983), in which acupuncture was found to be superior to mock TENS. Mock TENS has also been used in trials of acupuncture for post-herpetic neuralgia (Lewith et al, 1983) and migraine (Dowson, Lewith and Machin, 1985). The other, later, solution was 'minimal acupuncture' (Vincent and Richardson, 1986), a form of sham acupuncture that involves only minimal surface stimulation. In minimal acupuncture, needles are placed away from classical or trigger points, inserted only 1–2 mm and stimulated extremely lightly. Vincent (1989b) suggests that this procedure minimizes the specific effects of the needling while maintaining its psychological impact. The fact that the minimal acupuncture may have some physiological effect would make this control condition a somewhat sterner test of true acupuncture than a completely inert placebo. It might therefore be unsuitable as a control for a form of acupuncture where surface needling is used (Macdonald et al, 1983). However, this disadvantage is perhaps out-weighed by the fact that the treatment and control would be almost identical in the eyes of the patient. Minimal acupuncture has been used as a control condition in several studies, though not necessarily described in this way. True acupuncture was, for instance, found to be superior to minimal in a trial of the acupuncture treatment of migraine (Vincent, 1989b). Both mock TENS and minimal acupuncture have been shown to be credible control conditions, and each have their respective advantages and disadvantages (Vincent, 1993). The important point is that they are both near-perfect placebos, and that the original sham acupuncture condition is not. The importance of this distinction will become clearer when we separate out the small number of trials with an acceptable placebo control.

The Evaluation of Acupuncture Treatment

An enormous number of reports of the therapeutic efficacy of acupuncture have been published, but many are little more than rough descriptions of the immediate effects of acupuncture. For instance, Zang (Zang, 1990) treated 192 patients with bronchial asthma, reporting immediate improvement in 98.9% and clinical remission in 76.5%. These results appear impressive, but have not been matched in more careful studies. As Prance et al (1988) point out, such studies appear to be conducted by people who accept a priori the effectiveness of acupuncture and are only seeking to describe the results achieved. The acupuncture literature is overrun with descriptive studies, most of which are of such poor quality that nothing can be concluded from them. This is not to say that descriptive, or uncontrolled, studies do not have their place. If acupuncture has not been tried for a particular disorder, then it is perfectly reasonable to begin with an exploratory study. For instance, Filshie and Redman (1985) assessed the use of acupuncture for pain associated with malignancy by reviewing case notes. The study is by no means a controlled trial, but is certainly a useful preliminary report. Single case studies may also provide valuable information about the treatment process, but will not provide evidence of the efficacy of a treatment across a range of patients (Barlow and Hersen, 1984; Vincent, 1990a), which can really only be achieved with randomized clinical trials (Pocock, 1985). Several types of controlled trial can be distinguished:

1. *No-treatment or waiting list control*   Acupuncture has, for instance, been shown to be superior to waiting list control in the treatment of neck and back pain (Coan et al, 1980; Coan, Wong and Coan, 1982). These studies at least suggest that any changes observed are not simply due to the passage of time, but cannot tell us whether acupuncture is of real value as a treatment (Richardson and Vincent, 1986).
2. *Acupuncture as an addition to an existing treatment*   For instance, Gunn et al (1980) found that the addition of acupuncture to standard therapy produced a significant improvement in low back pain patients.
3. *Acupuncture compared to another treatment*   There are, for instance, a number of studies comparing acupuncture with TENS (Laitinen, 1976; Fox and Melzack, 1976).
4. *Acupuncture compared with placebo control*   These studies assess the crucial question of whether the effects of acupuncture are simply due to psychological factors. Although other types of controlled trials are considered, we will place most emphasis on those with a placebo control.

Acupuncture for Chronic Pain

Several reviews of the use of acupuncture in the treatment of chronic pain have now appeared (Lewith and Kenyon, 1984; Bhatt-Sanders, 1985; Richardson and Vincent, 1986; Patel et al, 1989; Ter Riet, Kleijnen and Knipschild, 1990a). All have commented on the poor quality of most of the studies, and all have stated that this severely limits the conclusions that can be drawn from the review. Richardson and Vincent (1986) reviewed all English language controlled trials of acupuncture published before 1986.

They concluded that there was good evidence for the short-term effectiveness of acupuncture for low back pain, mixed results for headache, and some encouraging preliminary results for cervical pain and arthritis. The proportion of patients helped varied from study to study, but commonly fell in the region 50 to 80%. Follow-up periods, however, were disappointingly short and evidence for longer term benefits was weak. They suggested that the response rate and degree of benefit obtained were higher than might be expected from a placebo response, but cautioned that very few studies used a satisfactory placebo control. The extent to which acupuncture was producing benefit by psychological mechanisms had not really been established.

In addition to the basic reviews, two meta-analyses of the literature on chronic pain have been reported. Meta-analysis is a discipline that critically reviews and statistically combines the results of previous research. The purposes of such a procedure include increasing overall statistical power, resolving uncertainty between conflicting reports and improving estimates of the size of the effect being investigated (Sacks et al, 1987). However, it should be emphasized that although these techniques have the potential for resolving questions of the efficacy of acupuncture, they cannot compensate for the poor quality of studies they set out to combine. For instance, if the placebo control is unsatisfactory in the original studies, then biased estimates will be produced in the final meta-analysis.

Patel and colleagues (Patel et al, 1989) reviewed all randomized controlled trials of acupuncture for chronic pain that measured outcome in terms of the numbers of patients improved. They attempted a statistical pooling of the results and concluded that the results favoured acupuncture, though various methodological problems precluded a definite conclusion. Combining the results of these studies, however, does not seem very sensible. There are only 14 trials, of very variable standard. They address the treatment of various chronic pain problems and they appear to use eight different control groups. It is not clear what any statement about the superiority of acupuncture over a control can mean in these circumstances.

A more comprehensive meta-analysis, and the most recent review available, was produced by Ter Riet and his colleagues (Ter Riet, Kleijnen and Knipschild, 1990). They decided not to attempt a statistical pooling of results, arguing that the studies were on the whole too poor and too disparate to allow their results to be combined. Their report is therefore perhaps best considered a critical review. They identified 51 reports of acupuncture for chronic pain that involved some kind of control or group comparison and had not been previously reported. Each study was scored on 18 methodological criteria, some weighted more heavily than others,

Table 9.1   Methodological criteria

Criteria	Weight
Comparability of prognosis	
(A) Homogeneity (1)	3
(B) Prestratification (2)	3
(C) Randomization	12
(D) Comparability of relevant baseline characteristics shown	2
(E) >50 patients per group	10
(F) <20% loss to follow-up (3)	5
Adequate intervention	
(G) Avoidance of DNIC (4)	2
(H) Adequate description of acupuncture procedure (5)	10
(I) Mentioning good quality of the acupuncturist	15
(K) Existing treatment modality in reference group	3
Adequate effect measurement	
(L) Patients blinded	10
(M) Evaluator blinded	5
(N) Follow-up after treatment >3 months (6)	5
(O) Pain (7)	3
(P) Use of medication	2
(Q) Activities of daily living	3
(R) Remark on side-effects	2
Data presentation	
(S) Reader is given opportunity to do inferential statistics	5

Numbers refer to points that were given if criterion was met; half of maximum (rounded up) was given if reviewers agreed that the report was unclear on this specific criterion. Maximum score is 100.

(1) This criterion was scored with great caution because it involves much knowledge about which factors are prognostically relevant. Opinions in this respect vary widely.
(2) This was always scored if authors mentioned it except in Lewith, Field and Machin, 1983 who prestratified on irrelevant variables.
(3) For cross-over designs a <10% criterion was used.
(4) DNIC means diffuse noxious inhibitory control and refers to extra-segmental counter-irritation phenomena that could cause sham acupuncture procedures to be active placebos.
(5) This was scored only if at least the acupuncture points used, the number of minutes per treatment, treatment interval and total treatment duration was mentioned.
(6) This was defined as the time period from the last treatment to the last effect measurement.
(7) Studies on migraine/tension headache could earn 4 points on this item, viz. 2 for frequency of attacks and 2 for severity of attacks. These could earn 2 points for social activities.

(From Ter Riet, Kleijnen and Knipschild, 1990a. Reproduced by permission of Elsevier Science Inc.)

with a maximum possible score of 100. The methodological criteria they used are reproduced in Table 9.1. Similar criteria were used by this team in their reviews of manipulative therapies, homeopathy, garlic and ginger, all of which are described later in the book. In the original review, minimal acupuncture control conditions were not distinguished from sham, though reference was made in the criteria to avoiding additional stimulation in the control condition.

Only 11 studies scored 50 or more points, with the best study obtaining 62% of the maximum score. Positive and negative results were approximately equally divided in the higher quality studies, where a cut-off score of 40 or 50 points was taken. The full list is shown in Table 9.2. Studies were also separated into four categories of pain: headache, musculo–skeletal (spine), musculo–skeletal (other) and miscellaneous. The pattern of results does not change, however. Results are equivocal for all four groups, though the treatment for musculo–skeletal problems of the spine (mostly low-back pain) show slightly more positive results (Table 9.3).

The overall conclusions of all reviewers are similar. Studies are generally methodologically poor. Acupuncture appears to produce some benefits for patients with chronic pain, but it is not clear how long they last or whether they are psychologically mediated. When acupuncture is compared with alternative treatments (such as TENS), the results are equivocal (Richardson and Vincent, 1986). When acupuncture is, crucially, compared with a placebo control the results are also equivocal. Flaws in the placebo control may bias some of these studies against acupuncture; studies with acceptable placebos are considered below.

Acupuncture for Other Disorders

Studies of acupuncture for chronic pain are poor. Studies of acupuncture for other disorders are, with some notable exceptions, generally worse. Vincent and Richardson (Vincent and Richardson, 1987) reviewed the use of acupuncture for asthma, deafness, hypertension, psychiatric disorders, smoking and obesity. They concluded that the studies on hypertension, obesity and psychiatric disorders were so poor that nothing could be concluded from them. Studies on asthma and deafness were of a higher standard; the studies on the treatment of smoking and drug addiction are also considered in a separate section. It should be noted that treatments for obesity, smoking and addictions generally are a rather special case as they tend to use auricular acupuncture. The mechanisms that may operate for musculo–skeletal pain may not have much in common with those mediating any effect of ear acupuncture.

Deafness

The treatment of sensori–neural deafness by acupuncture is interesting. It reads like a cautionary tale for researchers. Early studies from China claimed 80–90% success rates (Rosen, 1974). However, more careful studies

Table 9.2 Controlled trials of acupuncture

First author	Principal complaint	Control treatment	Total score for methodological criteria 100	Outcome
Baust	Migraine	Sham	45	−
Jensen	Headache	Sham	29	+
Ahonen	Tension neck pain	Physiotherapy	10	−
Loh	Migraine	Continued medical therapy	19	+
Ahonen	Myogenic headache	Physiotherapy	44	−
Doerr-Proske	Migraine	Relaxation programme	35	−
Hansen	Tension headache	Sham	29	+
Henry	Headache	Sham	62	−
Vincent	Migraine	Sham	57	+
Man	Rheumatoid arthritis	Hydrocortisone i.a.	45	+
Matsumoto	Chronic pain	Other acupuncture	33	+
Laitinen	Cervical syndrome	Historical (medical)	23	−
Weintraub	Musculo-skeletal pain	Sham	31	+
Lee	Chronic pain	Sham	20	−
Gaw	Osteoarthritic pain	Sham	55	−
Kepes	Chronic pain	Sham	19	−
Ghia	Chronic pain	Tender area needling	40	−
Laitinen	Chronic sacrolumbalgia and ischialgia	TENS	18	+
Edelist	Low back pain	Sham	41	−
Fox	Low back pain	TENS	21	−
Moore	Chronic shoulder pain	Sham	57	−
Godfrey	Musculo-skeletal pain	Sham	38	−
Co	Sickle cell anaemia	Sham	60	−
Mao	Chronic pain	Other acupuncture	13	?
Berry	Shoulder-cuff lesions	Steroids i.a. & analgesics	50	−

Author	Condition	Control	N	Result
Coan	Low back pain	Waiting list	40	+
Gunn	Chronic low back pain	Single point acupuncture	32	+
Boureau	Chronic pain	TENS	6	+
Gallacchi	Cervical and lumbar pain	Laser	60	−
Mazières	Chronic low back pain	Other acupuncture	22	+
Junnila	Osteoarthrosis	Analgesic	14	+
Junnila	Chronic pain	Minimal	44	+
Coan	Neck pain	Waiting list	21	+
Brattberg	Tennis elbow	Historical (steroid)	13	+
MacDonald	Chronic low back pain	Sham	38	−
Lewith	Post-herpetic pain	Sham	34	+
Petrie	Chronic cervical pain	Sham		
Mendelson	Chronic back pain	Sham	39	+
Hansen	Chronic facial pain	Minimal	35	−
Lundeberg	Chronic pain	TENS	28	−
Melzack	Chronic pain	Sham	27	−
Ballegaard	Chronic pancreatitis	Minimal	48	+
Junilla	Gonarthrosis	Arteparon i.a.	23	+
Ballegard	Angina pectoris	Minimal	51	−
Emery	Ankylosing spondylitis	Sham	27	+
Lehmann	Chronic low back pain	Sham	53	−
Petrie	Neck pain	Sham	41	−
Cheng	Chronic musculoskeletal pain	Acupuncture-like TENS	30	+
Helms	Dismenorrhea	Policlinic visit	57	−
Nordemar	Chronic pain	Other acupuncture	37	+
Ballegaard	Angina pectoris	Sham	43	−
Molsberger	Chronic tennis elbow pain	Sham	52	+

(Adapted from Ter Riet, Kleijnen and Knipschild, 1990a. Reproduced by permission of Elsevier Science Inc.)

Table 9.3   Relationship between methodological score and study outcome stratified according to the site of chronic pain ($n = 51$)

Site of pain	Outcome	< 29	Methodological score 30–39	40–49	50–59	60–69	No. studies/row
Headache	Positive	3	0	0	1	0	4
	Negative	1	1	2	0	1	5
Musculoskeletal	Positive	4	4	2	1	0	11
(spine)	Negative	3	1	3	0	1	8
Musculoskeletal	Positive	3	0	1	1	0	5
(other than spine)	Negative	2	3	0	3	0	8
Miscellaneous	Positive	1	1	0	2	0	4
	Negative	2	1	2	0	1	6

(From Ter Riet, Kleijnen and Knipschild, 1990a. Reproduced by permission of Elsevier Science Inc.)

undertaken later, involving audiometric evaluation, failed to find any effect. Finally, in 1982 a report appeared from the Beijing Research Institute of 1000 cases treated over 20 years, concluding that in the vast majority of cases acupuncture does not have any beneficial effect on deafness. Thus the earlier enthusiasm generated by reports based on subjective impressions of improvement has not been sustained when more careful studies have been carried out. Two controlled studies of acupuncture for tinnitus have also been carried out, but neither found it to be of any value (Vincent and Richardson, 1987).

Asthma

Several experimental studies have reported short-term effects of acupuncture on asthma (Vincent and Richardson, 1987), though not all have used a placebo control. Tashkin, Kroening and Bresler (1977) demonstrated the superiority of acupuncture over placebo in the treatment of metacholine induced asthma. It has proven more difficult to demonstrate the effects of acupuncture as a therapy for asthma. Tashkin, Kroening and Brester (1985) failed to demonstrate any effects of classical acupuncture on chronic asthma. Christensen, Laursen and Taudorf (1984) showed a modest effect on both subjective and objective measures, with true acupuncture proving superior to sham. Jobst et al (1986) showed an improvement in patient ratings of breathlessness and exercise tests, true acupuncture being superior to sham. All three of these studies are small—24 patients at most. The results are equivocal, perhaps because of the low power of the studies.

Similar conclusions were reached by Kleijnen, ter Riet and Knipschild (1991) in a review of 13 controlled trials of acupuncture for asthma, some looking only at short-term effects (which we have described as experimental). Methodological criteria were applied as in their previous reviews, with the authors concluding that the quality of most studies was mediocre. The results of the better studies were inconsistent.

Acupuncture in the Treatment of Addictions

Vincent and Richardson (1987) reviewed seven studies of acupuncture in the treatment of smoking. They concluded that acupuncture seemed to be as successful as many other techniques, but there was nothing to suggest it was of any special benefit.

Ter Riet and colleagues evaluated studies of acupuncture in the treatment of smoking, heroin addiction and alcohol addiction using very similar criteria to those in their previous reviews (Ter Riet, Kleijnen and Knipschild, 1990a, 1990b). As before, studies were of generally low quality, with the difference that low-quality studies were more likely to show that acupuncture was beneficial than high-quality ones. Only one of eight positive studies (Bullock, 1989) scored over 50 points out of 100. Only three of 15 studies on smoking showed positive results. Striking features in these studies were the inadequate numbers of patients, and lack of biochemical validation. Three out of five studies on heroin addiction claimed a positive result, but these studies are of very poor quality. A pilot study, and a later controlled trial, showed that acupuncture could help prevent relapse for alcoholics. These studies appeared to be carefully designed and implemented, but have been subject to a number of criticisms (Anon, 1990), in particular that drop-out rates were very high from the control group.

Studies with an Acceptable Placebo Control

This brief account of reviewers' conclusions makes depressing reading. Very few controlled trials of acupuncture meet acceptable methodological requirements. In our view, and that of other authors (Lewith and Machin, 1983; Ter Riet, Kleijnan and Knipschild, 1990a), an inappropriate placebo control is the most serious and completely invalidates many of the studies. It seems important therefore to separate out those studies with an acceptable placebo, to see if different conclusions can be drawn. Vincent (1993) has suggested that minimal sham acupuncture (in some form) and mock TENS are both plausible as control groups, though some reviewers have directed criticism at the mock-TENS control (Ter Riet, 1990). Lewith and Vincent (1995) identified only 11 studies with acceptable controls (Table 9.4), though others we have identified also meet these criteria (e.g. Tavola et al, 1992; Deluze et al, 1992)

Of the 11, six studies show a significant advantage of acupuncture over placebo, though some others show a non-significant advantage. However, the trials are very small, with four involving less than 20 subjects. It is doubtful if many of them have sufficient power to conclude that a non-significant result definitely shows acupuncture to be equivalent to a placebo. The probability of a Type II error—failing to detect an actual difference—is high. The difference between acupuncture and the control procedure in the study of Tavola and colleagues is quite marked, for instance, yet the results are not significant; with only 15 patients per group this is perhaps not surprising. The standard of the studies is also very variable, with methodology scores ranging from 28 to 57 on Ter Riet's ratings. A cautious interpretation of these studies is that the results of post-herpetic neuralgia and angina suggest that acupuncture is ineffective, that acupuncture may well be helpful for low back pain and that its efficacy for migraine remains to be resolved. The conclusions from a selective review of placebo-controlled studies are then similar to those of other reviews. Acupuncture may be effective for some types of chronic pain, but the results are equivocal in many cases.

Disappointingly little has been achieved by literally hundreds of attempts to evaluate acupuncture. Major methodological flaws are apparent in the vast majority of studies. Some tentative conclusions can be drawn, however. Acupuncture does not appear to be helpful for deafness and drug addiction and further investigations are probably unnecessary. There are a large number of pilot studies of the treatment of various disorders, some giving positive results and showing that acupuncture is possibly beneficial. Controlled studies have shown positive findings for low back pain and fibromyalgia, and equivocal results for migraine and asthma. Nevertheless, larger-scale studies are warranted for all these disorders, though other types of musculo–skeletal pain, tension headache and arthritis are also possible candidates.

MANIPULATIVE THERAPIES

This section is primarily concerned with the evaluation of osteopathy and chiropractic. As has been made clear in previous chapters, these systems of medicine have wider aims than simply the relief of musculo–skeletal and joint pains with which they are popularly associated. The views of individual practitioners on the scope and potential of their treatments

Table 9.4a Acupuncture for chronic pain: studies with acceptable placebo controls I

Authors	Population	N	Design	Control	Type of acupuncture	Dependent measures	Follow-up	Results
Hansen & Hansen	Facial pain	16	Cross-over	Minimal acupuncture	Classical 10 daily sessions	Daily pain ratings	4 week	66% patients improved. True acupuncture sig. > control
Macdonald et al	Low back pain	17	Group comparison	Mock TENS	Tender areas & trigger points. Some EA. Up to 10 sessions	Various pain VASs, mood, independent clinician's assessment	none	Acupuncture sig. > placebo for pain relief, activity, physical signs in pain area
Petrie & Langley	Cervical pain	13	Group comparison	Mock TENS	Classical. Twice weekly	8 self-ratings sessions	none	84% acupuncture group reported good pain relief. Acupuncture sig. > placebo
Lewith et al	Post-herpetic neuralgia	62	Group comparison	Mock TENS auricular	Classical & sleep, 6–8 sessions	Daily records	2 month moderation disturbance	Sig. improvement in only 7 patients in each group. No sig. sleep difference between groups
Dowson et al	Migraine headache	48	Group comparison	Mock TENS	Classical. 6 sessions	Frequency, duration, intensity, medication	24 week	56% acup. and 30% placebo showed 33% pain relief 44% acup. and 57% placebo less frequent headaches. No sig. difference between groups

(From Lewith and Vincent, 1995. Reproduced by permission.)

Table 9.4b Acupuncture for pain: studies with acceptable placebo controls II

Authors	Population	N	Design	Control	Type of acupuncture	Dependent measures	Follow-up	Results
Petrie & Hazleman	Chronic neck pain	25	Group comparison	Mock TENS	8 sessions, twice weekly	Daily diary: pain intensity disability, medication	1 month	45% of acup. group 30% of placebo group show sig. response. No sig. difference between groups
Lehmann et al	Chronic low back pain	53	Group comparison	Mock TENS	EA group and TENS group (all groups had additional treatment)	Physician assessment. VRS measures of pain & disability	6 month	EA sig. > TENS and mock TENS
Ballegaard et al	Severe angina	26	Group comparison	Minimal acupuncture	Classical. 7 sessions over 3 weeks	Exercise tests, pain diaries, medication	3 week	Acup. sig. > control for cardiac work capacity only
Vincent	Migraine	30	Group comparison	Minimal acupuncture	Classical acup. 6 weekly sessions	4 × daily ratings of pain and medication	1 year	43% reduction in weekly pain score for acup. group, 14% for control. Acup. sig. > control for pain levels, but not for medication reduction
Dickens & Lewith	Oesteo-arthritis	13	Group comparison	Mock TENS	Classical acup. 6 sessions	Diames. VAS pain scores medication sleep, grip, tenderness	3 week	76% reduction in pain in acup. group. 10% in control, but no sig. difference between groups
Ballegaard et al	Moderate angina	49	Group comparison	Minimal acupuncture	Classical. 10 sessions over 3 wks	Exercise tests, pain diaries, medication, well-being	6 month	Reduction of 50% in attacks & medication. No sig. difference between groups

(From Lewith and Vincent, 1995. Reproduced by permission.)

will naturally vary. Research on these therapies has, however, so far as randomized controlled trials are concerned, been largely limited to back and neck pain.

The term *manipulative therapies* covers a range of different techniques revolving around joint manipulation, soft tissue techniques and advice to the patient on posture and exercise (Curtis, 1988). Assessing whether manipulation works is complicated not only by the wide range of treatments, but also by the fact that surgeons, physicians, physiotherapists, osteopaths, chiropractors and others manipulate in different ways (Jayson, 1986). Studies have used a range of osteopathic, chiropractic techniques as well as the various systems (e.g. Cyriax) developed by orthopaedic physicians and surgeons. Most reviews have grouped all these trials together which, although it obscures differences between the treatments, seems the correct strategy at this stage. There are comparatively few controlled trials, and even fewer good ones, and to start breaking them down according to their particular manipulative techniques would render any general conclusions about manipulation impossible. If the efficacy of manipulation can be established, then further trials can compare different techniques.

A particular problem in this or any other area of physical therapy is defining an acceptable placebo control condition that is convincing to the patient. A bogus form of manipulation is likely to lack credibility to the patient, though non-forceful manipulation has been used in some studies. Short-wave diathermy or microwaves on very low settings have been used in most placebo studies. These appear to be credible treatments which could therefore have substantial psychological effects, but they are nevertheless completely different in form from the manipulations with which they are compared. Ideally, the perceived credibility of the treatments would be assessed (Vincent and Lewith, 1995), but the credibility of the treatments does not seem to have been checked in any manipulative trials.

Most trials compare a manipulative therapy with some simpler, cheaper therapy such as short-wave diathermy, massage or analgesics, though a few are comparisons of different manipulative techniques. Already one can see that a variety of different questions are being asked which are not always clearly distinguished, though the review of Koes et al (1991) does separate the placebo comparisons from the comparative treatment trials.

Reviews of Manipulative Therapies

A number of reviews have been published, with broadly similar conclusions, but confidence in the standard of the studies appears to have slowly increased over the years.

Brunarski (1984) identified 47 studies on spinal manipulation, most reporting substantial improvements, albeit usually in spontaneously remitting conditions. However, 15 of the studies were randomized controlled trials. Interventions were very variable, as were the control treatments. Control treatments ranged from no-treatment to any combination of: bed rest, detuned short wave, analgesics, heat, massage, corset, back school, physiotherapy or traction, and various placebo procedures. Of the 15 trials, 11 showed a significant advantage of manipulative therapies, but Brunarski cautioned that there were numerous methodological problems which precluded any firm conclusions.

These conclusions have been echoed by other reviewers such as Greenland et al (1980), Di Fabio (1986) and Curtis (1988). Curtis, for instance, while stating that there was evidence that manipulation gave some short-term advantage over other treatments, pointed to numerous methodological problems:

> Despite the thoughtful paper by Greenland et al (1980) concerning the elements required for an effective clinical trial of manipulation, none of the studies so far have dealt fully with the issues of subject selection, stratification, sample size estimations, standardized diagnostic categories, standardized manipulative procedures, the effects of confounding factors or optimal statistical analysis. (Curtis, 1988)

The most comprehensive review of spinal manipulation (Koes et al 1991) has come from the same source (Department of Epidemiology and Biostatistics, University of Limburg in The Netherlands) as some of the major reviews on homeopathy and acupuncture, although a different team was responsible for the review of spinal manipulation. Essentially the same methods were followed, however, with each trial being rated on key methodological criteria. They identified 35 randomized controlled trials, but no trial scored over 60 points out of a possible 100. The most common methodological problems were the proper description of drop-outs, the small size of the study population, the lack of a placebo group, the blinding of the patients and the blinded measurement of effects. A further crucial point, agreed on by all reviewers, is that there is a dearth of studies involving substantial long-term follow-up.

While the idea of scoring each study according to defined methodological criteria is clearly excellent, and while there are bound to be disagreements in the way these criteria are arrived at, the standard demanded in this particular review does seem particularly severe. The authors acknowledge that their ideal 100 points standard is difficult to reach in this area; a precisely defined trial is certainly easier to carry out with a drug or homeopathic treatment. The severity of scoring can be seen by considering where points are lost in one of the best trials. Meade et al (1990) attracted considerable attention with their finding that chiropractic treatment was superior to hospital out-patient treatment in an ambitious, large trial of 741 patients. As they chose to look at treatment given in its usual location (although patients were carefully randomized), they acknowledged that it was a pragmatic rather than a 'fastidious' trial, in which specific treatment techniques were compared. Points (from 100) were lost for: failing to specify the type of treatment (10) although it was a naturalistic trial with chiropractors specifying their own treatment; failing to exclude other therapies (5), again impossible in a naturalistic trial; failing to include a placebo condition (5), not the purpose of the trial; patients not being blind (5), impossible in this kind of trial; no blind assessment of outcome (10), again extremely difficult when patients are seen in different locations, though it is possible that the statistical analysis of the questionnaires could have been blind. The point of these remarks is not to quibble with the basic approach or the undoubted value of the review. We suggest that in the case of manipulative therapies (as compared with the reviews of homeo-pathy and acupuncture from the same department) that the best trials are of a somewhat better standard than a score of 50 out of 100 would suggest.

There were 30 trials concerning the treatment of back pain, and five neck pain. This produced 31 comparisons between spinal manipulation and another treatment and eight between manipulation and placebo, the 39 comparisons resulting from 35 trials as some involved more than one comparison. In 18 trials (51%) the authors reported better results for spinal manipulation than for the comparison treatment, usually some form of basic standard treatment such as physiotherapy (short-wave diathermy, massage, exercises) or drugs (generally analgesics) or placebo. In five studies spinal manipulation was more effective in a subgroup of patients or only at certain times after the treatment ended. In 11 studies there was no difference between the spinal manipulation and the comparison treatment or the comparison was superior. In the review these latter findings are referred to as *negative*, giving a slightly misleading impression in relation to the comparison of the two treatments. Generally this means that there was no difference between treatments; cases which might more strictly be described as negative, if spinal manipulation was worse than the standard treatment, are not distinguished or remarked upon. The term *negative results* is, however, completely appropriate in the case of placebo-controlled trials, discussed below, where no difference between groups suggests that spinal manipulation has only a placebo effect. The variation in comparison treatments means that it is very unlikely that the different groups were receiving equal amounts of time and attention in most trials; these studies are simply pragmatic in that they are concerned with the respective value of overall treatment strategies, rather than any attempt to identify key elements of the treatment.

Table 9.5 shows the 31 trials involving a comparison of treatments, of which 15 showed positive findings. Three trials scored 50 or more points, one positive and two positive in subgroups only; in eight trials scoring between 40 and 50, only two were positive, one with positive subgroup results and five found no difference. There was a tendency for trials with lower methodology scores to be more likely to report positive findings (Figure 9.1).

The details of the eight trials involving a placebo comparison are shown in Table 9.6. In most of the studies the placebo treatment consisted of detuned short-wave diathermy. Four studies reported a significant difference, one positive result only in a subgroup and three reported negative results. There are no clear differentiating factors between the positive and negative studies, though two studies by the same investigators, using similar designs and methods, found positive results for general practice patients but no effect for, presumably more chronically ill, hospital patients. The ratio of positive findings to negative/no difference is similar in the placebo and alternative treatment comparisons, which is curious. One would hope that spinal manipulation would be consistently better than placebo, even if it showed no great advantage over other standard (and presumably effective) treatments. Although the authors do not mention it, a possible interpretation of their findings is not that there is doubt about the efficacy of spinal manipulation, but there is also doubt about other standard treatments which appear no better (often less effective) than a treatment which is not clearly better than placebo in the studies conducted so far.

Overall, Koes and colleagues (1991) suggest that the results are promising, but not conclusive. Study populations are small, which makes it hard to detect differences between treatments—though detecting differences between treatment and placebo should be easier. A possible explanation of the inconsistencies in the findings is that manipulation is particularly effective for some subgroups of patients, and this fact is obscuring the results in trials with a large disparate group of patients. There is, however, little clear indication from the studies as to what those subgroups might be. It would seem possible that acute symptoms might be especially susceptible to early intervention by manipulation, which might in turn prevent the onset of a chronic condition, as the study of Meade et al (1990) might suggest. However, there are positive and negative findings for both acute and chronic conditions. As so often, further trials of a higher methodological standard are awaited.

Table 9.5 Randomized trials on the efficacy of manipulation for back pain and neck pain in order of stratified criteria score

Study	Total score 100	Indication	Conclusion
Back pain trials:			
MacDonald, Bell	56	Acute + chronic low back pain	Positive (only in patients with pain of 2–4 weeks' duration not those with <2 weeks or >4 weeks)
Hadler et al	53	Acute low back pain	Positive (only in patients with pain of 2–4 weeks' duration not those with >2 weeks)
Ongley et al	50	Chronic low back pain	Positive
Bergquist-Ullman, Larsson	49	Acute low back pain	Positive compared with placebo Negative compared with back school
Meade et al	48	Acute + chronic low back pain	Positive
Gibson et al	46	(sub)acute low back pain	Negative
Sims-Williams et al	45	Acute + chronic low back pain	Negative
Helliwell, Cunliffe	43	Acute low back pain	Negative
Doran, Newell	42	Acute + chronic low back pain	Negative
Matthews et al	41	Acute back pain	Positive (only in patients in whom straight leg raising was limited)
Evans et al	40	Chronic low back pain	Positive
Glover et al	39	Acute back pain	Negative
Coxhead et al	38	Sciatic symptoms	Positive
Waagen et al	37	Chronic low back pain	Positive
Hoehler et al	35	Acute + chronic low back pain	Positive
Sims-Williams et al	35	Acute + chronic low back pain	Positive
Zylbergold, Piper	33	Not mentioned	Negative
Postaccini et al	33	Acute + chronic low back pain	Positive (only in patients with acute back pain not those with chronic pain)
Rasmussen	33	Acute low back pain	Positive
Farrell, Twomey	32	Acute low back pain	Positive

continues overleaf

Table 9.5   *(continued)*

Study	Total score 100	Indication	Conclusion
Back pain trials: *(continued)*			
Nwuga	32	Acute low back pain (prolapsed disc)	Positive
Waterworth, Hunter	31	Acute low back pain	Negative
Arkuszewski	31	Acute + chronic low back pain	Positive
Buerger	31	Not mentioned	Positive
Tobis, Hoehler	30	Not mentioned	Positive
Bronfort	30	Acute + chronic low back pain	No conclusion
Kinalski et al	24	Not mentioned	Positive
Godfrey et al	22	Acute low back pain	Negative
Siehle et al	22	Not mentioned	Positive (only in patients with no nerve root compression not those with compression)
Rupert et al	20	Acute + chronic low back pain	Positive
Neck pain trials:			
Sloop et al	50	Chronic neck pain	Negative
Nordemar, Thörner	43	Acute neck pain	Negative
Brodin	39	Acute + chronic neck pain	Positive
Howe, Newcombe	29	Acute + chronic neck pain	Positive
Mealy et al	26	Acute neck pain (whiplash)	Positive

The labels acute and chronic are according to the authors of study. Classification might vary between the studies.

Conclusion of the author(s) of the study. Positive conclusion = manipulation better than the control treatment; negative conclusion = manipulation worse than or equally effective as control treatment.

(From Koes, Assendelft and van der Heijden, 1991. Reproduced by permission of the BMJ Publishing Group)

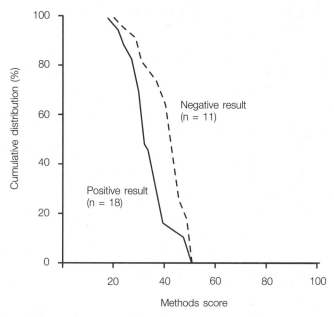

Figure 9.1 Relation between methods score of trials and their results (positive result shows manipulation is better than reference treatment, negative result shows manipulation is no better or worse than reference treatment) (*Source*: Koes, Assendelft and van der Heijden, 1991. Reproduced by permission of the BMJ Publishing Group)

Since the publication of their review Koes et al (1991) have published their own trial of manual therapy and physiotherapy, in which they try to avoid the flaws identified in previous reviews. The trial is certainly impressive in its scope, carefully conducted and comprehensively analysed. Two hundred and fifty-six patients with back pain of at least six weeks' duration were randomized into four groups receiving one of:

1. physiotherapy—exercise, massage, heat
2. manual therapy—manipulation and mobilization of the spine
3. placebo therapy—detuned short-wave diathermy or
4. continued treatment by their general practitioner.

At an initial six-week follow-up all four groups showed a considerable improvement (as expected in a self-limiting condition). Manual therapy and physiotherapy were significantly more effective than general practitioner treatment, which generally consisted of only a single visit, but non-significantly better than the placebo treatment. There was little difference between physiotherapy and manual therapy at any stage of the trial. The placebo therapy appeared convincing in subsequent checks of patient

Table 9.6   Details of trials comparing manipulation with placebo

Study	Placebo (no. of patients)	Methods score	Results
Ongley et al	Non-forceful manipulation (41)	50	Mean pain on visual analogue scale after 1, 3 and 6 months: (i) 2.1, 1.8, 1.5; (ii) 3.1, 2.9, 3.1. All differences significant.
Bergquist, Larsson	Short-wave diathermy at lowest intensity (75)	49	Mean no. of days until recovery: (i) 15.8; (ii) 28.7. Difference significant.
Gibson et al	Detuned short-wave diathermy (34)	46	% of patients free of pain after 4 and 12 weeks: (i) 28%, 42%; (34) (ii) 27%, 44%.
Sims-Williams et al	Microwave at lowest setting (46)	45	No. of patients improved after 4 and 12 weeks: (i) 29, 28; (ii) 25, 27. Not significantly different. Also no evidence that manipulation produced any long-term (1 year) benefit.
Glover et al	Detuned short-wave diathermy (41)	39	Mean pain relief (%) on visual analogue scale immediately after treatment and after 3 and 7 days: (i) 34%, 50%, 75%; (ii) 22%, 56%, 80%. Apart from slight immediate improvement after treatment no benefit from manipulation.
Sims-Williams et al	Microwave at lowest setting (47)	35	No. of patients improved after 4 and 12 weeks: (i) 39, 26; (ii) 32, 22. After 4 weeks the differences were of borderline significance. After 12 weeks the differences disappeared.
Postacchini et al	Antioedema gel (73)	33	Mean improvement on combined pain, disability, spinal mobility score (5–35) after 3 weeks, 2 months, and 6 months. In subgroup with acute pain: (i) 2.2, 2.6, 4.3; (ii) 0.7, 1.2, 2.0. Manipulation was significantly better only in subgroup with acute pain after 3 weeks.
Rupert et al	Sham manipulation, massage (–)	20	Improvement on pain visual analogue scale during treatment: more pain reduction in group receiving manipulation (data in graphs)

Results of the most important outcome measure according to the author(s) of the study. When not explicitly stated presentation of pain or a global measure of improvement. Significant means $p < 0.05$. Group (i) = treatment; Group (ii) = placebo.

(From Koes, Assendelft and van der Heijden, 1991. Reproduced by permission of the BMJ Publishing Group)

perceptions of the therapies, and was in fact remarkably effective. Koes and colleagues comment that the psychological component of physical therapies is large, although this does not affect their conclusion that both physiotherapy and manual therapies are valuable forms of treatment. At a one-year follow-up, many patients had opted to abandon general practice or placebo treatment for manual therapy or physiotherapy, an outcome measure in itself. In addition, manual therapy showed a slight advantage over physiotherapy, and both were now superior to placebo. The advantage of manual therapy over physiotherapy was considered a tentative finding in the discussion, with a number of possible explanations being advanced, but it may be that it confers a slight long-term advantage. One other fact is particularly worthy of mention. Patients receiving manual therapy received approximately half the number of treatments of those receiving physiotherapy—the therapists were free to choose the number of treatments within certain limits. This would suggest that manual therapy is certainly more cost-effective than physiotherapy in this particular condition.

Koes et al (1991) decided against a meta-analysis in their review of studies, because of the disparate nature of the studies both in terms of the techniques used and the standard of the studies. Anderson et al (1992) made similar observations after attempting a meta-analysis of 23 randomized controlled trials involving, because of some trials with several groups, 34 discrete comparisons between treatments. The paper contains a table describing the studies in some detail, and attempts a comprehensive evaluation of outcome at several time points after treatment. They concluded that spinal manipulation was consistently more effective than any of a range of comparison treatments, though there was some doubt as to whether these differences were clinically significant. As they point out though, comparing spinal manipulation to other treatments obscures its effectiveness. A small advantage over another treatment may still indicate that a change of treatment policy is a worthwhile long-term strategy for a clinic or department. However, their principal conclusion, which they acknowledge limits the possibility of a meaningful meta-analysis, is that: 'For the future, it is suggested that researchers strive for more consistent measures in terms of explicit descriptions of the nature of the manipulation, the times of post-treatment assessments and the nature of outcome measures. Only then can meta-analysis fulfil its potential in this clinical area' (Anderson et al, 1992).

Chapter 10

Evaluation of Herbalism, Homeopathy and Naturopathy

The scientific evaluation of herbal medicine, homeopathy and naturopathy is subject to many of the same difficulties that we outlined in the previous chapter regarding acupuncture and manipulation. However, trials of acupuncture for chronic pain and manipulation for back pain can be sensibly reviewed together to produce an overall assessment of efficacy, even though the basic techniques used vary for individual patients and different conditions. In the case of herbalism, homeopathy and naturopathy there are a multitude of different remedies targeted either singly or in combination at a wide variety of diseases. It is therefore not feasible to ask in general terms whether herbal therapy is or is not effective in some general sense. Individual herbal remedies must be evaluated in their own right and it is unlikely that any meaningful overall synthesis of results from scientific studies could be achieved. There are similar problems with overall assessment of homeopathy and naturopathy.

In one respect the evaluation of homeopathy and herbalism is simpler than the evaluation of acupuncture and other physical therapies which, as we have seen earlier, pose particular problems in the definition of a placebo control. In contrast, the placebo-controlled double-blind randomized clinical trial is well suited to the evaluation of ingested treatments and is certainly feasible both for herbal treatments and homeopathy. A more holistic approach to herbal medicine is less comfortably amenable to this methodology. To the extent that treatment is individualized to the patient, rather than the condition, the blinding of therapists may pose similar problems to those encountered in acupuncture outcome research.

HERBALISM

Medicines from Plants

Plants have long been and continue to be an important source of orthodox drug compounds, as a recent editorial in the *Lancet* makes clear:

In the UK and North America almost 25% of the active components of currently prescribed medicines were first identified in higher plants. Many of these compounds have been known for years but are still the drugs of choice in their respective areas of therapy—e.g. the Digitalis cardiac glycosides. Several recently introduced drugs that offer therapeutic advantages are extracted from plants. Thus taxoids derived from the yew are used in ovarian cancer, qing hao is otherwise known as annual or sweet wormwood and is the source of the antimalarial artemisinin and related compounds. (Anon, 1994)

Interest in herbs and herbalism has grown enormously in the last two decades, as has interest in other forms of complementary medicine. The attitude of the pharmaceutical industry to research into the effects of herbs and the uses of plant-based materials has also changed considerably: 15 years ago none of the top 250 companies had a research programme involving higher plants, but now over half of them have introduced such investigations. The upsurge of interest in plant-based medicines has, from an orthodox perspective, several explanations. The success of plant-derived anticancer drugs and other compounds is clearly important; other plants, while not clinically effective in themselves, can provide molecular templates for the design of more effective drugs; plants with their multiple actions can stimulate a much more wide-ranging enquiry than studies of isolated compounds; finally, plants are an inexpensive source of basic material for experiment (Anon, 1994).

The future of plants as sources of drugs seems secure. Less than 10% of the estimated 250 000 flowering plant species have been examined for their scientific potential. There is concern, however, that the loss of natural habitat could mean that some may be extinct before they can be examined. Another major difficulty is selecting plants for study from the enormous range available. Some directions can be derived from the discipline of ethnopharmacology, in which the plants used by different cultural groups for medical purposes are studied (Meserole, 1996).

Reviewing Research on Herbal Medicine

Herbal medicine involves the study of plant material for use as food and medicine, and for health promotion. This includes not only its use in the treatment of disease, but also for the enhancement of the quality of life, physically and spiritually (Meserole, 1996). The term *herbalism* is slightly misleading in that it implies that there is a single tradition giving rise to the huge variety of ways that herbs are used. In fact, the use of herbs in North America, Europe, Asia and Africa is often specific to a particular culture and tradition. Diagnosis and treatment with herbs in traditional Chinese medicine is very different in its approach to Western herbalism, though there are many shared themes as regards the basic underlying philosophies of wholeness and optimization of health. In contrast, orthodox medicine and pharmaceutical companies have shown very little interest in the philosophy and methods of herbalism. Herbs are increasingly valued and researched, but primarily as a means to producing more effective drugs, the ultimate intention usually being to isolate the active ingredients of the herbs. Our selective review of research adopts this orthodox perspective simply because there seems almost no research examining herbalism as actually practised (Mills, 1993a, and personal communication). Some of the difficulties of researching the actual practice of herbalism are discussed below.

The literature on the constituents, pharmacology and effects of herbal medicine is vast. Herbal medicine traditions exist in many countries of the world and a considerable volume of research is published in Europe, North America and Asia (Mills, 1993a; Tsutani, 1993). In the United Kingdom research on herbal medicine has little official recognition. In contrast, the German government treats herbal medicines much as they do pharmaceutical products and there are detailed government monographs on around 250 herbs. German pharmaceutical companies invest heavily in herbal medicine, and international conferences and meetings are of a similar size to equivalent pharmaceutical meetings (Mills, 1993b).

Many studies have been published on the effects of herbal treatment, but the majority appear to be of poor standard, often with major methodological flaws (Tsutani, 1993). There are relatively few properly conducted trials and those we have identified concern a variety of conditions and a number of different herbal products. Very few reviews or meta-analyses of herbal treatment appear to have been carried out, in part because few treatments have been sufficiently researched to permit a meaningful overview of the results for any one condition.

A complete review of herbal treatments and their effects on different diseases is clearly out of the question, requiring several books in its own right. As with other complementary therapies we are restricting our review to outcome studies, primarily randomized controlled trials, while acknowledging that other types of study, particularly those on mechanism of action, are equally important. We summarize reviews of the therapeutic properties of two particular herbs (garlic and *Ginkgo biloba*), and also describe studies of some other herbal treatments which have, at least in initial studies, been shown to be effective. Our review cannot, and is not intended to be, comprehensive. Its purpose is to show that there are at least some high-quality trials of herbal treatments in their natural form which suggest that effective treatments are available for some common conditions.

Examples of Controlled Trials of Herbal Medicines

We now look at some illustrative, carefully conducted trials of common herbal remedies, providing evidence both for and against their efficacy. We have not attempted to guide a comprehensive review, but have selected studies in which common conditions were treated by readily available, and generally widely used, herbal preparations.

Chinese Herbal Therapy in Adult Atopic Dermatitis

Atopic dermatitis is a common skin disorder, often first observed in childhood, which may become a serious handicap in adult life. A number of therapies are available, including ultraviolet light and corticosteroids, but the condition is often resistant to treatment. Sheehan, Rustin and Atherton (1992) compared a standard formula of Chinese herbs (described in their paper) with a placebo composed of inactive herbs, with a similar taste and smell to the original, in a five-month cross-over trial. Dietary treatment, which would be a standard part of the traditional therapeutic regime, was not instigated. Individual prescriptions of herbs were not used, but the standard formula was derived after discussion of the basic components of treatment with a Chinese herbalist. Objective improvements in erythema and surface damage were greater for the herbal treatment than for placebo, and patients reported less itching and sleep disturbance during the active phase of the trial. The authors discuss the likely active ingredients of the concoction, but comment that understanding of the mechanism of action is limited at present. In a further trial with a similar design, Sheehan, Rustin and Atherton (1992) report that a Chinese herbal preparation was superior to placebo in the treatment of atopic eczema in children. In both trials the response was clinically valuable and there was no evidence of toxicity, suggesting the wider therapeutic potential for traditional Chinese medical plants in skin diseases.

Feverfew in the Treatment of Migraine and Arthritis

Feverfew was, as the name suggests, used as an antipyretic in medieval times, and more recently it has become popular as a lay remedy for migraine prevention. The cause of migraine is not fully understood, but abnormal platelet behaviour has been implicated. During an attack platelets release serotonin and a pathogenic role for this process is supported by the value of serotonin antagonists in migraine prevention. In vitro studies have shown that feverfew extract inhibits serotonin release from platelets, which could explain the reported clinical benefits of feverfew (Murphy, Heptinstall and Mitchell, 1988). There have also been encouraging results from a previous study of feverfew withdrawal in migraine sufferers (Johnson et al, 1985).

Murphy, Heptinstall and Mitchell (1988) compared feverfew with placebo in a double-blind cross-over study. After a one-month single-blind placebo run-in, 72 volunteers received four months of treatment with either dried feverfew leaves or matching placebo, before switching to the other treatment. Treatment with feverfew was associated with a reduction in the mean number and severity of attacks in each two-month period and in the degree of vomiting; duration of individual attacks was unaltered. Some side-effects, particularly mouth ulceration, were reported in each group, but there was no overall excess of side-effects in the feverfew group. No serious adverse effects were reported, but the authors note that a four-month study is insufficient to assess any long-term adverse effects, which is particularly important in conditions such as migraine that could require lifelong treatment.

Feverfew has also been used in the treatment of rheumatoid arthritis and its efficacy tested in a small trial of 41 patients (Pattrick, Heptinstall and Doherty, 1989). Patients received either dried feverfew or a comparable placebo once daily for six weeks. Multiple assessments included stiffness, pain, grip strength, articular index, full blood count, a variety of biochemical parameters and functional capacity and the opinions of both patient and observer. However, no important differences emerged between the groups either on laboratory or clinical variables. It is possible that differences might have emerged in a longer and larger study, but preliminary results were not encouraging.

Ginger—A New Antiemetic

Nausea and vomiting are regarded as some of the most unpleasant sequelae of anaesthesia; effects range from the simply annoying to life-threatening electrolyte disturbances and aspiration of stomach contents. There has been no real reduction during the last 50 years in the incidence of nausea and vomiting after anaesthesia, despite the continued introduction of new antiemetics. No available antiemetic is both effective and without side-effects (Bone et al, 1990).

In their study Bone et al (1990) compared the preoperative administration of ginger with metaclopramide in a double-blind trial, in which patients received both a capsule and an injection in a three-way comparison. Group 1 received ginger and placebo injection; Group 2 placebo capsule and metaclopramide injection; Group 3 placebo capsule and injection. Ginger was shown to be as effective as metaclopramide, with the significant advantage of being, as far as is known, free of side-effects—and presumably much cheaper.

Urtica dioica *(Stinging Nettle)* in the Treatment of Allergic Rhinitis

Urtica dioica (stinging nettle) has long been considered a nutritive herb, used both as a food and medicine in North America, Europe, Asia and Africa. Histamine, betaine, choline, acetylcholine, serotonin and formic acid have all been identified as constituents, and the herb is available as a proprietary treatment for allergic rhinitis (Mittman, 1990).

Mittman (1990) assigned 98 hayfever sufferers to two groups, one group taking freeze-dried *Urtica dioica* and the other a placebo. Participants were instructed to take two capsules at the onset of symptoms and record the effects within one hour. Assessment was based on daily symptom diaries with a global assessment at the end of the one-week study period. The 69 participants who completed the study took an average of 18 doses during the week. No statistical analysis was reported, but the results appear to show a clear advantage for the *Urtica dioica* group.

Assessment of a Proprietary Herbal Remedy for Premenstrual Syndrome

Turner and Mills (1993) compared a proprietary herbal remedy (*Vitex agnus-castus*) with placebo in the treatment of premenstrual syndrome. In the three-month double-blind study, 600 volunteers were entered though only 217 completed it—105 in the *Vitex* group and 112 on placebo. Substantial improvements were noted in the first month in both groups, assessed by standard questionnaire, with relative stability over the next two cycles. There was, however, no significant difference between *Vitex* and placebo on a variety of measures, with the exception of feelings of restlessness where *Vitex* showed an advantage. The overall conclusion was that *Vitex* showed little advantage over placebo.

Reviews of Herbal Treatments

Carefully conducted controlled trials of herbal preparations are comparatively rare, and so it is difficult to provide a comprehensive review of the various effects of a particular herb or preparation. However, in some instances thorough literature searches have been carried out allowing a more definite assessment of efficacy to be made than is possible from single trials.

Ginkgo biloba

Extract from the leaves of *Ginkgo biloba* (maidenhair tree) has been used therapeutically for centuries. In China the leaves are used to make tea for the treatment of asthma and bronchitis. The main indicators for *Ginkgo* in the West are peripheral vascular disease, such as intermittent claudication and 'cerebral insufficiency'. Cerebral insufficiency is an imprecise term that describes a collection of symptoms in elderly people including difficulties with concentration and memory, confusion, lack of energy and tiredness, depressive mood, dizziness and headache. These symptoms have been associated with impaired cerebral circulation and are sometimes thought to be early indicators of dementia (Kleijnen and Knipschild, 1992).

The effects of *Ginkgo* could be caused by single active ingredients or by the combined action of the many active agents found in extracts. The most important substances are flavonoids (ginkgo-flavone glycosides) and terpenoids (ginkgolides and bilobalide). Experimental studies suggest that *Ginkgo* has effects on skin perfusion, blood viscosity and cerebral metabolism. Pharmacokinetic studies, to identify the therapeutically active ingredients, are difficult because of the many active ingredients. Interactions (synergistic, additive or antagonistic) are likely because of the multiple sites in the body where various compounds are active, often by different mechanisms (Kleijnen and Knipschild, 1992).

Kleijnen and Knipschild (1992) reviewed 40 trials of *Ginkgo* for cerebral insufficiency, mostly published in France and Germany. Only eight trials were of good quality, the others having various methodological shortcomings. However, all but one of these eight trials showed positive effects of *Ginkgo* compared with placebo on the symptoms described above. The only negative trial concerned patients who already had dementia of vascular origin. Effects large enough to be of clinical relevance were apparent after treatment for six weeks to three months. The authors conclude that the evidence is strong enough to recommend *Ginkgo* for patients with mild to moderate cerebral insufficiency, though many questions remain about dose, duration of effects and the effect of stopping treatment with *Ginkgo*. No serious side-effects have been noted in any trial.

For intermittent claudication 15 trials have been published (Kleijnen, Knipschild and ter Riet, 1991), but only two are of good quality. All trials showed positive effects, with the two best trials showing improvements in walking distance and pain relief for *Ginkgo* as compared with placebo. While the evidence is not strong enough to recommend routine clinical use, preliminary results are encouraging.

Garlic

Garlic (*Allium sativum*) was used as a remedy for a wide variety of ailments from as early as 1500 BC. Recently most attention has been paid to the possible cardioprotective actions of garlic; these include a lipid-lowering action, antioxidant activity, antiplatelet action, favourable haemostatic effects and haemodynamic properties (Mansell and Reckless, 1991; Silagy and Neil, 1994a). Allicin, the principal active compound in a garlic bulb, is thought to be responsible for most of the pharmacological activity, but a variety of other potentially active compounds have been extracted.

The first clinical trials appeared in the late 1970s, but many suffered from significant methodological shortcomings, such as lack of controls, short duration and inadequate patient numbers. In 1989 Kleijnen, ter Riet and Knipschild (1989) published a review of 12 controlled trials on the efficacy of garlic supplements on cardiovascular risk factors. The size of the effect found on cholesterol and triglycerides was not consistent across trials, varying from no effect at all to a difference of almost 20% as compared with placebo. The majority of the trials reported positive results.

Since then several other randomized controlled trials have been conducted. Silagy and Neil (1994b) identified a total of 25 randomized controlled trials, though 9 were excluded as being of too short duration or with insufficient data to permit meaningful comparisons. A total of 16 trials, involving 952 subjects, were reviewed, each of which examined levels of cholesterol, triglycerides and high-density lipoprotein cholesterol before and after treatment. Garlic therapy achieved a 12% greater reduction in cholesterol than that achieved by placebo alone. The reduction was evident after one month and persisted for at least six months. The quality of many of the trials was poor, however, leading to only a tentative conclusion about garlic's efficacy. Similar conclusions were reached by Warshafsky, Kamer and Sivak (1993) who reviewed 28 studies and selected five high-quality placebo-controlled comparisons of garlic with placebo for detailed analysis. They concluded that the best available evidence suggested that garlic decreased total serum cholesterol levels by about 9% in the groups of patients studied.

Silagy and Neil (1994b) conclude:

> Garlic is not a licensed medication and there is not enough evidence to recommend garlic therapy as a lipid lowering agent for routine clinical use. However, there is also no evidence to suggest it is harmful. The currently available data support the likelihood of garlic therapy being beneficial, at least over a few months. Resolving this situation will require further trials that avoid the methodological problems of earlier studies and, in particular,

last long enough and have adequate statistical power to detect whether any clear cut benefits arise from the use of garlic.

In a similar review, of eight randomized controlled trials of the use of garlic for hypertension, Silagy and Neil (1994b) found that garlic reduced systolic blood pressure in three of the trials that compared garlic to placebo and diastolic blood pressure in four trials. They concluded that garlic might be of some clinical use for hypertension, but as yet there was insufficient evidence to recommend it.

Research Issues in Herbal Medicine

Many of the difficulties encountered in researching herbal medicine, such as the emphasis on an individual treatment strategy, are common to research into other complementary therapies and, as we have argued earlier, common to research into many orthodox therapies. There are, however, some particular difficulties associated with researching herbalism which inevitably complicate any enquiry.

The first is that many medicinal plants are complex mixtures of a variety of different, and potentially active, compounds. The presence of multiple constituents means that they are likely to have multiple actions, in contrast to drugs which aim at least to have a single specific action. In practice, as Meserole (1996) points out, drugs are bound to act in various ways in the body and the benefit of a drug is always a balance between the desired effect and the various unwanted effects it may have. Herbs are also available in many forms: dried or fresh, as leaves, flowers or root, preserved in syrups or as concentrates. Routes of administration and delivery include pessaries, suppositories, creams, ointments, gels, enemas, snuffs, steams, inhaled smokes and oils.

Herbs have also traditionally been applied in a qualitatively different way from conventional drugs. Whereas drugs are primarily designed to directly affect a specific disability, herbal remedies aim to support the individual's recuperative capacities. The emphasis with herbal medicines is on gradual, long-term restoration of health rather than on the desired rapid action of a drug. Traditional views of herbal remedies emphasize their primary influence on transient body functions, that is they are classified as diaphoretics, expectorants, circulatory stimulants, diuretics, digestive stimulants and so on (Mills, 1993a). Many drugs of course could be similarly classified. Mills argues that ideally research into herbal medicine should reflect this emphasis on the supportive action of herbs, which in practice would mean an emphasis on monitoring a variety of transient clinical effects, which in turn might have an effect on diseases. 'Thus it might be more valid to say that a herb, for example, in certain individuals at least, changed the constitution of phlegm or urine, or altered circulatory activity to one or other tissues or over the body as a whole, rather than that it is statistically likely to be effective against bronchitis, urinary stones, or other disease states' (Mills, 1993a).

The argument is in effect to examine mechanism and transient effects on body function in parallel with research on outcomes. The suggestion is not that herbal treatment will not affect bronchitis, but that this is not exactly the spirit of the intervention and provides an incomplete picture of the action of the herbs and the herbalist. A further complicating factor is that some herbalists consider that the action of the herbs will vary with the patient and the nature of the disturbance.

Pharmacologists might well agree that the action of any drug or herb might vary according to the condition of the patient and a greater understanding of the multiple actions of any product would be very useful. It is not clear how far there is a real divergence of opinion on research strategy between those herbalists who are advocates of research into herbalism and doctors who are interested in the action of herbs. Probably all would agree that measuring individually-based transient effects in the course of a trial as Mills (1993a) suggests, though useful, would be complex and difficult.

Meserole (1996) has called for herbalists to undertake and become involved in research in order to preserve the holistic spirit of their practice in the research. She argues for a greater respect for traditional knowledge and for documenting the existing traditional uses of plants as part of the research process. She also argues for the importance of considering the action of a complete plant and not rushing too quickly to isolate a single active ingredient.

> Retaining a holistic context in medicinal plant research also involves addressing differences in paradigm. Involving traditional herbalists as research design consultants would protect against inadvertently eliminating a critical element of the paradigm in which the herb is used . . .

> British sailors were cured of scurvy with limes, originally presumed to be therapeutic against the disease solely because of their vitamin C content. However limes and citrus proved more effective against scurvy than vitamin C supplementation; this was largely explained by the presence of bioflavonoids, later isolated and discovered to be prevalent in citrus pulp. The desirability of performing bioassays and clinical efficacy studies on whole herbs and herbal formulas, as well as on identified active constituents is clear. (Meserole, 1996)

Many of the studies we have reviewed have followed these recommendations to the extent that whole herbs, such as garlic or *Ginkgo*, have been evaluated for their effects. Experimental studies on the constituents of the herb and their various actions may follow outcome research or proceed in parallel with it. From the point of view of the researcher, though, a central question remains. Herbalists would presumably argue that the individual approach of not only using complete plant products (rather than single constituents) but prescribing individually based combinations of natural products is somehow preferable, at least for some conditions, than the possibly more dramatic but potentially harmful actions of a drug. How this question might be addressed is not at all clear.

The difficulties of holistic enquiry mount if one wishes to examine the actual practice of herbalism. All the studies we have examined have considered single compounds in isolation, rather than the combinations that herbalists adapt to individuals. The aim of most research appears to be to provide preliminary evidence of efficacy in order that the active ingredients may be isolated. Researching herbalism as practised may be a still more complex undertaking than the already difficult task of isolating, identifying and evaluating the active constituents.

Some research in Asia has attempted to take the take the traditional diagnoses into account, but as yet without much success (Tsutani, 1993). Tsutani points out that such diagnoses could, as we have earlier discussed (see Chapter 8 and Wiegant, Kramers and van Wijk, 1993) be incorporated in standard trials particularly as many traditional diagnoses are in fact subdivisions of recognized orthodox Western diagnoses.

> In this context it is useful to understand that the zheng and sho (Chinese and Japanese traditional diagnoses) have layered structures. At the bottom each patient has a different zheng or sho and is to be treated differently, whereas at the higher level each patient conforms to a population group. Theoretically, the clinical trial could be done at the higher level without serious deviation from the individual zheng or sho diagnosis. (Tsutani, 1993)

Tsutani also points out that trials could combine orthodox endpoints, such as blood pressure in hypertension studies or blood glucose in the case of diabetes, with endpoints based on the *zheng* or *sho*. Quality of life measures appear to have some common ground with the traditional concept of better balance in the body.

In conclusion, therefore, it is clear that many herbs have therapeutic benefits either in their natural form or as sources for drugs. However, very little research has been carried out on herbalism as it is practised or on the specific claims made by herbalists concerning the value of natural products and combinations of remedies adapted to the individual.

HOMEOPATHY

In keeping with the aims and limitations of this chapter the purpose of this section is primarily to review the clinical evidence for homeopathy in the form of controlled trials. Two substantial reviews have been published (Kleijnen, Knipschild and ter Riet, 1991; Hill and Doyon, 1990) which will form the basis of our discussion, and the bulk of the material in this section is derived from these sources. We are particularly indebted to the paper by Kleijnen, Knipschild and ter Riet (1991).

Although a discussion of the mechanisms underlying complementary therapies is beyond the scope of this book, and beyond the knowledge and abilities of the authors, some discussion of the possible mechanisms that might underlie homeopathy is important because views about the probability or improbability of the mechanism have undoubtedly affected the assessment of the clinical literature. As we shall see, opinion is divided on the merits of homeopathy, but it seems fair to say that if the trials concerned an ordinary drug there would, at the very least, be no argument that further trials were warranted. The story of recent investigations into a possible mechanism for homeopathy is also illuminating in that it shows what strong feelings can be aroused within the scientific community by findings that are incompatible with accepted scientific knowledge. In this homeopathy is unusual among the major forms of complementary medicine; acupuncture, herbalism, manipulation and at least some aspects of naturopathy could, if proved effective, be explained in orthodox terms. This is not to say that the theories advanced by their practitioners could necessarily be substantiated in orthodox terms, only that the action of the therapy (needles, herbs, manipulation, dietary measures) is at least potentially explicable. Much of homeopathy, like some of the avowedly alternative practices such as radionics, is a good deal harder to explain in conventional terms.

A Mechanism for Homeopathy?

The Beneviste Affair

Homeopathy is a system in which a diluted (*potentized*) agent is used as a treatment, either singly or in combination with other agents. On the principle of *similia similibus curantur*, the agent used produces, when undiluted, complaints similar to those being treated. Potentiation is a combination of dilution and shaking of a substance. A plant—for example, *Arnica montana*—is macerated and dissolved in alcohol. One part of this *mother tincture* is mixed with nine parts (D1 potency) or 99 parts (C1 potency) of 90% alcohol and then vigorously shaken. This process may be repeated many times, resulting in very high dilutions (potencies): D6 means one molecule of the original substance in 10^6 molecules of alcohol; C6 means one molecule in 10^{12} molecules. In potencies of D24 or C12 it is very unlikely that even a single molecule of the mother tincture is present (Ullman, 1991; Kleijnen, Knipschild and ter Riet, 1991). Gibson and Gibson (1988) remind us, however, that homeopathic remedies are frequently prescribed in material doses, and that although the high dilutions are of great clinical value they are not essential to the practice of homeopathy. The idea that homeopathy principles 'strike at the very basis of chemistry' is therefore not entirely correct (Gibson and Gibson, 1988).

The idea that dilute remedies, let alone very high dilution potentized agents, should be effective treatments for a large number of disorders and complaints clearly goes against orthodox medical thinking and is arguably incompatible with the very foundations of scientific knowledge. Homeopaths and others, impressed by observations of the clinical effectiveness of homeopathy, have speculated on a possible mechanism for such an action. As Fisher (1993) has observed there has been no shortage of theories, but little in the way of substantiated experimentation. However, in June 1988, after apparently almost two years of successive referees' reports, requests for replication and initial rejections, *Nature*, the world's premier scientific journal, published a paper offering evidence that very high dilution antiserum could retain a biological action (Davenas et al, 1988). In essence the paper reported that when a type of human white blood cell, with certain antibodies of the immunoglobulin E (IgE) type, is exposed to anti-IgE antibodies, they release histamine and change their staining properties. At usual concentrations this is an ordinary finding; at dilutions of 1×10^{120} it was remarkable.

The report generated a flood of correspondence in succeeding weeks, which makes fascinating but rather depressing reading. The main themes of the correspondence were later summarized by the editor of *Nature* (Maddox, 1988). Some advocates of investigation into homeopathy welcomed it as the first step in unravelling the mechanisms of homeopathy. Most, however, were sceptical. Various suggestions were offered to explain how the findings might be in error, (contamination, human error, experimental artefacts of various kinds) but some correspondents appeared outraged that *Nature* had published the report in the first place.

A condition of publication was apparently that the Beneviste laboratory offer to replicate the experiments in the presence of a team from *Nature*. On 28 July 1988 a report by the team stated that the experiments were 'statistically ill-controlled, from which no substantial effort has been made to exclude systematic bias, and whose interpretation has been clouded by the exclusion of measurements in conflict with the claim'. Beneviste (the head of the laboratory where the research was conducted) and others were outraged by the fact that the team included a magician expert in detecting scientific fraud (although no fraud had been suggested), and saying that the team's report contained numerous inaccuracies and asking, not unreasonably, why the paper was published and then rubbished by the very same referee only a few weeks later (Beneviste, 1988). Perhaps the most important correspondence in the subsequent few weeks were two brief, non-inflammatory, reports appearing on 18 August from laboratories in New Mexico and Rome in which the experiment was repeated by other investigators who failed to replicate the results.

Some thoughtful correspondence in later weeks commented on the tone of the debate and the investigation:

> Yet the tone of the investigation . . . has been that of a grand jury looking for evidence of a crime. The elaborate security precautions taken by the Nature team on the expedition to the Beneviste laboratory are inconsistent with a simple inquiry into human error. Rather, they are the precautions of people who expect to encounter deliberate falsification. (Petsko, 1988)

The original paper was not presented as an investigation of homeopathy. It contained only a single reference to the results possibly being related to a recent double-blind study of hayfever patients treated with a high dilution of grass pollen. However, the spectre of homeopathy clearly lurked behind at least some of the furore. The editor of *Nature* raised the question in the editorial accompanying the paper; some correspondents regretted that the press would immediately claim scientific support for homeopathy, but that any subsequent negative findings were unlikely to attract the same attention. The investigative team regretted the fact that two members of Beneviste's research team were funded by a homeopathic company, a completely unwarranted criticism. The results of the majority of drug trials would have to be dismissed if those funded by pharmaceutical companies were eliminated. Beneviste, in his final comment on the affair in that particular sequence of correspondence, asked why,

> after scrutinizing the paper for two years, having urged confirmation of our initial work in independent laboratories, which was done in Canada, Israel, and Italy. Nature, short of any valid objection, published it hastily, then went to these extreme lengths to deNature it. The answer is to be found in (two

reports in Nature) . . . both of which emphasize warnings against homeopathy. (Beneviste, 27 October 1988)

It is not clear quite why such passions were aroused, although the actions
of the investigative team are some explanation; the whole affair seems to
have been both damaging and dispiriting to all concerned. However, it is a
salutary reminder of the difficulties facing anyone who seeks to convince
scientists of the virtues of homeopathy or other complementary therapies.
The tone of the 'debate' is curiously reminiscent of the correspondence after
the Bristol Cancer Help Centre study (see Chapter 11). With this in mind,
we turn to the reviews of clinical studies of homeopathy.

Clinical Trials of Homeopathy

A tremendous number of descriptive studies have been published in the
homeopathic literature, but there have been comparatively few controlled
trials carried out. As before, we will concentrate on the findings of the
controlled trials, which are of varying standard and design. They also ask a
variety of different questions. Some are comparisons of homeopathy with a
placebo (the majority), others compare homeopathy with a standard treatment and a few are comparisons between different forms of homeopathy.
It is regrettable that the two reviews (Hill and Doyon, 1990; Kleijnen,
Knipschild and ter Riet, 1991) do not always clearly distinguish the three
types of study, as clearly the implications of significant or non-significant
findings are different in each case. Non-significant differences between
homeopathy and a standard treatment could be seen as a positive finding
for homeopathy, if it proved itself as effective as a standard treatment. The
problems of defining an appropriate placebo control do not arise to the
same extent as with acupuncture, as inert capsules or solutions can be
employed. It is also both feasible and desirable to employ a double-blind
methodology.

The most comprehensive review is by Kleijnen, Knipschild and ter Riet
(1991), representing a herculean effort to track down all known controlled
trials of homeopathy. As well as the standard searches they checked
references of articles, corresponded with researchers and manufacturers
and visited several specialist libraries over a period of three years. A total
of 107 controlled trials was identified, dealing with a variety of different
conditions: diseases of the respiratory system (19 trials on respiratory
infections, 5 on hay fever and 1 on asthma); 27 trials on pain of various
kinds; gastrointestinal complaints (7 trials); diseases of the vascular system

(9 trials, 4 on hypertension); recovery of bowel movements after surgery (7 trials); psychological problems (10 trials) and a variety of other diagnoses.

The trials were of varying standard and in the next stage each study was blind-rated for methodological soundness by two of the authors. Their system, similar to that employed for acupuncture, is described in their paper and examples of the scoring given (Kleijnen, Knipschild and ter Riet, 1991). Maximum score was 100, with different methodological criteria being weighted for importance. Particular importance (30 points/100) was attached to numbers of participants in the study. Most of the conditions under treatment would improve spontaneously in any case, and large numbers would be needed to give a trial adequate power to detect a small difference between groups, in addition to the greater likelihood of equality of prognostic factors in unmatched groups. They also argued that publication bias (failure to publish negative results) was less likely in large trials as they would be deemed worthy of publication whatever the findings. Other major criteria for methodological soundness were randomization and double-blindness. Few would argue with the basic list of criteria, but it is worth noting that Hill and Doyon (1990) took a more radical view on randomization, refusing to consider any trial in which the subjects had not been satisfactorily randomized—arguing that such a major flaw invalidated a trial. The implications of the two different strategies are discussed below. It is also noteworthy that the adequacy of double-blinding (essentially asking the patients to guess which group they were in) was apparently not checked in any homeopathic trial.

Kleijnen, Knipschild and ter Riet (1991) report that overall the methodological quality of the studies was disappointing, although some good studies were reported. More than half of the publications (63) were of trials in which fewer than 25 patients per group were treated. Of the trials 68 were randomized, but only 17 described the process of randomization. The intervention was adequately or reasonably well described in 80 trials. There were 75 that were double-blind, but the placebo was described as indistinguishable in only 31 trials. In 67 publications the measurement of effect was judged to have been sensible and well described, and sufficient data were given for the reader to check the analysis in 65 trials. Some of these problems may reflect inadequacies in the reporting of the trials, rather than inadequacies in the trials themselves, but the authors point out that clarity of description is itself an important methodological consideration—especially if replication is contemplated.

Overall the findings were positive: of the 105 trials with interpretable results 81 indicated positive results, and 24 trials had negative findings when homeopathy was compared with (mostly placebo) controls (Table 10.1).

Table 10.1 Clinical trials of homeopathy grouped according to diagnoses from conventional medicine

	Indication	Score max = 100	Result
Diseases of the vascular system:			
Bignamini et al 1987	Hypertension	58	Negative
Wiesenauer & Gaus 1987	Hypertension	58	Positive
Savage 1977	Stroke	55	Negative
Gauthier 1983	Flushing	53	Negative
Savage & Roe 1978	Stroke	53	Negative
Hitzenberger et al 1982	Hypertension	48	Negative
Dorfman et al 1988	Venous perfusion	35	Positive
Hadjicostas et al 1988	Bleeding	35	Positive
Master 1987	Hypertension	13	Positive
Respiratory infections:			
Ferley et al 1989	Influenza	88	Positive
Bordes & Dorfman 1986	Coughing	70	Positive
Ferley et al 1987	Influenza	68	Negative
Maiwald et al 1988	Influenza	65	Positive
Wiesenauer et al 1989	Sinusitis	60	Negative
Gassinger et al 1981	Common cold	58	Positive
Lewith et al 1989	Influenza	55	Negative
Lecocq 1985	Respiratory infections	50	Positive
Lewis 1984	Whooping cough	49	Negative
Schmidt 1987	Bronchitis	45	Positive
Chakravarty et al 1977	Tonsillitis	38	Positive
Mössinger 1985	Otitis media	38	Positive
Davies 1971	Influenza	35	Positive
Mössinger 1973	Pharyngitis	35	Positive
Mössinger 1982	Common cold	35	Negative
Hourst 1982	Respiratory infections	28	Positive
Mössinger 1976	Pharyngitis	25	Positive
Masciello & Felesi 1985	Influenza	18	Positive
Bungetzianu 1988	Influenza	0	Negative
Other infections:			
Valero 1981	Postoperative infection	80	Negative
Valero 1981	Postoperative infection	50	Positive
Ustianowski 1974	Cystitis	45	Positive
Mössinger 1980	Furuncles	43	Positive
Subramanyam et al 1990	Filariasis	38	Positive
Carey 1986	Vaginal discharge	35	Positive
Castro & Noguiera 1975	Meningitis	13	Positive

continues overleaf

Table 10.1   (*continued*)

Indication	Score max = 100	Result
Diseases of the digestive system:		
Ritter 1966 — Gastritis	58	Positive
Rahlfs & Mössinger 1979 — Irritable colon	50	Positive
Owen 1990 — Irritable colon	35	Positive
Rahlfs & Mössinger 1976 — Irritable colon	35	Positive
Mössinger 1976 — Abdominal complaints	23	Negative
Mössinger 1974 — Cholecystopathy	15	Positive
Mössinger 1976 — Abdominal complaints	13	Negative
Pollinosis:		
Reilly et al 1986 — Pollinosis	90	Positive
Wiesenauer & Gaus 1985 — Pollinosis	85	Positive
Wiesenauer & Gaus 1986 — Pollinosis	80	*
Wiesenauer et al 1983 — Pollinosis	75	Positive
Reilly & Taylor 1985 — Pollinosis	50	Positive
Reilly et al 1990 — Asthma	35	Positive
Recovery of bowel movements after surgery:		
GRECHO 1989 — Lieus	90	Negative
Aulgnier 1985 — Lieus	75	Positive
Valero 1981 — Lieus	70	Positive
Chevrel et al 1984 — Lieus	58	Positive
Valero 1981 — Lieus	50	Positive
Estrangin 1979 — Lieus	48	Negative
Castelin 1979 — Lieus	20	Positive
Rheumatological disease:		
Shipley et al 1983 — Osteoarthritis	50	Negative
Fisher et al 1989 — Fibromyalgia	45	Positive
Gibson et al 1980 — Rheumatoid arthritis	40	Positive
Audrade et al 1988 — Rheumatoid arthritis	38	Negative
Fisher 1986 — Fibrositis	38	Positive
Gibson et al 1978 — Rheumatoid arthritis	33	Positive
Trauma or pain:		
Zell et al 1988 — Ankle sprains	80	Positive
Brigo 1987 — Migraine	68	Positive
Bourgois 1984 — Haematoma	53	Positive
Casanova 1981 — Myalgia	45	Positive
Pinsent et al 1986 — Dental extraction	45	Positive
Berthier 1985 — Dental extraction	40	Positive
Albertini et al 1984 — Dental neuralgia	38	Positive
Campbell 1976 — Bruising	38	Negative
Hildebrand & Eltze 1983 — Myalgia	38	Positive
Hildebrand & Eltze 1983 — Myalgia	38	Positive

Table 10.1 *(continued)*

	Indication	Score max=100	Result
Hildebrand & Eltze 1983	Myalgia	38	Positive
Hildebrand & Eltze 1983	Myalgia	38	Positive
Leaman & Gorman 1989	Minor burns	38	Negative
Geiger 1968	Oedema	35	Positive
Kubista et al 1986	Mastalgia	35	Positive
Michaud 1981	Oedema	35	Positive
Mergen 1969	Oedema	33*	
Caspar & Foerstel 1967	Oedema	28	Positive
Campbell 1976	Bruising	28	Positive
Khan 1985	Hallux valgus	15	Positive
Anon 1980	Cystitis	13	Positive
Mental or psychological problems:			
Delaunay 1985	Behaviour in children	48	Positive
Carlini et al 1987	Insomnia	45	Negative
Heulluy 1985	Depression	45	Positive
Ponti 1986	Travel sickness	40	Positive
Tsiakopoulos et al 1988	Vertigo	35	Positive
Vu Din Sao & Delauney 1983	Nervous tension	30	Positive
Dexpert 1987	Seasickness	25	Positive
Alibeu & Jobert 1990	Agitation	23	Positive
Davies 1988	Aluminium deficiency	23	Negative
Master 1987	Aphasia	23	Positive
Other diagnoses:			
Arnal-Laserre 1986	Duration of delivery	80	Positive
Skaliodas et al 1988	Diabetes	50	Positive
Coudert-Deguillaume 1981	Duration of delivery	45	Positive
Kennedy 1971	Postoperative complications	43	Negative
Paterson 1943	Gas poisoning	41	Positive
Basu 1980	Myopia	35	Positive
Hariveau 1987	Cramps (dialysis)	35	Positive
Kirchoff 1982	Lymphoedema	33	Positive
Kienle 1973	Respiratory insufficiency	30	Positive
Paterson 1943	Gas poisoning	28	Positive
Ventonskovskiy & Popov 1990	Complications of delivery	22	Positive
Schwab 1990	Skin diseases	20	Positive
Schwab 1990	Skin diseases	20	Positive
Mössinger 1976	Cramps (legs)	13	Negative
Khan & Rawal 1976	Verruca plantaris	0	Positive

* Comparison of homeopathic treatments.

(From Kleijnen, Knipschild and ter Riet, 1991. Reproduced by permission of the BMJ Publishing Group)

However, the methodology of many of these trials is quite poor with 83 scoring 55 or below and only 16 scoring 60 or above. Most worrying is the fact that in 42 trials there was insufficient data to check the authors' interpretation of the outcomes; it is not clear if there was just no data at all or whether there was insufficient data to check the statistical analysis. Mindful of the fact that more positive findings can be associated with poorer methodology the authors separated out the best studies, those scoring at least 60/100. Their table of these studies is shown in Table 10.2.

Ten of the best studies show an advantage for homeopathy against four negative findings (and one which is inapplicable in that it was a comparison of homeopathic treatments). If the cut-off is set a little lower at 55 points, the finding is similar at 15 positive and seven showing no difference between groups. The important possibility of publication bias is carefully considered. Negative findings might not be reported in complementary journals but, on the other hand, might be more readily accepted in a mainstream medical journal. There was no relation between the results and the place of publication. The authors tried to decrease the effect of publication bias by making many attempts to discover any unpublished trials: very few unpublished studies emerged.

The discussion of the paper is thoughtful and especially interesting in the light of the authors' own avowed scepticism about homeopathy. Their scepticism appears to have been at least dented, in that they conclude that 'we would be ready to accept that homeopathy can be efficacious, if only the mechanism of action were more plausible'. Before considering this conclusion further, we will summarize the rather different approach and conclusions of Hill and Doyon (1990).

Hill and Doyon restricted their review to randomized controlled trials; any non-randomized trials, pseudo-randomized with a predictable assignment before inclusion in the trial, such as alternate assignment, and any trials showing an obvious misunderstanding of randomization were excluded. This left 40 trials whose results were summarized.

A variety of different disorders was considered. Trials were generally a straightforward group comparison, except for seven which used a cross-over design. Most were placebo controlled, with the exception of four in which the comparison was a standard therapy. These four trials are asking a different question, and it is not clear that they should be grouped with the placebo-controlled trials. All except seven trials were stated to be double-blind, though there were doubts about the adequacy of the blinding in one trial. Few trials used a clearly defined main endpoint. Only three

Table 10.2 Characteristics and results of best trials of homeopathy

	Score for methodology (max-100)	Indication (No. of patients/No. of controls)	Results (No. of patients/ No. of controls)
		Homeopathic combinations v. placebo	
Ferley et al 1989	88	Treatment of influenza (H v P)	Recovery rate within 48 hours (17.1%/10.3%)
Arnal-Laserre 1986	80	Duration of delivery (H v P)	Duration of delivery: (5.1/ 8.5 hours); 'Dystocie' [problems with dilation] (11.3%/40%)
Zell et al 1988	80	Ankle sprains (H v P)	No. of patients without pain after 10 days: (28/13)
Aulagnier 1985	75	Bowel movements after abdominal operation (H v P)	Days until first flatus (2.5/ 3.2); days until first faeces (4.0/4.9)
Bordes & Dorfman 1986	70	Dry cough (H v P)	Very good or good result after 1 week (20/8)
Ferley et al 1987	68	Prevention and treatment of influenza (H v P)	Incidence (6.5%/7.2%); duration of symptoms (7.0/ 6.8 days)
Maiwald et al 1988	65	Influenza (H v Aspirin)	Positive result within 4 days (29%/23%)
Wiesenauer et al 1989	60	Sinusitis (H, H, H, P)	Combination score of 6 symptoms (no difference between the 4 groups)
		Same formula in all patients	
GRECHO 1989	90	Bowel movements after abdominal operation (4 groups of 150) (H, H, P, NT)	Time until 1st faeces: (1)96 hours; (2)99 hours; (3)94 hours; (4)95 hours. Similar results for 1st peristaltic sounds and 1st flatus
Wiesenauer & Gause 1985	85	Pollinosis (H, H, P)	Improvement of nasal symptoms after 4 weeks: (1)78%; (2)51%; (3)58%. Similar results for ocular symptoms
Valero 1981	80	Postoperative infections (H v P)	No. of patients with infection (15/20)
Valero 1981	70	Bowel movements after abdominal operation (H v P)	Time until 1st flatus (53.3/ 58.6 hours)
Wiesenauer et al 1983	75	Pollinosis (H v P)	Improvement of symptoms after 4 weeks: (1)81%; (2)57%

continues overleaf

Table 10.2 *(continued)*

	Score for methodology (max-100)	Indication (No. of patients/No. of controls)	Results (No. of patients/No. of controls)
		Single remedy v placebo	
Reilly et al 1986	90	Pollinosis (H v P)	Change in 100 mm visual analogue scale symptom score after 5 weeks (–17.2mm/–2.6mm)
		Classical homeopathy v placebo	
Brigo 1987	68	Migraine (H v P)	Change in 10cm visual analogue scale symptom score after 4 months (–6.2cm/–0.6cm). Similar results for frequency and duration of attacks

H = Homeopathy; P = Placebo; NT = No treatment

(From Kleijnen, Knipschild and ter Riet, 1991. Reproduced by permission of the BMJ Publishing Group)

trial reports specified a sample size calculation. The number of patients varied enormously, between 10 and almost 600 per group with a median of 28 per group.

Clearly a possible criticism of some of the smaller trials is that they were not large enough to reliably detect any differences in treatments. Imbalances in group size were reported in a number of trials. Statistically this is not in itself important, but Hill and Doyon are concerned that it could indicate unreported exclusions of certain patients or disguise early dropouts. Half of the reports conclude that homeopathy is effective, and seven others conclude that the results are promising but the sample size is too small to permit valid conclusions. None of the trials mention any side-effects. Hill and Doyon single out the three largest trials for special mention; they are well conducted and clearly of an adequate sample size (unless homeopathic effects are so slight as to be clinically meaningless). The trials found one negative and one positive result in the treatment of influenza (Ferley et al, 1987; 1989) and the third (Mayaux et al, 1988) found no effect on postoperative bowel problems. These trials also score highly on Kleijnen's methodological criteria.

Hill and Doyon preface their summary by suggesting that there are numerous sources of bias in most of the trials and conclude that there is insufficient evidence for the efficacy of homeopathy. Apart from the three largest trials, most of the others had major flaws: most had only a very small number of patients, and hence could only detect very large effects, and many others were biased by the exclusion of patients during the analysis. They conclude, reasonably, that the therapeutic value of homeopathy has not been demonstrated. Less reasonably they conclude that there is no justification for further expensive trials. This is a curious piece of logic. If the trials are too small to detect differences between treatments, and yet there are a considerable number of positive findings, then surely there is a possibility that larger trials may detect significant differences. Admittedly, tighter methodology may reveal that earlier positive findings were due to design flaws, but there is certainly evidence that suggests that there might be a positive effect.

Disputed Findings: Improbable Mechanism

It is a very curious feature of both these reviews that homeopathic treatments for all manner of different problems are grouped and evaluated together. Under no circumstances would the results for drug treatment of digestive, respiratory, allergic psychological symptoms be grouped together. The relatively small number of trials in each grouping means that no other strategy is possible at the moment, but it should at least be borne in mind that homeopathy might be effective in only some of these conditions.

The reviews have different strengths as well as different conclusions. That of Kleijnen and colleagues is very much more thorough in its approach, with an admirably exhaustive search and a clear assessment of methodological criteria. There is no doubt that the weighting of the criteria could be disputed, as acknowledged by the authors, but it seems unlikely that the ranking of trials would be greatly changed. Of greater concern is the fact that other factors may weaken the strength of the conclusions. For instance, the high scoring trial of Reilly et al (1986) was criticized for excluding patients from the analysis; Colquhoun (1990) claimed that the result was in fact negative on reanalysis. Even if such criticisms were valid, it seems improbable that this would apply to all Kleijnen's high-scoring trials.

An acknowledgement in Doyon and Hill's review makes it clear that they began with Kleijnen and colleagues' list of trials; in fact each set of authors acknowledges the other. Doyon and Hill's evaluation strategy was different, essentially to treat adequate randomization as an essential criteria of an adequate trial. This meant that at least one of Kleijnen's top trials was excluded from their analysis (Baum, 1991). It is unfortunate that they did not then go on and develop methodological criteria of their own to examine the quality of trials in relation to outcome.

Kleijnen, Knipschild and ter Riet (1991), in spite of the generally positive nature of their conclusions, state that the evidence is probably not sufficient for most people to form a definite view. They do suggest that the evidence is sufficiently positive to warrant further large-scale trials, under rigorous double-blind conditions, with human subjects. The series of papers on recovery of bowel function seems to have been brought to an end by a large collaborative trial with negative findings (GRECHO, 1989) and similar large studies might resolve other conflicting findings. It would also be helpful if studies on animals or plant material, where at least some sources of bias are reduced, could be conducted; existing studies appear to be unsatisfactory (Scofield, 1984).

Kleijnen, Knipschild and ter Riet (1991) are surely right to suggest that collaboration between advocates of homeopathy and sceptics is likely to lead to the most trustworthy trials; the ubiquitous experimenter effects should at least be balanced equally in terms of bias. The question, as they say, is how many trials would be needed before the weight of evidence became convincing. The evidence, while disputed, would certainly warrant continuing investigation of any drug with a similar weight of trial results behind it. The methodological problems do not appear to be very different from those found in many other treatment trials. Yet again, it comes back to the implausibility of the mechanism: 'Are the results of randomized double blind trials convincing only if there is a plausible mechanism of action? Are review articles of the clinical evidence only convincing if there is a plausible mechanism of action? Or is this a special case because the mechanisms are unknown or implausible?' (Kleijnen, Knipschild and ter Riet, 1991).

There is no absolute answer to these questions. However, given its extensive use, and the positive findings in at least a proportion of trials, we consider like Kleijnen and colleagues that the problem needs resolving with larger trials. Even if homeopathy is unlikely to replace, or even supplement, more conventional medication there is still an argument for serious trials. If homeopathy is a placebo, then patients need to know this—as a matter of fact not simply opinion. Unless trials are carried out to resolve this question, then any informed person can say that it is still an open question whether homeopathy works and, furthermore, that the reluctance of the medical profession to carry out or even recommend clinical trials is hardly evidence of a clear-sighted, even-handed attitude. If the evidence mounts opinions may soften and (the logical consequence) the search for a mechanism would become imperative. Conversely, the question of mechanism will die should the larger trials not be supportive.

NATUROPATHY

More than any other complementary system, the essence of naturopathy is therapeutic eclecticism. Doctors of naturopathic medicine may use any of a wide range of techniques spanning lifestyle advice, dietary instruction and detoxification through breathing exercises, hydrotherapy and other complementary techniques, to the orthodox use of conventional prescription drugs and even surgery. The developmental history of the naturopathic movement is marked by the sequential adoption of a variety of therapeutic schools of thought with their associated practices. These have included the nature cure movement, vegetarianism, the hygienic school, autotoxicity and colonic revitalization, Thomsonianism, homeopathy, Christian Science and the physical culture movement. More recent influences include clinical nutrition and clinical ecology. A naturopathic physician may therefore use a variety of different approaches and methods. The very diversity of the elements of a naturopathic approach means that conventional outcome studies, in which patients might be randomly allocated to a naturopathic physician or to some other control condition and their progress compared, are unlikely to yield much in the way of understanding the therapeutic potential of the many different ingredients of the naturopathic programme (Micozzi, 1996).

The American Association of Naturopathic Physicians (AANP) expresses this problem as follows:

> Naturopathic physicians typically administer several treatments simultaneously, on the principle that treatments acting through different mechanisms may be more effective than any one of them used alone. They tailor groups of treatments to fit the individual needs of the patient. These complex protocols have only rarely been formally tested, although many of the individual treatments have been subjected to controlled trials. The orthodox approach of only testing single agents and the need for controlled conditions comes into conflict with the naturopathic practice of using protocols and adapting them to the patient's needs. Financial constraints also make the costs of evaluation of complex protocols prohibitive in some cases. (Bergner, 1991)

The potential range of naturopathic techniques is long and, for this reason, the range of research that is potentially relevant to the evaluation of the naturopathic approach is vast. These research areas include clinical nutrition (any dietary treatment of chronic disease), herbal medicine, hydrotherapy, manipulative therapies, oriental medicine including acupuncture, homeopathy and various psychological techniques. We have already examined the efficacy of some of these techniques and it is not feasible to examine all the others in similar depth. However, evidence on dietary manipulation and food supplements, using naturopathic techniques, will be briefly examined.

Dietary Manipulation

It is well known that lifestyle factors such as smoking, alcohol intake, exercise levels, and fat and salt consumption can affect the risk of developing cardiovascular disease, cancer and a variety of other diseases. However, a considerable number of different studies suggest that dietary manipulation can also have a therapeutic effect on diseases that have already developed. For instance, several epidemiological studies suggested that a vegetarian diet was associated with reduced blood pressure. These initial observations were confirmed, and therapeutic effects of a vegetarian diet demonstrated, in a controlled cross-over trial with normal subjects during a 14-week trial (Rouse et al, 1983), and in a further study of patients with hypertension by Margetts et al (1986). Stamler et al (1987) reported a four-year controlled study of patients with hypertension which found that a combination of reduction of weight, salt intake and alcohol intake brought about considerable reductions in hypertension, sufficient to replace drug therapy in many patients.

Early reports of dietary changes for rheumatoid arthritis suggested that it could be beneficial for at least a proportion of patients. However, Panush et al (1983) found no evidence of improvement in a small controlled trial of a restricted diet and Skolstan et al (1979) found no effect from a vegetarian diet in another small controlled trial. In contrast, Darlington, Ramsey and Mansfield (1986), in a larger study comparing a much stricter dietary regime with placebo, found evidence of significant objective improvements compared with placebo particularly among 'good responders'. They suggest that the reason that early studies failed to find effects might be that only a proportion of patients are helped. It would be unlikely that effects on a subset of patients would be discerned in a small trial. Darlington and colleagues commented that:

> it is one thing to describe improvement . . . and quite another to explain how it may work. There are several possible mechanisms which, singly or in combination, could explain improvement on dietary therapy in rheumatoid arthritis. It may be due to reduction in genuine intolerance of foods or perhaps to correction of abnormalities of absorption of food or bacterial antigens, particularly in patients on non-steroidal anti-inflammatory therapy. The weight losses during the study may also have had beneficial effects on disease activity.

Open trials of exclusion diets have also shown pronounced benefits with irritable bowel syndrome, with a wide range of foods being identified during subsequent challenge as possible triggers of symptoms (Nanda et al, 1989).

Food Supplements

Supplementation with vitamins and minerals is also frequently advocated by naturopaths. Supplements where there is clear vitamin or other nutritional deficiency, from whatever cause, is not disputed in orthodox circles. The use of vitamin supplements, perhaps in high doses, by people who would be considered to have an adequate diet is more contentious. Kleijnen and colleagues have published several reviews of the more common uses of vitamin supplements. For instance after reviewing 11 controlled trials of the use of vitamin C for the common cold, they concluded that there is no prophylactic (preventative) effect of vitamin C on the common cold, but as a therapy it might exert some small effect (Kleijnen, ter Riet and Knipschild, 1989). Bielory and Gandhi (1994) found that there were some promising and positive studies of a therapeutic effect of vitamin C on asthma, though there were a number of negative findings. Most trials, however, were of too short duration to permit meaningful conclusions and they recommend the monitoring of long-term supplementation, especially given the large sums expended on vitamin supplements. In a later review of six controlled trials of vitamin E in angina pectoris and five of vitamin E in intermittent claudication, Kleijnen and colleagues concluded that vitamin E probably had a positive effect, especially on intermittent claudication (Kleijnen, ter Riet and Knipschild, 1989). After a review of 53 controlled trials of niacin, vitamin B6, and multivitamins on mental functions they concluded that virtually all trials showed serious shortcomings (Kleijnen et al, 1991). There were some positive effects for autism, but little indication for any effect for hyperactivity, Down's syndrome, schizophrenia and on other measures of psychological functioning in adults. A search for studies on the use of vitamin B6 on premenstrual syndrome yielded 12 trials, most with too few patients to permit meaningful conclusions. Evidence for the therapeutic efficacy of vitamin B6 was assessed as weak, at least until better designed trials were conducted (Kleijnen, Knipschild and ter Riet, 1991).

Researching the Naturopathic Approach

There is then some evidence for a number of the specific approaches used by naturopaths. A few of the techniques, especially those concerning dietary changes, are quite firmly embedded in orthodox medicine, although not quite given the status and importance attached to them by naturopaths. The essence of the naturopathic approach, however, and what most clearly distinguishes it from other complementary approaches, is its therapeutic eclecticism. Is it possible to assess the efficacy of the naturopathic approach rather than the efficacy of specific techniques and regimes?

The AANP has approached this question by summarizing scientific evidence for a variety of techniques used by naturopaths in the treatment of otitis media (middle ear infection), hypertension and rheumatoid arthritis. We will illustrate their approach by discussing rheumatoid arthritis before considering a trial which, although not designated as naturopathic, does embody many naturopathic principles and does consider the impact of the combination of a number of different therapeutic approaches.

In rheumatoid arthritis the principal objectives of naturopathic protocols include the reduction of pain with non-toxic and/or non-pharmacological agents, the reduction of inflammation, enhancing various lifestyle factors including improving diet, increasing exercise and, where appropriate, reducing weight. As with all naturopathic approaches special emphasis is placed upon the natural homeostatic self-healing mechanisms of the body. Despite this naturopaths do not claim to 'cure' rheumatoid arthritis but to assist the body in combating the disease. The contrasting approaches of naturopathy and orthodox medicine are shown in Box 10.1.

In reviewing the available scientific evidence for the effectiveness of naturopathic medicine for the treatment of rheumatoid arthritis, Bergner (1991)—in a document prepared on behalf of the AANP—identified 18 'suggestive' studies and a further 18 controlled trials which he considers to be supportive of the approach (Table 10.3). The suggestive studies include uncontrolled, epidemiological and animal studies, none of which has a strong bearing on the evaluation of therapeutic outcome. The controlled studies cover 10 broad domains of activity including dietary adjustment, fasting, exercise, hydrotherapy, homeopathy and acupuncture.

The four double-blind trials include two studies of homeopathy, one of acupuncture and one of dietary supplement (with Omega-3 fatty acids). Given the diversity of this list of interventions it is difficult to know exactly what it is one might be evaluating in examining the evidence for the effectiveness of the naturopathic approach. For example, homeopathy and acupuncture are widely varying techniques with substantially different therapeutic rationales. With this in mind, it could be argued that any evidence for the effectiveness of any complementary medicine approach or technique in any area of health care is *de facto* evidence for the value of the naturopathic approach.

Box 10.1 Contrasting approaches to the treatment of rheumatoid arthritis

	Naturopathic protocols	Orthodox treatment
Approach	The naturopathic strategy is to reduce pain with non-toxic or non-pharmacological agents as much as possible, reduce inflammation, and to instill positive lifestyle factors such as weight reduction, increased exercise (especially water exercises), and improved diet. Special attention is put on the digestive and eliminative processes, to encourage the body's own self-healing mechanisms. See accompanying protocol for more details and scientific backing for each treatment	Conventional treatment consists of drug therapy to manage pain, reduce inflammation, and slow progression of the disease Most patients are treated with non-steroidal anti-inflammatory drugs (NSAID). About 25% of patients require stronger drugs, such as gold injections, penicillamine, and methotrexate
Rate of success	Naturopathic medicine does not claim to cure arthritis. Many studies (see, for example, Table 10.3) show that naturopathic methods can improve both subjective and objective measures of the severity of the disease. Success may be limited by patients' willingness to make lifestyle changes. Naturopathic physicians refer cases of uncontrolled rheumatoid arthritis to MD specialists	There is no known cure for rheumatoid arthritis. Conventional drug therapy can reduce both subjective and objective measures of the disease. About 10% of patients progress to severe crippling despite any known treatment
Adverse effects and risks	No significant adverse effects to naturopathic treatments are known	Potentially life-threatening side-effects from gastrointestinal bleeding occur on 2–4% of patients taking NSAID. Other side-effects are more dangerous and more frequent in patients taking stronger drugs
Long-term effects	The need for naturopathic treatment may decline over time, as lifestyle changes are implemented. Naturopathic treatment lowers risk factors and the costs associated with subsequent heart disease, cancer, stroke, and other chronic diseases	Conventional treatment is considered permanent, although the disease tends to remit naturally and joint damage slows down within six years for about two-thirds of patients. The life expectancy of patients with rheumatoid arthritis is reduced by about five years. Drug-induced infection and gastrointestinal bleeding are major contributors to the increased mortality rate

(Adapted from Bergner, 1991. Reproduced by permission.)

Table 10.3 Scientific support for naturopathic protocols: rheumatoid arthritis

Protocols	Scientific support		
After routine history, physical, lab work and diagnosis, individualized treatment might include:	Double-blind clinical trials	Other controlled studies	Suggestive studies including uncontrolled trials
Examine nutritional status for either primary or secondary nutrient deficiencies		Helliwell	McDuffie
Adjust diet or supplement with appropriate vitamins or minerals		Balough Simkin Svenson	
Screen for food allergies or sensitivities		Hicklin Darlington	Marshall
Increase exercise to appropriate level		Lyngbert Minor	
Treat pain with natural anti-inflammatory agents, e.g. bromelain, licorice root, turmeric		Cohen	Ghatak Tangri Kuroyanagi Arora Okimasa Srimal
Consider supplementing or increasing dietary Omega-3 fatty acids	Cleland	Kremer Sperling	
Consider appropriate fast		Uden Skoldsam	Kroker Marshall
Treat with hydrotherapy		O'Hare	
Treat with homeopathy	Gibson Gibson		
Treat with acupuncture (only NDs specializing in this procedure)	Ruchkin		Junnila Xi

Table 10.3   (*continued*)

Protocols	Scientific support		
After routine history, physical, lab work and diagnosis, individualized treatment might include:	Double-blind clinical trials	Other controlled studies	Suggestive studies including uncontrolled trials
Treat deficient digestion (achlorhydria, hypochlorhydria) with bitter tonics			DeWitte Hartung
Treat symptomatically with salicylate-containing plant medicines, e.g. willow bark or poplar buds			Lewis
Treat with sedative plants, e.g. valerian, scullcap			Boeters Kurnakov

(Adapted from Bergner, 1991. Reproduced by permission.)

(References can be found in the original document of the American Association of Naturopathic Physicians)

Researching a Combination of Therapeutic Measures

Similar diversity of potentially relevant therapeutic ingredients is very much a feature of psychotherapy. In this context, Shapiro (1981) argued that to compare the overall performance of two global approaches to psychotherapy in a randomized treatment trial was metaphorically tantamount to comparing the performance of two pharmacies by sweeping all the pills off the shelves of each into two separate sacks and randomly distributing them to patients. If the two sacks yield different results one is none the wiser about what was and was not therapeutic. Shapiro suggested that a more rational approach would be to study clearly identifiable elements of the therapies. This is difficult where composite therapies, like naturopathy, are concerned.

The counterargument to this view is that in simply evaluating the individual components one loses any perception of the overall value of the approach. This is especially true if the therapeutic force of the naturopathic approach derives from the fact that the individual elements of the approach interact with each other. It may also be very important to examine how powerful the combination of measures is. Isolating these elements in a tightly controlled study will not provide a fair test of their therapeutic potential. Clearly it is difficult to assess an overall approach if it varies widely for each patient. The problems alluded to by Shapiro then become insuperable. However, successful trials have been conducted not of naturopathy *per se* but of combinations of methods based on lifestyle changes rather than orthodox, more invasive and dramatic interventions. An example of such an approach, which might be described as naturopathic in spirit, is the Lifestyle Heart Trial.

Lifestyle Heart Trial: Naturopathic in Spirit

The Lifestyle Heart Trial was the first randomized controlled trial to determine whether cardiac patients outside hospital could be motivated to make and sustain comprehensive lifestyle changes and, if so, whether regression of coronary atherosclerosis could occur as a result of lifestyle changes alone. Other trials evaluating treatments for atherosclerosis primarily involve drugs and surgery. In this trial 28 patients were assigned to the lifestyle intervention, described below, and 20 to a usual-care control group. Progression or regression of coronary artery lesions was assessed in both groups by quantitative coronary angiography after one year and a variety of other indices were routinely monitored (Ornish et al, 1990).

The intervention was comprehensive, systematic and demanding. We will only summarize the main points:

> The intervention began with a week-long residential retreat at a hotel to teach the lifestyle intervention to the experimental-group patients. Patients then attended regular group support meetings (4 hours twice a week).
>
> Experimental group patients were asked to eat a low-fat vegetarian diet for at least a year. The diet included fruits, vegetables, grains, legumes and soybean products without calorific restriction. No animal products were allowed except egg white and one cup per day of non-fat milk. Salt was restricted for hypertensive patients, caffeine eliminated and alcohol restricted.
>
> Stress management techniques included stretching exercises, breathing techniques, meditation, progressive relaxation and imagery. The purpose of each technique was to increase the patient's sense of relaxation, concentration and awareness. Patients were asked to practice their stress management techniques for at least 1 hour per day.

Patients were individually prescribed exercise levels (typically walking) according to their baseline treadmill tests and trained to identify their own exertion levels. They were asked to exercise for a minimum of 3 hours per week and for a minimum of 30 minutes each session.

The twice weekly group discussions provided social support to help patients adhere to the lifestyle change programme. The sessions were led by a clinical psychologist who facilitated discussion of strategies for maintaining adherence to the programme, communication skills, and expression of feelings about relationships at home and at work.

The programme showed that patients with coronary heart disease could be motivated to make comprehensive lifestyle changes. The reductions in blood cholesterol (serum lipid levels) were similar to those obtained with medication. The intervention appeared safe and compatible with other forms of treatment.

After a year the patients who had undergone the programme showed significant regression of their atherosclerosis as measured by coronary arteriography (i.e. the narrowing of their arteries was reduced permitting greater blood flow). Even small changes can produce marked effects on overall mobility and functioning. In contrast, the patients receiving the standard coronary care, which included a 30% fat diet, showed progression of their coronary heart disease. There was a strong relationship between adherence to the programme and improvements in clinical condition. Since degree of stenosis (narrowing) was associated with extent of lifestyle change, small changes in lifestyle may slow the progression of atherosclerosis, but major changes in lifestyle may be required to halt or reverse coronary atherosclerosis.

Ornish and colleagues comment that many important questions remain unanswered. It is not clear whether such comprehensive lifestyle changes can be sustained in a larger group of patients with heart disease, especially as it appears that adherence must be very good for substantial change to occur. This is clearly an important issue for any naturopathic regime. They also comment that further research is needed to determine the respective contributions of the various components of the programme. Though there is already at least suggestive evidence for the efficacy of most of the components, but it is not clear which ones make the most substantial contribution.

The study identified 1133 (3.7%) of patients with disabling injuries caused by medical treatment (adverse events). Errors in management were identified in 58% of adverse events, of which nearly half were judged to have been caused by negligence. In 27.6% the injury was judged to be the result of negligent care, thus about 1% of admissions resulted in some negligent treatment. In more than 70% of injured patients the injuries led to minimal or moderate disability of less than six months' duration, but in 7% it was permanent and 14% of patients died in part as a result of their treatment. Standards of care varied considerably, with hospital rates of adverse events varying tenfold. Nearly half (48%) of the events were associated with an operation, but drug complications were the most common problem (19%) overall.

The authors concluded that medical injury in hospitalized patients is more frequent than is generally recognized, and that reduction of iatrogenic injury requires both improved methods of detection and the development of mechanisms to prevent errors (Leape et al, 1991). If their results are extrapolated to Britain, with approximately eight million hospital admissions per annum in England alone (DHSS, 1991) they suggest that about 320 000 injuries are sustained in England per annum, with 80 000 being due to negligence.

Another important cause of adverse events stems from inappropriate use of drugs, either by patients or staff, or unforeseen side-effects of medication. A substantial proportion of hospital admissions are drug related. Drug-related admissions can be caused by numerous factors, such as adverse drug reactions (ADRs), drug interactions, erroneous drug use, inadequate or improper therapy, and exacerbation of or complications to disease resulting from non-compliance with prescribed therapy. Einarson (1993) examined 36 studies, covering 49 hospitals, of rates of drug-related admissions to hospital. Drug-related admissions accounted for approximately 5% of all admissions in industrialized countries, though Einarson suggests that the true percentage may be much higher. Cook and Ferner (1993) found that only about half of potential adverse reactions to drugs known by patients were recorded in the medical notes. The prevalence of reported admissions resulting from ADRs ranged from 0.2% to 21.7%, partly accounted for by wide variations in methods of reporting and assessment. Of these ADRs 71.5% were side-effects, 16.8% excessive effects, 11.3% hypersensitivity reactions and 0.4% idiosyncratic; 3.7% of patients admitted for ADRs died. Eleven of the reports suggested that on average 22.7% of ADRs were induced by non-compliance by patients.

The point of describing these rather unnerving findings is not to denigrate the achievements of modern medicine, still less to recommend a wholesale move towards complementary forms of treatment. Our aim is, as before, to provide a context for any discussion of the dangers of complementary forms of treatment. The risks and benefits of any treatment must be assessed in relation to the risks and benefits of alternative treatments, or in relation to the risks and benefits of not intervening at all. The potential adverse effects of orthodox medical treatment may also be important in another way, as a reason for patients turning to complementary medicine. It is not clear what appreciation the general public has of these risks. However, even this cursory survey of iatrogenic disease suggests that a substantial number of people may have suffered adversely from their medical treatment at one time or another, which could provide a motivation to seek other safer (even if less effective) forms of treatment.

ADVERSE EFFECTS OF COMPLEMENTARY MEDICINE

Randomized controlled trials and clinical audit are less well developed in complementary than in orthodox medicine, and the same applies to the auditing of adverse effects. There are almost no studies which examine the rate of adverse effects. The literature consists mainly of isolated case reports, usually made by doctors who have seen the patient after the complementary practitioner. A number of reviews have attempted to draw this scattered literature together, but they can only give an indication of the kind of problems that may arise, not the overall safety of a procedure. With this proviso in mind we turn to the individual therapies.

Adverse Effects of Acupuncture

The reported adverse effects of acupuncture mainly concern damage caused directly by the insertion of needles. There are few reports of adverse effects of the treatment *per se*, in the sense that the treatment caused a deterioration in a patient's condition or interacted adversely with some other concurrent treatment. In this latter, iatrogenic sense acupuncture appears, on the extremely limited evidence available, to be very safe. There are, however, a considerable number of case reports of damage of various kinds, which have been reviewed by Rampes and James (1995). The following account is derived from their comprehensive article.

Rampes and James reviewed all English language papers reporting adverse effects of acupuncture between 1966 and 1993, using standard computer databases (e.g. Medline) and extensive cross-referencing. There were a total of 395 cases of complications. These are summarized in Table 11.1. Some

Table 11.1 Complications of acupuncture

Complication	Cases
Bleeding	1
Bruising	2
Burns (eschars, scars)	3
Cardiac trauma	4
Compartment syndrome	1
Contact dermatitis	5
Deep venous thrombophlebitis	2
Drowsiness	79
Endocarditis	3
Erythema	4
Granuloma	2
Haematoma	1
Haemothorax	2
Hepatitis	126
Herpes zoster reactivation	1
Koebner phenomenon	1
Multiple lymphocytoma cutis	1
Osteomyelitis	1
Pain	2
Perichondritis	12
Peripheral nerve injury	3
Pneumothorax	32
Renal injury and calculi	17
Retained needle (X-ray findings)	12
Septicaemia	3
Spinal cord injury	19
Spinal infection	1
Subarachnoid haemorrhage	2
Syncope	53

(From Rampes and James, 1995. Reproduced by
permission of the British Medical Acupuncture Society)

were minor, such as bleeding, lightheadedness or fainting, bruising, pain during treatment, drowsiness after treatment (over half the patients in one study) and minor burns from the use of moxibustion (a technique in which acupuncture points are warmed by burning herbs on the skin). There have also been reports of various allergic reactions to the metals used in the needles.

After excluding some speculative reports and minor complications, Rampes and James reported a total of 216 instances of serious complications worldwide over a 20-year period. They comment that, considering the large numbers of people receiving acupuncture treatment each year, these figures are reassuring. Nevertheless, some of the complications were undoubtedly serious. There have been many reports of pneumothorax, resulting from puncturing the pleura and lung when the needle is inserted in the thorax, particularly in the intercostal spaces. All the cases reported were admitted and treated with chest drains leading to successful recovery. Only one fatality due to acupuncture was reported, in which a needle penetrated the pericardium of the heart. This was a case of self-administered acupuncture, a practice which has also led to two cases of deep venous thrombosis. There have been several reports of trauma to the spinal cord, particularly from Japan, and various other injuries.

Infections from needles are, of course, a major concern. Press needles are small needles or studs which are left in place during treatment for days or weeks. They are often used in the treatment of addictions. They may cause local infections, which can become more serious. Three cases of bacterial endocarditis and several cases of septicaemia have been associated with this technique. There have a number of definitive reports of Hepatitis B, and other forms of hepatitis. The first report in the United Kingdom in 1977 was influential in encouraging a shift to the use of disposable needles. There has been much speculation about the transmission of AIDS through acupuncture, but no proven cases. There were very few reports of any interactions between acupuncture and drug treatments, though they caution against bleeding in patients on anticoagulants.

Rampes and James point out that most of these problems can be avoided by competent practitioners. Pneumothorax is easily avoided with some basic anatomical knowledge and a degree of caution. The use of disposable needles minimizes risk of cross-infection provided a proper sterile procedure is followed for disposal of the needles. They suggest that there are certain contraindications for acupuncture, primarily for patients on anticoagulants (for fear of bleeding) and that press needles should not be used on patients with prosthetic or damaged cardiac valves, because of the risk of infection. Overall, however, acupuncture appears to be a basically safe technique in the hands of a competent practitioner.

A summary of individual case reports gives a very useful indicator of the types of complications that may occur, but cannot tell us how often they occur. Given the number of acupuncture treatments that take place worldwide, the reported rate of complications seems low. There does not appear to have been a direct study of the rate of complications, but additional information comes from a study of 1135 Norwegian doctors and 197 acupuncturists (Norheim and Fonnebo, 1995) who were asked if they had encountered adverse effects of acupuncture in their practice.

Adverse effects were reported by 12% of doctors and 31% of acupuncturists (see Table 11.2), the higher rate among acupuncturists probably

Table 11.2 Adverse effects of acupuncture reported by Norwegian doctors and acupuncturists

Type of adverse effect	Number of patients with adverse effects reported by acupuncturists	Number of patients with adverse effects reported by doctors
Mechanical organ injury		
Pneumothorax	8	25
Burns from moxa	1	3
Paraesthesia/numbness	1	0
Nerve injury	0	3
Forgotten needle	0	1
Infections		
Local skin infection	2	66
Perichondritis	0	16
Arthritis/osteomyelitis	0	4
Endocarditis	0	2
Hepatitis B virus	0	1
Myostitis	0	1
Peritonitis	0	1
Pleural emphysema	0	1
Other adverse effects		
Psychiatric problems	0	20
Fainting during treatment	132	10
Increased pain	25	31
Menstruation disturbance	1	2
Lymphoedema	2	0
Insomnia	1	0
Malaise	1	0
Angina pectoris	1	0
Epileptic seizure	1	0
Nausea/vomiting	25	0
Delayed doctor-contact	0	10
Chylothorax	0	3
Sweat hypersecretion	0	1
Granulomatous infection	0	1
Total number of patients reported with adverse effects	201	202

(From Norheim and Fonnebo, 1995. Reproduced by permission of The Lancet Ltd.)

being explained by their greater volume of acupuncture treatments. Pneumothorax, fainting, local infections and increased pain were fairly common, whereas hepatitis, arthritis, osteomyelitis and endocarditis were rarely encountered. Since only 10% of doctors were questioned, a minimum estimate of 250 cases in Norway to date seems warranted. The authors comment that conventional medical education alone does not seem to

Table 11.3   Nature of complications in manipulative
therapy

Vertebral artery injury	84	(65.1%)
Cervical fracture and/or dislocation	6	(4.7%)
Cervical fracture and metastasis	2	(1.6%)
Cervical pre-existing tumor	2	(1.6%)
Cervical disc rupture	2	(1.6%)
Tracheal rupture	1	(0.7%)
Diaphragmatic paralysis	1	(0.7%)
Thoracic disc rupture	3	(2.3%)
Meningeal haematoma	1	(0.7%)
Lumbar disc rupture	8	(6.2%)
Cauda equina syndrome	16	(12.4%)
Femoral compression neuropathy	1	(0.7%)
Lumbar vertebral fracture	1	(0.7%)
Complications by osteomyelitis	1	(0.7%)

(From Patijn, 1991. Reproduced by permission.)

prevent pneumothorax as 50% of previously reported cases were caused by
doctors.

Adverse Effects of Manipulative Therapies

Patijn (1991) reviewed 93 case reports of complications during manual
therapy, involving a total of 129 cases. Table 11.3 shows the nature of the
different complications. The most frequent kind (65.1%) were those involving the vertebro–basilar vascular system, with complications involving
intervertebral discs accounting for a further 22.5%. In 16 of the cases of
vertebral artery injury the patient died and in a further 55 there were
permanent neurologic deficits. Patijn notes that 65% of the cases involved a
chiropractor, but this may only reflect the greater number of treatments
given by chiropractors rather than the inherent safety of their techniques.
Nevertheless, Patijn cautions against the use of high-velocity thrust
techniques, particularly in cases where there has been a recent trauma. He
further suggests that most of the complications could have been avoided
with proper diagnostic procedures, such as a full clinical history, examination and X-rays.

As with other complementary therapies, the rate of complications is
impossible to ascertain, though it appears to be small. Patijn (1991) cites
estimates of serious complications occurring in approximately 1 in 400 000
manipulations, but it is not clear how this figure was arrived at. To obtain
an estimate of the frequency of complications, Lee et al (1995) surveyed all

members of the American Academy of Neurology in California and enquired about the number of patients presenting over the previous two years with a neurologic complication of chiropractic manipulation. They surveyed 486 neurologists, but only 177 replied. Of these 51 (about 10% of the total sample surveyed) reported 102 complications. Most injuries followed cervical manipulation, leading to stroke (56 cases), myelopathy (16) and radiculopathy (30) and other injuries. Lee and colleagues admit to a number of problems with their study, such as the low response rate and the high frequency of injuries reported by a small number of neurologists. Nevertheless, the study highlights the dangers of cervical manipulation which, however rare the complications, carries a risk of serious long-term deficits.

Some caution is needed when interpreting the literature on the adverse effects of spinal manipulation as being due specifically to chiropractic or osteopathic manipulation. Terret (1995) reviewed recent cases of injury from chiropractic manipulation reported in the medical literature with the specific purpose of ascertaining the profession of the practitioner concerned. A survey of publications, autopsy reports and coroner's findings revealed 535 cases of injury after cervical spine manipulation. Of these, 494 were in English, but 375 were anecdotal, leaving a total of 119 cases of actual reported cases in the English language (1934–94). Of these 78 had led to a death or serious neurologic deficit. All had been attributed to chiropractors who, admittedly, carry out much more manipulation than the medical professions. However, only 50 actually resulted from manipulation by a chiropractor, the remainder being due to osteopaths (8), medical practitioners (7), physiotherapists (3), unnamed practitioners in 6 cases and 3 single cases due to a wife, the patient, and a barber! The barber and patient produced only neurological deficits, but the wife accidentally caused the death of her husband. Terret also notes that once a case has appeared in the literature, it may subsequently be misrepresented as a chiropractic injury. He cites 24 cases in which subsequent reports misrepresent the original findings and 12 where, on inspection or after correspondence with the author, the 'chiropractor' turns out to be a member of another profession. Terret wryly notes that there do not appear to be any cases reported in which an injury caused by a chiropractor is wrongly attributed to a medical practitioner.

Adverse Effects of Herbalism

Medicines derived from plants formed the majority of the earlier materia medica because chemically synthesized compounds were not available.

Many drugs and herbal preparations clearly have effects on the body and so have a potential for harm as well as therapeutic benefit. The active ingredients of many herbal preparations have now been synthesized and are used by orthodox medicine. Drugs such as curare, digoxin, ephedrine, morphine, quinine and reserpine all entered orthodox medicinal use by this route (D'Arcy, 1991).

The most comprehensive account of the adverse reactions and interactions with herbal medicine is contained in two papers by D'Arcy (1991, 1993). He describes some of the more obvious examples of toxicity attributed to herbal medicines, while warning that information is sparse and the review cannot be comprehensive. We will primarily rely on his papers, selecting some of the more important cases he describes as examples of adverse effects; readers needing a more complete and authoritative account are referred to the original papers.

Toxic Herbal Extracts

Herbal teas have a variety of therapeutic uses being given as analgesics, diuretics, hypnotics, tonics and used locally as compresses or wound dressings. Some herbal teas are toxic, the most important being comfrey, used as a demulcent in chronic catarrh, and as a treatment for gastro-intestinal and other problems. The presence of certain alkaloids makes comfrey potentially damaging to the liver, though this depends on the total dose ingested, route of exposure and the susceptibility of the person concerned. There have been numerous case reports worldwide and D'Arcy suggests, citing a comprehensive review by Winship (1991), that the balance of risk is no longer acceptable for the oral use of comfrey.

A number of herbs, such as cannabis, khat and hallucinogenic fungi (magic mushrooms), are used for their psychoactive effects as recreational drugs. However, we are only concerned here with herbs with psychoactive properties that are used therapeutically, primarily as sedatives. MacGregor et al (1989) described four women who sustained liver damage after repeated use of proprietary herbal remedies for relieving stress; the ingredients of the remedies were not precisely defined but valerian and skullcap, which are common components of herbal remedies, were thought to be the most likely hepatotoxic components. None of these women appeared to have been seeing a herbalist; these particular hazards are due to self-medication.

Various reports have appeared attributing toxic effects to a number of other herbal products. D'Arcy cites three in which ginseng allegedly produced side-effects because of its oestrogenic activity, though the effects may have been due to other substances which are used to adulterate some of the cheaper forms of ginseng. High doses of liquorice and mistletoe extract have also been reported to produce hepatotoxicity. It must be stressed, however, that these are isolated case reports.

Adverse Interactions between Herbal Medicines and Drugs

Predicting, or even understanding, interactions between herbal preparations and drugs is very difficult because many herbal preparations contain a mixture of compounds each of which may itself be pharmacologically complex. Furthermore, where such interactions are reported it appears that many of the adverse interactions may not have been due to the herbs themselves but to the substitution or contamination of the herb by a more toxic herb, a poisonous metal or a potent non-herbal drug substance (D'Arcy, 1993). In that paper, D'Arcy classifies herbs into twelve major groups, based on their use and pharmacological properties and considers each group in turn for actual and potential drug interactions. In many cases, such as herbs containing cardiac glycosides, the interactions are potential and not based on case reports. The purpose is to alert both herbalists and doctors to possible interactions. Definitive information on adverse interactions is extremely sparse and even case reports are rare. The few case reports include an interaction of liquorice with hypertensive treatment, a possible interaction of ginseng with antidepressants and the potentiation of other drug effects, such as sedation, when used in combination with herbal sedatives.

Adulterated Herbal Mixtures

The final problem described by D'Arcy concerns the purity of some herbal preparations, particularly those from Asia and East Africa which have a high mineral content, sometimes containing oxidized heavy metals such as arsenic, mercury, tin, zinc and lead. D'Arcy comments that 'few of these mixtures have been satisfactorily tested for efficacy but their toxicity has been more than adequately demonstrated'. He cites a number of case reports, such as that of Dolan et al (1991) describing a man who developed lead poisoning after being treated for impotence with a herbal preparation. The problem of lead poisoning appears to be specific to certain ethnic preparations. These reactions are not characteristic of herbal treatment *per se*, but rather a reaction to impurities in the preparations. Such reactions cannot therefore be considered an argument against herbalism.

As with investigations into the adverse effects of other complementary medicine, there is very little information on the frequency of adverse reactions. The only study of the incidence of complications known to us is that of Chan and colleagues in Hong Kong (Chan, Chan and Critchley, 1992). As part of a prospective study on hospital admissions due to adverse drug reactions, 1701 patients were examined over an eight-month period. In only three patients (0.2%) was the admission due to the adverse effect of Chinese herbal medicine in a community where the use of herbal medicines is common. However, even low rates such as this could present a considerable problem in, for instance, the United Kingdom with 8 million hospital admissions per annum. However, the true state of affairs is simply unknown:

> The sparse reports of adverse reactions associated with herbal medicines that have been published in the medical or pharmaceutical press cannot confirm their relative safety nor indeed suggest the true incidence of such reactions. The simple fact is that the incidence of such reactions to herbal remedies in the self-medicating community is not known, indeed such reactions are probably often unrecognized by patient and doctor alike. (D'Arcy, 1991)

The objective of most authors reporting the adverse effects of herbal preparations has not been to condemn the use of herbs but to caution against misuse and unwanted side-effects and interactions. Herbs are, of course, potentially dangerous if misused, just as drugs are. However, drugs are treated, both by the public and professionals, with a great deal more caution. The particular danger of herbal preparations comes rather from the belief that they are natural and therefore necessarily safe because they act in harmony with the body's own functions.

> However the reality is that plants elaborate the chemicals found within them for their own purposes and not for ours. Plants have evolved in the presence of continual assault from animals, insects, parasites and bacteria and have survived by developing sophisticated chemical defenses. A Victorian poet talked of 'nature being red in tooth and claw' but the truth is that it is the green rather than the red in nature that poses the greatest threat. (Huxtable, 1992)

The message of these case reports of adverse effects of herbs is therefore to treat herbs with greater respect and caution. Both herbalists and doctors need to be aware of the potential for adverse interactions between herbal preparations and prescribed drugs. Atherton (1994), describing a conference on the safety of herbal medicines with participants from very diverse backgrounds, including doctors, pharmacologists and herbalists from several different traditions, reported a 'reassuring consensus' about the action needed. Atherton suggests that herbalists participate in a formal system of reporting of adverse reactions and interactions as exists for prescribed drugs.

Although this could be seen as another attempt to control complementary medicine and restrict its use, such a system could be of great benefit to herbalists concerned about the quality and safety of herbal medicines. D'Arcy (1991) emphasizes, as do herbalists, the need to monitor the quality of herbal remedies, a theme which has recently been highlighted by the Committee for Proprietary Medicinal Products of the European Union. Specifically, it suggests that herbs should be tested for microbiological quality and for residues of pesticides and fumigation agents, radioactivity, toxic metals and likely contaminants.

Homeopathy and Naturopathy

Acupuncture, manipulation and herbal medicine are clearly all capable of having some effect on the body, whether or not they are thought to be therapeutically effective. There is also, by the same token, the potential for harm. With homeopathy the central debate, between advocates and critics, is about whether tinctures with such extreme dilutions can have any effect at all. Even the most ardent critics do not suggest that homeopathy has any direct adverse effects, and there are almost no reports of such effects in the orthodox medical literature. Reviews of controlled trials of homeopathy either do not even mention adverse effects (Kleijnen, Knipschild and ter Riet, 1991) or state that no side-effects were reported in the trials they reviewed (Hill and Doyon, 1990). Whereas a critic of herbalism, for instance, may properly draw attention to the harmful constituents of some herbal preparations, it would be curiously illogical for someone who believes homeopathic preparations to be inert also to claim that they are harmful. As we have discussed, the adverse effects of homeopathy that are adduced concern its role in preventing orthodox treatment being instituted, rather than direct adverse effects of the homeopathic preparations.

The difficulties in specifying the nature of naturopathic treatment closely enough to allow formal evaluation of its effects also extend to examining its adverse effects. A number of therapeutic techniques are employed, each of which may have adverse effects as well as benefits. Acupuncture, manipulation and herbal treatment, which have already been reviewed, may all be used by naturopaths, who often train in several techniques and therapies. There are very few case reports citing any adverse effects of a naturopathic regime *per se*, apart from isolated examples of bizarre regimes, such as the giving of coffee enemas (Eisele and Reay, 1980). Changes in diet and lifestyle are unlikely to have any adverse effects unless carried to extremes. Reports of the adverse effects of rigorous dietary regimes in the context of naturopathic treatment are largely anecdotal.

However, one well-known example that involved a strict dietary regime which was alleged to be very harmful to patients was that of the Bristol Cancer Help Centre.

A Cautionary Tale: the Bristol Cancer Help Centre

The best-known example of a complementary approach being castigated as harmful is the study of the Bristol Cancer Help Centre (BCHC) (Bagenal et al, 1990). The purpose of relating the saga of the research into the efficacy of its approach is to illustrate the difficulty of a sober assessment of complementary medicine. We are not concerned with providing our own assessment of the methodology of the study, which has been amply commented on, but with the initial impact of the results and the subsequent recognition of the study's various methodological problems.

The Centre was set up in 1979 to offer a range of complementary treatments to patients with cancer. Central features of the approach were adherence to a strict diet of raw and partly cooked vegetables with proteins from soya and pulses (this diet has since been modified). The Centre also placed great emphasis on the patients' ability to help themselves, using a range of psychological, healing and spiritual methods to foster a positive approach to the disease. The Bristol approach incorporates a number of different therapies, but could certainly be described as broadly naturopathic.

The study was initiated by the BCHC who felt a need to validate scientifically the results they had obtained. They invited a team of scientists and doctors to discuss how this should be done. A randomized trial was apparently suggested, but the BCHC felt that it would be unethical to withhold the BCHC treatment from women who had expressed a wish to attend the Centre. The study carried out was therefore a comparison between patients attending the BCHC, who would also have had conventional treatment, and patients only attending NHS cancer centres.

In the study the survival of 334 women with breast cancer attending the BCHC were compared with the survival of 461 women with breast cancer attending a specialist cancer hospital or two district general hospitals. A parallel study on quality of life was also planned, but never progressed beyond the pilot stage. The interim results of the first study, not in fact the full results according to the initial protocol (Bourke and Goodare, 1991), were published in the *Lancet* and stated that: 'For patients metastasis-free at entry, metastasis-free survival in the BCHC group was significantly poorer than in the controls (relapse rate ratio 2.85). Survival in relapsed cases was

significantly inferior to that in the control group (hazard ratio 1.81)'
(Bagenal et al, 1990).

These figures were obtained from regression analyses after a number of
prognostic factors were taken into account in an effort to provide a control
for the inevitable differences in the two groups of patients. Raw data in fact
suggested a lower relapse rate at the BCHC, and some commentators
suggested that the complete reversal of the basic findings after the
regression analysis 'defied common sense' (Bourke and Goodare, 1991).
The study authors responded that it would not be correct to rely on raw
data in a study with unmatched groups (Chilvers, Bagenal and Harris,
1991).

The study report was reasonably cautious stating quite clearly that the
difference in survival could be due to the result of a difference in disease
severity at the time of entry and to various other differences between the
two groups. Nevertheless, the possibility had to be faced that 'some aspect
of the Bristol regime is responsible for their decreased survival'. This latter,
tentative conclusion was seized on and generated substantial, and often
sensational, media coverage. Even the *British Medical Journal* in an otherwise fairly sober news piece on the study entitled their report 'Death from
complementary medicine' (Richards, 1990).

The study generated a great deal of correspondence in the *Lancet*'s pages.
One of the key themes of the correspondence from a number of different
sources was the possibility that the two groups differed substantially on
some important prognostic factor that had not been taken into account,
such as the fact that the BCHC group, although roughly matched to the
controls at the time of entry to the study, had a much worse previous
disease history (Hayes, Smith and Carpenter, 1990).

In spite of the many questions raised about the methodology of the study,
the message that emerged to the public at large was, at least in the short
term, extremely negative. From the BCHC, Sheard (1990) wrote in a letter
to the *Lancet*:

> The study is seriously flawed and entirely inconclusive, yet it has been
> published as demonstrating that attendance at BCHC worsens prognosis. The
> consequences have been far-reaching. Many cancer patients have been very
> distressed by the publicity, some concluding that activities such as relaxation
> or visualization may have seriously damaged their health . . . the number of
> patients attending the BCHC has dropped substantially.

The authors of the study reacted again, responding to queries in detail,
answering many of the criticisms but stating in a letter to the *Lancet*:

> We broadly agree with much of the comment generated by our report on breast cancer patients attending the BCHC, which indicated that they had higher risks of recurrence and mortality than similar patients. . . . We did not claim and do not believe that our findings constitute strong evidence that some aspects of BCHC management was the direct cause of the observed difference in outcome.

The letter concludes:

> We regret that our paper has created the widespread impression that the BCHC regimen directly caused the differences that we observed in recurrence and survival. This was never stated. In our view it is much more likely that the differences could be explained by increased severity of disease in BCHC attenders. . . . The important conclusion to be drawn from our study is not that the BCHC regimen is harmful but that there is as yet no evidence of anti-tumour effect. Ultimately the only definitive way to evaluate complementary therapeutic methods will be by means of randomized, controlled trials, and we welcome news that such studies are being planned. (Chilvers, Bagenal and Harris, 1991)

These remarks are substantially in accord with the study's conclusions, though somewhat different in tone, being much more emphatic about the differences in the characteristics that emerged. The effect of the study, or rather of the furore that followed it, was that the BCHC nearly went into receivership and has barely survived. One would imagine that for the researchers it was also a terrible experience, to be exposed to such a high level of media attention and the fury of the patients at the BCHC, who felt frustrated and betrayed. One of the authors of the study committed suicide a few months after its publication, though the role of the study in this tragedy is not known. The editor of the *Lancet* was apparently quoted as saying that when he dies the words 'Bristol Cancer Help Centre' will be found tattooed on his heart (Smith, 1994).

We are not describing this study in order to criticize the research team. With the benefit of hindsight it is easy to say that a randomized controlled trial (as first suggested) should have been carried out, which would have meant that the patients in the two groups would have been much more likely to have been comparable, making interpretation of the results much more straightforward and avoiding the major flaws of the study. (There would certainly have been considerable ethical problems associated with such a trial.) As a first step, the study must have seemed entirely reasonable. Although the results were interim findings and arguably should not have been published at that stage, one can sympathize with the authors saying that they would surely have been criticized if they had waited another three years to publish.

If two types of orthodox treatment were being compared, there would probably have been the same questions about the comparability of the patient groups, especially as the results were so remarkable. The debate would have generated less heat, though, and more light; it would have been conducted without the pressure of media coverage and without such furious criticism. The strong feelings aroused by complementary medicine, both advocates and critics, fuelled the controversy to an extraordinary degree.

The worst aspect of the whole affair, clearly never intended by either the BCHC or the researchers, is the wariness it has probably induced in the complementary medical community about being involved in research. If inviting researchers into your Centre alienates your patients and nearly destroys your work, it is hardly likely to foster a productive relationship between complementary practitioners and researchers. On the positive side, it may alert all sides to the need for a gradual approach to evaluation which is usually the result of a long series of studies and, curiously, it may promote randomized controlled trials. Although doubts have been expressed about randomized controlled trials by complementary organizations they may, in the end, provide a fairer assessment of complementary therapies. Finally, the affair highlighted the extent to which patients who take part in trials are ignored once their participation is complete. Many learnt of the results through the media, hearing on the evening news that those who had been to the BCHC were twice as likely to die and three times as likely to relapse. This was, of course, not what the study said, but the damage was done. A number of initiatives are underway to protect the rights of patients taking part in research (Goodare and Smith, 1995), whether into orthodox or complementary medicine.

Chapter 12

A Research Agenda

The principal aim of this book has been to review research, from a variety of perspectives, on the main systems of complementary medicine. We have touched on broader sociological and political issues, but largely confined ourselves to an examination of research on the use, practice and efficacy of the therapies themselves. Others have discussed such issues as changing conceptions of health, the rationing of orthodox care, the impact of a consumer culture on medicine, the increasing professionalization of complementary medicine, the case for statutory registration of complementary therapies and the broad sociological and political context of complementary medicine (e.g. Salmon, 1985; Saks, 1992; Sharma, 1992).

There are certain findings which we would now regard as straightforward and uncontentious. With the proviso that there are many differences between the various branches of complementary medicine, certain general conclusions can be drawn. Complementary medicine is extremely widely used throughout Europe, North America and Australasia, even allowing for the variations in the definitions used. Complementary therapies are generally used for chronic conditions as an adjunct to orthodox treatment, rather than as a replacement for it. Patients of complementary practitioners tend to be quite well educated and the great majority do not appear to be ill-informed, credulous, naïve or bankrupted by the cost of treatment.

The cost of complementary medicine is usually quite modest, certainly compared with private medicine, with the incomes of most complementary practitioners probably also being rather modest. In our experience, complementary practitioners might be accused of being romantic idealists in some cases, but seldom of being materialistic quacks knowingly peddling bogus remedies. This is not to say that such people do not exist, but we doubt that they are heavily represented in the ranks of complementary therapists. There is also considerable interest in complementary medicine in the medical, nursing and allied professions, with some health professionals undergoing formal training. Nurses especially see complementary medicine as a route back to a more caring form of medicine and 'putting the heart back into nursing' (Wright, 1995). Some advocates of a holistic approach to medicine see complementary medicine at the vanguard of a new concept of health, embracing psychological, social and spiritual aspects of health (see Salmon, 1985, for discussion of this issue).

In this final chapter, the emphasis on research will be maintained. We review the major topics again, in part to highlight key themes, but principally to put forward suggestions for what we hope will be fruitful and important avenues of research in the future. In doing so, we will be returning again to themes considered in the Introduction to this book in the description of a woman's experience of cystitis and the various treatments she received. That single account raised questions about the characteristics of patients receiving complementary treatment, their attitudes to and experience of orthodox medicine, the difficulty of assessing the efficacy of treatments, the role of the practitioner and the therapeutic encounter, the appeal of the philosophy and language of complementary medicine, and the importance of the actual experience of treatment. Before discussing research on these topics, we will briefly consider the demarcation between orthodox and complementary medicine, and argue that the quality of evidence for a therapy should now be the marker of its value rather than its label as orthodox or complementary.

THE QUALITY OF EVIDENCE

There is no sharp dividing line between orthodox and complementary medicine. Most of the defining features we have discussed are represented, in some degree, on both sides of the orthodox/complementary divide. Some complementary practitioners aspire to be scientific in their approach, much orthodox medicine is preventative, work on the evaluation of quality of life is a move towards a broader orthodox view of health, a holistic approach is certainly not the sole province of complementary practitioners, and so on. Perhaps it is time to turn to a different kind of demarcation, between therapies that have empirical support for their efficacy and underlying concepts and approach, and those that do not. 'It is more fruitful to regard the demarcation as determined by scientific philosophical considerations . . . If this is agreed, then we must accept that it is not so much the treatment on offer that determines whether the medicine is orthodox or alternative, but the quality of evidence adduced in its favour' (Anon, 1989).

Within both complementary and orthodox medicine there is a huge variation on this score, which highlights the fact that the lines between complementary and orthodox medicine are not quite as sharp as some suggest. Much orthodox medical treatment has not been subjected to empirical testing, and on the above definition might qualify as alternative medicine. Complementary medicine embraces therapies such as osteopathy and chiropractic, which have quite reasonable empirical backing, but also many entirely unresearched therapies.

This approach also highlights the differences between the complementary therapies. They should not all be tarred with the same brush when attacks are being made on some of the more doubtful practices. It would surely now be more fruitful to pay less attention to definitions and demarcations of what is orthodox and what is complementary, and begin to examine the various therapies and techniques individually and on their own terms. The crucial question is surely the quality of the evidence, rather than the origin of the therapy, or which profession practises it. Thus the status and importance of a therapy, whatever its origins, is underpinned by research. Just as evidence-based medicine is coming to the fore, so must evidence-based complementary medicine.

Is Complementary Medicine Scientific?

Even if evidence is not available, or not yet available, this does not necessarily mean that a complementary therapy can be immediately dismissed as 'unscientific'. Briskman (1987) has examined this question in relation to medicine in a paper entitled 'Doctors and witchdoctors: Which doctors are which?' In the paper he considers Francis Bacon's inductivist solution to the problem of demarcation between science and pseudoscience, but argues that, in medicine at least, Popper's radical solution to the problem of demarcation is to be preferred.

> According to Popper, what demarcates the theories of empirical science is not that they have been reached from observation by some special method of inference, or even that they are especially well supported by observation, but rather that they are open to observational and empirical criticism and refutation and that severe attempts have been made to discover their falsity by such means. Thus for Popper the distinguishing mark of empirical science is its insistence that only theories that are falsifiable—and hence testable—by empirical evidence should be admitted. (Briskman, 1987)

On this view pseudoscience results from the desire to find empirical support; a genuine empirical method results only if we relinquish this desire and instead look for empirical refutations. There is therefore nothing inherently unscientific about putting forward hypotheses or claims about the efficacy of a therapy, provided one is willing to submit it to empirical test and, furthermore, able to formulate hypotheses in such a way that they can be put to the test.

Briskman suggests that Popper's solution can explain the rationality of our preference for Western medicine over superstitious medical practices. There are observations to support many kinds of medical treatment; patients have been observed to improve under almost any kind of regime. What distinguishes the scientific approach is a willingness to question this evidence. The clinical trial is seen, in this light, as an attempt to provide a refutation of the claim that the treatment is effective. Briskman (1987) writes:

> What is wrong with, say, faith healing is not that it does not have a 'scientific basis' if this means that we cannot at present give any scientific explanation of its effectiveness. After all, it is perfectly possible that such practices are regularly effective in, say, curing cancer (just as the old wives' tale that milkmaids did not get smallpox turned out to be true). If this were the case then the fact that we cannot explain it within present medical science would not mean that faith healing is ineffective but rather that our present scientific knowledge is defective. But if the assertion that faith healing does not have any scientific basis means that the claims made on its behalf are incapable of being tested empirically, or have been subjected to such tests and have failed, this is quite a different matter. Of course, the defenders of faith healing may respond to any such negative findings by rejecting altogether the appropriateness of empirical tests for evaluating their claims; but in that case they are asking the rest of us to treat them as oracles, with an unimpeachable hotline to the truth.

We are aware that philosophers of science are not agreed on the precise demarcation of science from pseudoscience and that these remarks reflect only a fragment of a complex debate. However, we would argue that advocates of complementary medicine maintain a scientifically respectable position if they can (a) formulate their claims in a manner which allows empirical testing and (b) encourage research aimed at testing such claims. The fact that in many cases evidence is not yet available need not in itself indicate that a therapy is inherently unscientific. Having argued for the primacy of evidence and empirical research, we now consider what form research on the complementary therapies might take in the future.

PATHWAYS TO COMPLEMENTARY MEDICINE

Early speculation about patients' pathways to complementary medicine was orthodox in orientation, in the sense that the primary aim was to explain why people turned their backs on orthodox care. From the patient's perspective it is, as we have seen, rather different. Patients, especially well-informed patients, behave as consumers faced with a choice of therapeutic possibilities of which orthodox medicine, in its various forms, represents one approach. Patients very seldom turn their backs on orthodox medicine, rather they will use the therapy that they perceive as most appropriate for their particular condition. Furthermore, they are likely to progress through a range of therapeutic options, with advice from friends and self-medication often preceding consultation with a general practitioner.

There is now a certain amount of information about the factors that bring people to complementary medicine. However, the studies have not distinguished the reasons for beginning the treatment from the reasons for continuing it, nor have they assessed the relative importance of the different factors. Sharma (1992) is surely right to stress that the way forward in this area is longitudinal research. At present no longitudinal studies of evolving attitudes have been carried out and for the most part we cannot say which factors are likely to be uppermost at any particular time. It seems likely that previous experience of orthodox medicine, the opinions and experience of others and perhaps attitudes to science and orthodox medicine are most important in an initial decision to try complementary medicine. The decision to continue will presumably be based on an assessment of the treatment and practitioner involved. Multiple factors will then be involved, including the nature of the therapeutic encounter, efficacy of the treatment and the explanation given for the illness. Clearly these various factors are not mutually exclusive and several may operate simultaneously. Different patterns may exist for clients of the different branches of complementary medicine. The task of research is to track these decisions about therapies over time and discern the influences at decision points.

KNOWLEDGE, ATTITUDES AND BELIEFS

Our own studies examined a number of possible distinguishing characteristics of patients of complementary practitioners. As might be expected, they tend to perceive complementary therapies as more effective, relatively speaking, than do general practice patients, though orthodox medicine is still preferred for serious illness. They appear on the whole, again compared to general practice patients, to have better biological knowledge, to be more health conscious and to believe more strongly that people can influence their own state of health, both by physical means and through maintaining a psychological equilibrium. They tend to have less faith in the ability of orthodox medicine to treat disease and maintain health.

In the early stages, this sampling of the beliefs of complementary and general practice patients was a reasonable one. After all, if no differences emerged in straightforward comparisons, there would be little to understand about complementary patients. They might simply have chronic problems and the money to experiment with private treatments. Now, however, as some differences have emerged, there is a need to integrate the various findings, initially by exploring the interrelationships of the various characteristics in more complex analyses. It is possible, for instance, that greater biological knowledge of complementary patients simply reflects a higher lever of education rather than knowledge of biology *per se*. In one of our recent studies (Vincent and Furnham, 1997), we found that attitudes to science and medicine were a more powerful predictor of perceived efficacy than provider of locus of control. The early findings on locus of control may reflect not a general pessimism about the role of medicine, as the original scale intends, but more specific attitudes to orthodox medicine.

In addition, patients attending different types of therapy, and different styles within the same therapy, may be more or less strongly distinguished from, say, general practice patients. There will be degrees of 'complementarity' as regards views on medicine, personal responsibility for health and so on. Patients attending an osteopathy clinic in the City of London, primarily dealing with sports injuries, are likely to have very different views from those attending an acupuncturist practising with a group of complementary therapists above a health food store. Assessment of the philosophy of a centre and its practitioners throws additional light on the characteristics of the patients who attend if, and this is of considerable interest in itself, they are aware of the philosophy underlying the treatment they are receiving and the views of their practitioner.

The Consultation

There has been a great deal of speculation about consultations with complementary practitioners, but remarkably little in the way of hard evidence. From the limited research available, it appears that patients attending complementary practitioners do tend to find the consultations more satisfactory than those with their own general practitioner. However, being a self-selected group there is an element of bias in this comparison, in that this finding does not automatically mean that general practice consultations are 'worse' than complementary ones. It might be that other general practice patients, if given the chance to sample complementary medicine, would prefer the more businesslike ten minutes of a general practice consultation.

Nevertheless, there appears to be something important about the complementary consultation for at least a proportion of patients, though it is not at all clear what aspects influence patient trust and satisfaction, perceptions of competence and so on. It might simply be that longer consultations are more satisfying. Future studies should perhaps compare consultations with complementary practitioners with longer orthodox consultations, rather than the necessarily brief visits to a general practitioner. In addition, the key elements of the consultation, especially touch and physical examination, should be monitored and related to satisfaction and other variables. The exploration of complementary practitioners' views on the key components of the consultation, and their relationship with their patients (Choi and Tweed, 1996, unpublished, personal communication) is a fascinating extension to this work and needs to be explored further.

Emotional Issues

Complementary practitioners may also be more willing to discuss emotional issues, in terms of being supportive and offering informal counselling. The emphasis on emotion may have an additional importance in that complementary therapists may be seen as being more attuned to the way patients themselves perceive their emotional lives and the relation of their emotions to their physical health. This possibility is expressed by Salmon (1985) as follows:

> Disease according to scientific medicine is a disorder of the biological state, described in terms of physical sciences and treated generally independently from social behaviour and intrapsychic processes, let alone larger cosmological forces. When given attention, such factors are too often isolated under the rubric of psychological problems or referred to a separate practitioner who is not usually concerned with the physical aspects of the problem.

This is too strongly stated in that there are many doctors who try, within the time available, to give attention to their patients' emotions and the broader context of the illness. However, it is possible that complementary practitioners, for whatever reason, give this larger context of health a higher priority and that this is especially valued by some patients. This is, of course, speculative, but would appear to be a topic worthy of research.

Explanations of Illness

A further area of importance is the diagnosis and explanations offered to patients. General practitioners are faced with a large number of patients who are by no means well, but who have no clearly diagnosable condition. This 'undifferentiated illness' has been considered to be especially fertile ground for complementary medicine both by sceptics and adherents (Lewith, 1988). As we have seen, a complementary diagnosis can be made whatever the malaise in question. This in itself may provide hope, comfort and legitimization for the patient—just as, of course, a diagnosis from a doctor will. The most striking aspect of the complementary diagnosis, however, is that it usually provides a radically different explanation of the patient's symptoms than an orthodox diagnosis. We have seen that there are parallels between lay concepts and descriptions of illness and, for instance, the concepts used in traditional Chinese medicine. This may be less surprising than it seems, in that systems with prescientific origins may be more apt to derive their concepts from people's actual experience of illness. The conceptual framework might then be very closely related to the way in which people naturally think about their illnesses. Thus it is possible, as Sobell (1979) has suggested, that 'Western scientific medicine is largely concerned with the objective, non-personal, physiochemical explanations of disease as well as its technical control. In contrast, many traditional systems of healing . . . are aimed principally at providing meaningful and understandable explanations of illness experience'.

We suggest, therefore, that the nature of the explanation provided by complementary practitioners may be an important part of their appeal if, for some reason, their explanation is especially meaningful to the sick person. The suffering of chronic illness is perhaps slightly more easy to bear if one feels acknowledged and understood by one's practitioner and that one's disease makes sense in their terms of reference. This is a completely unresearched area, again, yet potentially of enormous importance for the understanding of complementary medicine, patients' conceptions of illness generally and the nature of a successful consultation.

THE EFFICACY OF COMPLEMENTARY THERAPIES

There is now a substantial amount of research on the major complementary therapies. There are certainly major methodological flaws in many of the studies, but it is clearly feasible to assess the efficacy of complementary medicine. The time is past when the major complementary therapies could be dismissed on the grounds that there was no evidence available. In each area there are important studies showing positive effects of the therapy in question, though there may also be conflicting findings. This is not to say that the evidence for efficacy is necessarily strong, only that the attempts to evaluate are now thoroughgoing and serious. We would say that the jury is still out as regards the overall value of most of the systems we have reviewed, though clearly evidence varies markedly according to the condition being treated and the therapy in question.

Acupuncture and Manipulative Therapies

For acupuncture there are a large number of preliminary studies of the treatment of various disorders, some giving positive results and showing that acupuncture is possibly beneficial. Controlled studies have shown positive findings for low back pain and fibromyalgia, and equivocal results for migraine and asthma. Larger scale studies are warranted for all these disorders, though other types of musculo–skeletal pain, tension headache and arthritis are also possible candidates. For the manipulative therapies, results are promising, but not yet conclusive. Study populations are small, which makes it hard to detect differences between treatments, though detecting differences between treatment and placebo should be easier. It would seem possible that acute symptoms might be especially susceptible to early intervention by manipulation, which might in turn prevent the onset of a chronic condition. As so often, further trials of a higher methodological standard are awaited.

Herbalism

Herbalism is slightly unusual in that, while the therapeutic approach of its practitioners may not be orthodox, many of the remedies contain active therapeutic ingredients which may have already been incorporated in the orthodox pharmacy. Research on herbal medicine is a vast field and our review has only been illustrative. There is, for example, preliminary evidence, from placebo-controlled trials, for the efficacy of Chinese herbal therapy of atopic dermatitis in adults and atopic eczema in children, and for feverfew in the treatment of migraine. In the case of *Ginkgo biloba*, where there are sufficient trials for a formal review, evidence is strong enough to recommend *Ginkgo* for patients with mild to moderate cerebral insufficiency, and possibly, after further study, for intermittent claudication. Garlic again requires further study, but it seems that it may be of value as a lipid-lowering agent, and perhaps in the treatment of hypertension.

There is, however, a sense in which herbalism is almost entirely unresearched. All the studies we have examined have considered single compounds in isolation, rather than the combinations that herbalists adapt to individual patients. The aim of most research appears to be to provide preliminary evidence of efficacy in order that the active ingredients may be isolated. This is entirely reasonable from a pharmacological point of view, but tells us very little about the possible value of herbalism as a therapy rather than simply as a staging post to an improved and enriched orthodox pharmacopoeia.

Homeopathy and Naturopathy

There are some positive results from high-quality studies of homeopathy, but we would agree with Kleijnen, Knipschild and ter Riet (1991) that the evidence is probably not yet sufficient for most people to form a definite view. The evidence is sufficiently positive to warrant further large-scale trials, under rigorous double-blind conditions, with human subjects. The series of papers on recovery of bowel function seems to have been brought to an end by a large, collaborative trial (GRECHO, 1989) and similar large studies might resolve other conflicting findings, either positively or negatively. The eclecticism of naturopathy makes an overall evaluation of the therapeutic approach, even for a single condition, a difficult undertaking. The Lifestyle Heart Trial (Ornish et al, 1990) demonstrated that such trials are feasible, but there do not appear to be any trials that have evaluated a complete naturopathic treatment regime or compared such an approach with a more orthodox regime (Bergner, 1991). In this sense naturopathy, like herbalism, is unevaluated as a system of medicine. There is, however, some supportive evidence for many components of naturopathic practice, including dietary measures and the various individual complementary therapies that we have already discussed.

Mechanisms of Action

A serious discussion of the mechanisms of action of the major complementary therapies is beyond the scope of this book (and beyond the knowledge and abilities of the authors). However, the issue of mechanism is relevant to all the systems of complementary medicine that we have discussed. The mechanism of action of a therapy, whether actually established or just presumed, may affect the interpretation of the controlled trials that we have reviewed. The mode of action of many herbs, even those studied in controlled trials, is often unknown, though a list of potentially active ingredients may have been identified. However, the idea that herbs could potentially produce therapeutic effects is not really at issue. Again, it is clearly plausible, even if one were to find the trial evidence unconvincing, that manipulation could relieve chronic pain problems. The position is less clear in the case of acupuncture. The discovery that acupuncture released endorphins and enkephalins, naturally occurring opiates in the body (see, for example, Clement-Jones et al, 1980), certainly made it more plausible that acupuncture might be of value in the treatment of chronic pain and hastened its acceptance in pain clinics. The lack of evidence for meridians and much acupuncture theory was counterbalanced by experimental evidence from another quarter. However, most of the mechanisms postulated concern relatively short-term effects and it is not clear how these might translate into long-term therapeutic benefit (Price et al, 1984; Vincent, 1989b). The general point is clear, however; the plausibility of the postulated mechanism influences how one views the results of controlled trials.

This problem finds its clearest expression in the case of homeopathy, though other branches of complementary medicine have equal or greater problems in this regard. In the case of the diagnostic system iridology, for example, described in Chapter 1, it is not at all clear how the body might be mapped on to the eye or, in the case of auricular acupuncture, on to the ear. Kleijnen, Knipschild and ter Riet (1991) asked whether review articles of clinical evidence could only be convincing if there is a plausible mechanism of action. Should trial results be considered in isolation and taken on their own terms, or viewed as part of a more general attempt to understand the therapy in question? There seems no doubt that the evidence is stronger when some mechanism seems at least plausible even if, as in the case of many herbs, it cannot be identified.

Although controlled trials are viewed as the gold standard, they should surely be seen as only one aspect of the research endeavour and one part of the general attempt to understand a therapy in scientific terms. In practical terms, the question might be how long one is prepared to carry on with clinical trials, in an effort to resolve the issue of efficacy, before calling a halt to the process. As clinical evidence mounts, opinions may soften and (the logical consequence) the search for a mechanism then becomes imperative. Conversely, the question of mechanism will die should the larger trials not be supportive. However, it is also surely correct that any supportive experimental evidence, in the form of work on plant materials on animals, would greatly assist homeopathy's case and lend considerable weight to the case for funding of further clinical trials. The same arguments apply to other forms of complementary medicine, and indeed to therapies of all kinds.

METHODOLOGY OF EVALUATION

Some have argued that the individualized, holistic approach of the complementary therapies means that they can never be satisfactorily evaluated in controlled trials (e.g. Heron, 1986). We have argued that, with some important provisos, complementary medicine is not a special case. Certainly randomized controlled trials into complementary therapies present many difficulties, but few are specific to complementary medicine, though alternative diagnostic systems do present special problems. There is no special reason to abandon the controlled trial in favour of a more fluid, subjective approach supposedly more suited to complementary medicine. In fact, many of the particular concerns of complementary therapists could be incorporated in controlled trials or standard experimental studies. McGourty (1993), for example, calls for a greater use of multiple measures, a greater use of subjective measures, and research on the treatment process and choice of therapist, and the impact of length of consultation and personal qualities of therapists.

There are clearly major methodological problems with many of the trials, as clearly demonstrated by the ratings of methodological criteria of many of the reviews. A central problem, which must be resolved, is the size of trials. Much larger trials are needed, which in turn require a much higher level of funding. The definition of an appropriate control group, certainly for acupuncture and the manipulative therapies, creates particular problems. Agreement on a standard methodology in regard to these issues would be of immense value. A further difficulty, at least for the complementary medicine community, is that, in the interests of standardization, few trials have allowed therapists to work as they would in actual practice. It is at least arguable that attempts to restrict a therapy too closely may be detrimental to its efficacy; a compromise needs to be worked out in each case to allow reasonable flexibility while ensuring sufficient standardization on key issues (such as number and length of sessions) to ensure comparability between treatment groups.

A Pluralism of Methodologies

As Canter and Nanke (1993) point out, different methodological approaches are required for different questions and different therapeutic situations. Here again, useful lessons can be learnt from psychotherapy; Kazdin (1984) has emphasized that progress in psychotherapy research has come from employing a 'pluralism of methodologies'. For example, qualitative methods would allow a much deeper exploration of the subjective experience of patients and practitioners than has been possible with questionnaire surveys, which might find a particular resonance with complementary practitioners. This might be complemented by a greater use of subjective or patient-centred measures in quantitative work. Employing different methods of enquiry, including the controlled trial where appropriate, allows a sophistication of approach and should not be seen as second-rate research. Controlled trials should not be abandoned, but allowed to find their place in a more comprehensive enquiry into complementary medicine.

The use of single case designs merits special consideration, because of their potential for examining efficacy with small patient numbers and their relatively low cost. They allow an individual approach to each patient and are not generally disruptive of the clinical situation. Single case studies can be very straightforward and an ideal introduction to research. There are differing levels of formality and experimentation, varying from close observation of the clinical situation with some simple measures, to a tightly controlled experimental design in which the management of the patient's illness is systematically varied (Aldridge, 1993). Placebo treatment, for instance, can be intermixed with standard treatment (e.g. Vincent, 1990b). With diary data though, especially when they have a fluctuating pattern, quite complex statistics may be needed to discern the impact of a treatment (Chatfield, 1985).

STUDIES OF THE THERAPEUTIC PROCESS

A greatly neglected area, but one with immense possibilities for research by complementary practitioners and organizations, is the study of the components of the therapeutic process itself. Complementary journals are full of case descriptions and discussions of how to treat particular conditions, just as the more practice-oriented medical journals are. Such discussions of the therapeutic process are clearly valuable and necessary, but not what we have in mind. Rather we are suggesting a systematic evaluation of the components of treatment to ascertain their validity and relationship to the outcome of treatment. We believe, for instance, that it would greatly enhance the validity of complementary therapies, and not necessarily threaten the overall enterprise, if the reliability and validity of some of the diagnostic techniques were examined. The example we consider has been discussed by one of us previously (Vincent, 1992).

The pulse diagnosis is a means of assessing the energy state of the twelve main acupuncture meridians. It provides both an index of the health of the patient and a guide to the most appropriate form of treatment. There are many different systems of pulse diagnosis (a worry in itself) and many claims are made for the different qualities that can be distinguished. To complicate matters further, the same disease may manifest as several different pulse pictures. This method of diagnosis was the subject of a series of small studies (Cole, 1975) in which experienced acupuncturists' claims about what they could and could not tell from the pulse diagnosis were subjected to empirical test. The results were, in summary, that none of the claims made were substantiated. Acupuncturists could not, for instance, tell whether a person's bladder was full or empty. They could not distinguish a pulse change, as predicted, when a treatment had been given by another acupuncturist. There was little consistency in the pulse diagnoses of experienced practitioners on different occasions and little relationship between the diagnoses of different practitioners. They had some success at distinguishing ill and healthy people, but not much more than an anaesthetist only accustomed to orthodox pulse taking.

Cole (1975) was aware of the subtleties and complexities of the pulse diagnosis, and obviously sympathetic to acupuncturists and their values. Her studies were, if anything, an attempt to provide empirical support for a system that she clearly found both appealing and important. Her conclusion, however, was that the pulse diagnosis 'is not apparently a means of objective analysis, but offers subjective meaning to the practitioner and is a vehicle for a meaningful and helpful interaction with the patient'. There are certainly problems with the studies. For one thing, the numbers involved are certainly too small for the results to be regarded as a definitive test of the pulse diagnosis. However, they offer a challenge, in that they point to the need to establish the validity of this system of diagnosis more firmly, if it is to continue to be used.

Simple experimental studies of the reliability and validity of complementary diagnostic methods could readily be carried out. The results would be illuminating and of immediate clinical interest and relevance. If the pulse diagnosis, for instance, did not withstand critical scrutiny, then perhaps it should be abandoned and an effort made to develop more reliable indicators for the choice of treatment. In each case, research results, if followed through, could have definite implications both for the individual practitioner and the profession as a whole. Such studies are likely to be mainly of interest to complementary practitioners, not because they are inherently of less value but simply because they are the people with most interest in the practice of their particular discipline. Studies of other aspects of the treatment process, such as within session changes or patient and practitioner variables, are more difficult, especially when process measures are linked to outcome. A look at the vast psychotherapy literature examining parallel questions should make one cautious about making quick progress in this notoriously difficult field (Bergin and Garfield, 1994).

ADVERSE EFFECTS, PHYSICAL AND PSYCHOLOGICAL

Complementary therapies appear, on the limited evidence available, to be remarkably safe. Orthodox treatment is associated with a much higher level of risk, though clearly this must always be offset against the benefits of treatment for serious or life-threatening illness. Reports of adverse responses to the main complementary therapies, deterioration in the patient's condition, or actual injury, are very rare. The evidence is, however, sparse, consisting almost entirely of case reports. There is undoubtedly a need for serious audit of the nature and frequency of adverse responses to all forms of complementary medical treatment. In the case of herbal medicine, some form of adverse incident reporting is also indicated, not so much because herbal medicine *per se* is dangerous, but because of concerns about the contamination of some herbal preparations.

At various points we have discussed other, indirect, adverse effects. One of the most serious accusations levelled against complementary medicine is that its practitioners act, intentionally or not, to withhold orthodox treatment from patients in need. The most disturbing reports concern cancer patients who, while they might not have recovered, would certainly have been spared the more gruesome and painful stages of unchecked, advanced cancer. A survey of complementary practitioners to ascertain what advice they give in relation to orthodox medicine would be a start, followed by surveys of patients to ascertain if they have ever been actively persuaded not to have important orthodox treatment. Clearly this is a difficult area to research sensitively and fairly; for a chronic condition such as arthritis, it would seem very reasonable for a complementary practitioner to suggest a trial of acupuncture, say, before a trial of medication. The risks are probably minimal, and it is in the end the patient's decision. On the other hand, it would be alarming if patients were being actively persuaded against receiving potentially important orthodox treatment for serious, acute illness. Similar surveys might also be conducted on the advice doctors give about potentially useful complementary therapies.

Medicalization of Distress and Unhappiness

A more subtle concern is that complementary medicine might first attract, and then encourage, patients who are overly concerned with their health, if not frankly hypochondriacal. Private medicine of all kinds allows access to medical treatment for lesser, sometimes trivial, complaints. There is nothing necessarily wrong with this. Whether or not any effective treatment can be given, be it orthodox or complementary, the advice and support of an experienced professional can be invaluable when dealing with the misery of chronic illness or simply with general unhappiness. Of more concern is what has become known as the 'medicalization' of ordinary distress and unhappiness (Illich, 1976).

Illich was primarily objecting to the interference of medicine and medical institutions in aspects of life that were best faced by people alone or simply with the support of others. Illich's critique was wide ranging and only one aspect concerns us here, which is that medicine can encourage people to turn to experts when they might better draw on their own resources to face and deal with sickness, distress and unhappiness. This criticism may apply especially powerfully to complementary medicine, in that it tends to draw more emotional and physical malaise into the medical arena than orthodox medicine. Striving for optimum health and monitoring slight imbalances also means paying more attention to slight malaise. The psychological effects of considering any symptom to be something that requires treatment are not necessarily beneficial. This theme would appear to us to be worthy of research, not in the spirit of finding something else to criticize about complementary medicine, but to discover what meaning the philosophies of the complementary therapies have for people and how they understand and react to the detection of very subtle changes in their vital energy, as it might be expressed to them.

Personal Responsibility for Health

A criticism sometimes made of those who espouse a strongly holistic view of health is that they exaggerate the links between emotional development and physical illness. If one believes, for example, that 'Illness occurs when people don't grow up and develop their potentials or when they become blocked by a crisis or a series of events' (Blattner, 1981), then one is likely to be burdened by a sense of personal responsibility, shame and failure for succumbing to cancer or heart disease. This echoes Sontag's description of the way certain types of illness, such as tuberculosis and cancer, become associated with certain personality types, weak, sensitive and imaginative in the case of tuberculosis, emotionally withdrawn and stunted in the case of cancer (Sontag, 1983). The illness becomes a metaphor for a whole array of personal characteristics with which it may have no real connection at all. The philosophy of personal responsibility for illness is often linked to complementary medicine, but is in fact just as prevalent, if not more so, in certain areas of humanistic psychology and is also espoused by some nurses and doctors.

Wikler (1985) in a critique of holistic concepts of personal responsibility for health, points out that the notion of personal responsibility can take on a number of different meanings, which are not always sufficiently distinguished. It has received several interpretations in the holistic literature, but the differences are rarely noted and seldom explained. In an obvious way we are all responsible for the amount of exercise we take, whether we smoke, drink and engage in other healthy or unhealthy behaviours. There is clearly a positive sense of responsibility which encourages an active approach to health, with a strong emphasis on exercise, relaxation, coping with stress and so on. What is controversial is not the concept of responsibility, but the holist's account of what actions lead to what consequences, the extent to which people are responsible for the onset of their illnesses and what measures patients should take to promote recovery.

We do not pretend to be able to disentangle all the different senses of personal responsibility, or to adequately have explored the various ways in which the term is used by complementary therapists and psychologists of various persuasions. The issue of blame is also extremely complex, even in far simpler cases, such as whether one blames a cancer sufferer for having continued to smoke as the evidence for its harmful effects mounted over the last two decades. The most important point is that, while the possible harmful effects of personal responsibility have been amply alluded to, we do not know how common such burdensome feelings of self-blame are among those with chronic illness or whether these feelings of self-blame are more prevalent amongst patients of complementary therapists of various kinds. Even then it could be that such people are attracted to complementary therapists rather than deriving such ideas from them. Some sensitive interviewing, followed by a survey of patients with cancer and other serious illness, attending orthodox and complementary centres, would shed some welcome light on this difficult but important area.

This completes our review of the themes of the book and ideas about the directions future research might take. In the remainder of the chapter we consider some of the difficulties, both personal and practical, that researchers in this area face, whether they are from academia, medicine or the complementary professions.

WHY MIGHT COMPLEMENTARY THERAPISTS WANT TO CONDUCT RESEARCH?

Many complementary practitioners now consider that it is important that research into complementary medicine is carried out. Acupuncturists, for example, believe that research would increase acceptance in the medical and scientific community, help acupuncturists evaluate their own treatment, increase public awareness, improve the efficacy of the treatment and lead to a greater understanding of the way acupuncture works (Vincent and Mole, 1989; Fitter and Blackwell, 1993). There are some complementary practitioners, however, who have no interest in research, who are frankly suspicious, or even contemptuous. In one survey of acupuncturists, the most common reason for this scepticism was, in essence, 'What's the point, we know it works' (Vincent and Mole, 1989). Presumably these practitioners never consider that they might be mistaken in their assessment of acupuncture's efficacy or that any effect might be primarily psychological. Others would say, more reasonably perhaps, that they too were doubtful about some aspects of acupuncture, but as long as people got better what did it matter? For an individual patient, it perhaps does not matter how acupuncture is working or whether it is actually the treatment that is responsible for the improvement. However, these questions are crucial when the overall value and efficacy of a treatment is being assessed.

One's own clinical impressions are a useful source of information about treatment and its effectiveness. However, it is difficult for an individual practitioner, faced with a very varied set of patients, to draw any general conclusions about a therapy's effectiveness. It is more or less impossible to decide whether the treatment (whether acupuncture, drugs or whatever) is effective for psychological reasons. That question can only be answered by formal studies. A number of studies, for instance, have carefully examined the effect of acupuncture on sensorineural deafness, and found that it has no effect whatever. It seems doubtful whether any practitioner should offer treatment to someone with this problem. On the other hand, acupuncture may well be beneficial for migraine, though it is not yet clear why this is. If acupuncture helps migraine by the action of needles, future clinical research and practice should concentrate on refining methods of treatment. If, on the other hand, the effect of acupuncture appears primarily psychological, future advance is more likely to come from examining the psychological aspects of acupuncture and developing explicitly psychological treatments. Either way, the assessment of the relative contribution of psychological and physical factors is of considerable importance.

The results of formal studies will eventually affect both the assessment of its value and the extent to which it will be funded and used in the orthodox arena, where evidence of efficacy is increasingly demanded when funding decisions are made. Research is crucial if complementary medicine is to be taken seriously and its value clearly discerned. Therapies that are content to remain on the margins will perhaps survive without benefit of research, which ultimately means that they may be of less benefit to patients.

Personal Perspectives: The Process of Questioning

All research, all science, involves asking questions. The answers are sometimes awkward, even shocking, and can shatter deeply held beliefs. At a less grandiose level, it is always annoying to find that research findings do not support one's own personal beliefs or hypotheses. In clinical work it is very important to be able to question whether one's treatment of an individual patient is correct and to review and adapt one's formulation if necessary. To be able to examine the treatment more generally requires a more formal and co-ordinated approach, but the initial process of questioning is an essential preliminary. This inevitably involves a capacity to doubt, or at least to suspend belief in, the validity of the treatment the practitioner is giving. The process of questioning, if it involves fundamental assumptions about the therapy and the way it works, can be painful, difficult and disruptive of practice (Vincent, 1992).

Doubt creates major problems for a practitioner of complementary medicine, particularly when it extends to the whole of his or her therapeutic endeavours. This is seldom, if ever, acknowledged by critics of complementary practitioners in their calls for research. Some critics of complementary medicine make great play of their willingness to test out their own theories (Baum, 1987) and face the consequences of having them disproved. However, there is a crucial difference. If you are a doctor or a psychologist, and your pet theory is disproved, it may be painful, but seldom leads you to doubt that medicine or psychology is fundamentally flawed, nor does it threaten your livelihood. You simply shift to another area of activity, or perhaps you start a research project to examine your concerns in more detail.

For a complementary practitioner to entertain serious doubts about the overall effectiveness of the therapy they have trained in is difficult. However, to begin to question some aspects is feasible and hopefully valuable. It is often forgotten that research is not necessarily just an academic exercise, but that it may spring from questions of personal relevance to the researcher. Research can, at least in time, resolve some of these questions and assist the process of reflection about one's own work and provide a way forward. The process of research, and the findings of the research, may lead to a different view of the complementary medicine, cooler but perhaps more valid.

WHAT SHOULD THE PRIORITIES BE?

Although many complementary therapists now have an interest in research, they usually have no experience of the research process and no time to conduct studies. Most medical research is carried out by paid staff, or at least by people who are able to take some time away from clinical posts to conduct research. Medical researchers and academics also have considerable, usually free, facilities in the form of libraries, computers, advice from colleagues and so on. The practical difficulties for most complementary practitioners, again usually neglected by critics, of undertaking research are immense, especially as most are necessarily working in private practice. While individual practitioners may carry out small studies and perhaps take part in larger research projects, substantial research programmes can only really be developed by the complementary professional organizations or by university or medically based researchers.

The lack of funding for medical research generally means that research into complementary medicine is likely to be low on the list of priorities for any of the major established funding organizations. The funding of $2 million in 1992, rising to $7.4 million in 1996, from the National Institute of Health (NIH) in the United States to establish research into complementary medicine is the envy of many European complementary therapy researchers, although it is a tiny fraction of the total NIH budget. In Germany, the government has initiated a project to at least build the infrastructure for research into complementary medicine. One of the key tasks has been to find researchers interested in complementary medicine and complementary therapists interested in becoming the scientists/practitioners that complementary therapy so badly needs.

The priorities for research depend, in our view, on whether the researchers are working from within the complementary community or from an academic or hospital environment. This is partly because the medical and complementary communities will have different priorities, but also because of the different levels of expertise available. Very few complementary practitioners have experience of research and many of the main organizations are only just beginning to develop the necessary expertise. Research programmes are developing from an almost complete absence of knowledge about research findings and methods. Priorities must therefore be modified in the light of this basic fact. It is no use, at the moment, berating complementary groups for failing to carry out controlled trials, though it would be fair to criticize some of the professional associations for failing to initiate a research programme that might ultimately include formal trials.

Need for Education and Training in Research

The most urgent need is therefore educational. In Germany, attempts to initiate research into complementary medicine have quite explicitly included an educational component and have anticipated a long time-scale. A series of seminars over three years has been established at one medical school, with help at every stage of the research design and application, with the long-term aim of training a core of serious and experienced complementary medical researchers (Aldridge, 1990). Most osteopathic and chiropractic colleges in Britain now have a basic introduction to research methodology and the findings of research into their discipline (BMA, 1993). Such courses could be instituted relatively quickly and inexpensively by simply bringing in sympathetic academics who teach similar courses.

There is no reason, or need, for all complementary practitioners to take a long-term interest in research—certainly many psychologists and doctors do not. We have remarked on the absence of interest shown by many psychotherapists in research or research findings, which is one reason why most forms of psychotherapy are not taken as seriously as they might be. However, some training in basic research findings and methods would at least ensure a basic understanding of the nature and purpose of research and help to inculcate a climate of interest in research. One purpose of writing this book was the hope that it might be a useful overview for colleges of complementary therapies setting up courses on research.

We suggest that experienced complementary practitioners who wish to begin research in their institutions should make contact with sympathetic researchers and academics in a collaborative exchange of views and experience. This does not imply that complementary practitioners do not have the ability to carry out research; there are very many able people in the complementary fields. It is simply that there is no point in reinventing the wheel; where a researcher already has experience with trial methodology or knowledge of the complementary field in question, it is much quicker and more efficient to use their expertise. Obviously in time complementary practitioners will develop their own knowledge and expertise in these areas. Because most complementary practitioners work in quite small groups, research is perhaps best co-ordinated by the colleges and professional associations. There is also the practical point that if research is not based in a hospital or general practice, the complementary colleges are likely to be the only places with a sufficient throughput of patients for many research projects.

The type of studies initiated by complementary practitioners is likely to be different from those carried out by academic or medical researchers, though substantial studies have been undertaken in some complementary institutions. It would seem better to begin with audits of practice, surveys of the use of complementary medicine and of patient satisfaction. Such work would provide valuable basic information as well as a foundation for later, more tightly controlled clinical research. There is certainly a great deal of scope for experimental research on the treatment process. Large controlled trials are more likely, for the moment, to be the province of experienced researchers, hopefully in collaboration with complementary practitioners. The questions they need to address concern the efficacy, cost-effectiveness, the durability of treatment effect, the extent to which treatment is psychologically mediated and the advantages and disadvantages of complementary therapies in relation to standard treatment.

INTEGRATION OF ORTHODOX AND COMPLEMENTARY RESEARCH

Finally, we would like to make a plea for a different attitude to research on complementary medicine from within the research community. Just as we hope that complementary practitioners will come to take a greater interest in both the findings and practice of research, so we hope that the research community will come to take a greater interest in complementary medicine.

The first reason for this is straightforward and concerns, among other things, the way in which people build a career in research. At the moment we suspect that researching complementary medicine is regarded in most academic and medical departments as maverick, fringe, methodologically suspect and so on—in fact, labelled in the same way as complementary practitioners themselves. It is therefore risky for many academics to devote much time to the area. In part this is just a plea for tolerance and a recognition that, whatever one's private views about complementary medicine, it is a subject of legitimate scientific enquiry both because of its inherent interest and its enormous importance to a very large proportion of the population.

However, there is a more fundamental argument. The field of complementary medicine is potentially an important domain of research for enquiries into more general theories and principles. At many points in the book we have remarked on the need to link research on complementary medicine to theories and empirical work on patient choice, the nature of the consultation, the reasons patients seek particular forms of treatment and so on. In controlled trials it is possible that innovative methodology might be developed within complementary medicine on, say, changes in patients' subjective experience during treatment, which might then find a place in trials of orthodox treatment. The main point is that research on complementary medicine, of whatever form, needs to be drawn into the general research enterprise, which would be of benefit both to complementary medicine and to many aspects of medical, psychological and sociological research. The fact that there is a divide professionally between orthodox and complementary practitioners does not mean that there has to be a divide when basic scientific questions are at issue.

We will end with a plea for patience from both advocates and critics of complementary medicine. Clarifying the therapeutic value, mechanisms, internal consistency and coherence of even the major systems of complementary medicine is a substantial project. Kazdin (1986) has emphasized that progress in psychotherapy research, a similarly difficult area both conceptually and practically, has been slow and difficult, even with considerable resources being devoted to the enterprise. It would be as well to be cautious about the speed of resolution of the fascinating and important problems in the arena of complementary medicine.

References

Aakster, CW. 1989. Assumptions governing approaches to diagnosis and treatment. *Social Science and Medicine* **29**(3):293–300.

Aldridge, D. 1990. Pluralism of medical practice in West Germany. *Complementary Medical Research* **4**:14.

Aldridge, D. 1993. Single case research designs. In: Lewith, GT and Aldrige, D, eds. *Clinical Research Methodology for Complementary Therapies*. London: Hodder and Stoughton.

Anderson, E. and Anderson, P. 1987. General practitioners and alternative medicine. *Journal of the Royal College of General Practitioners* **37**(295):52–5.

Anderson, R, Meeker, WC, Wirick, BE, Mootz, RD, Kirk, DH and Adams A. 1992. A meta-analysis of clinical trials of spinal manipulation. *Journal of Manipulative Physiological Therapy* **15**(3):181–94.

Anderson, W, O'Connor, BB, MacGregor, RR and Schwartz, JSl. 1993. Patient use and assessment of conventional and alternative therapies for HIV infection and AIDS. *AIDS* **7**(4):561–5.

Anon. 1987. New Zealand cancer patients and alternative medicine. Clinical Oncology Group. *New Zealand Medical Journal* **100**(818):110–13.

Anon. 1989. Psychosocial intervention and the natural history of cancer [editorial]. *Lancet* **2**(8668):901.

Anon. 1990. Bristol Cancer Help Centre [letter]. *Lancet* **336**:743-4.

Anon. 1994. Pharmaceuticals from plants: great potential, few funds. *Lancet* **343**(8912):1513–5.

Anthony, HM. 1987. Some methodological problems in the assessment of complementary therapy. *Statistics in Medicine* **6**:761–71.

Anthony, HM. 1993. Clinical research: questions to ask and the benefits of asking them. In: Lewith, GT and Aldridge, D, eds. *Clinical Research Methodology for Complementary Therapies*. London: Hodder and Stoughton.

Argyle, M. 1972. *The Psychology of Interpersonal Behaviour*. Harmondsworth: Penguin.

Argyle, M, ed. 1981. *Social Skills and Health*. London: Methuen.

Atherton, DJ. 1994. Towards the safer use of traditional remedies. *British Medical Journal* **308**:673–4.

Baer, HA. 1989. The American dominative system as a reflection of social relations in the larger society. *Social Science and Medicine* **28**(11):1103–12.

Bagenal, FS, Easton, DF, Harris, E, Chilvers, CE and McElwain, TJ. 1990. Survival of patients with breast cancer attending Bristol Cancer Help Centre. *Lancet* **336**: 606–10.

Bakx, K. 1991. The 'eclipse' of folk medicine in western society. *Sociology of Health and Illness* **13**:17–24.

Barlow, DH and Hersen, M. 1984. *Single Case Experimental Designs*. New York: Pergamon.

Baum, M. 1987. Science versus non-science in medicine. *Journal of the Royal Society of Medicine* **80**(6):332–3.

Baum, M. 1989. Rationalism versus irrationalism in the care of the sick: science versus the absurd [editorial]. *Medical Journal of Australia* **151**(11–12):607–8.

Baum, M. 1991. Bridging the gulf. *Complementary Medical Research* **5**(3):204–8.

Beaven, DW. 1989. Alternative medicine a cruel hoax—your money and your life? *New Zealand Medical Journal* **102**:416–17.

Beecher, HK. 1955. The powerful placebo. *Journal of the American Medical Association* **159**:1602–6.

Bensoussan, A. 1991. Part 1: Acupuncture meridians—myth or reality? *Complementary Therapies in Medicine* **2**(1):21–6.

Bensoussan, A. 1994. Part 2: Acupuncture meridians—myth or reality? *Complementary Therapies in Medicine* **2**(2):80–5.

Benveniste, J. 1988. Benveniste on the Benveniste affair. *Nature* **335**:759.

Bergin, AE and Garfield, SL. 1994. *Handbook of Psychotherapy and Behaviour Change.* New York: Wiley.

Bergner, P. 1991. Safety, effectiveness and cost effectiveness in naturopathic medicine. [Report] American Association of Naturopathic Physicians.

Bergner, M, Bobbitt, RA, Carter, WB and Gilson, BS. 1981. The sickness impact profile development and final revision of a health status measure. *Medical Care* **19**(8):787–805.

Beutler, LE, Machado, PP and Neufeldt, SA. 1994. Therapist variables. In: Bergin, AE and Garfield, SL, eds. *Handbook of Psychotherapy and Behavior Change.* New York: Wiley.

Bhatt-Sanders, D. 1985. Acupuncture for rheumatoid arthritis: an analysis of the literature. *Seminars in Arthritis and Rheumatism* **14**(4):225–31.

Bielory, L and Gandhi, R. 1994. Asthma and vitamin C. *Ann Allergy* **73**(2):89–96.

Bishop, G. 1987. Lay conceptions of physcial symptoms. *Journal of Applied Social Psychology* **17**:127–46.

Black, N. 1996. Why we need observational studies to evaluate the effectiveness of health care. *British Medical Journal* **312**(7040):1215–18.

Blanchard, EB and Andrasik, F. 1982. Psychological assessment and treatment of headache: recent developments and emerging issues. *Journal of Consulting and Clinical Psychology* **50**:859–79.

Blattner, B. 1981. *Holistic Nursing.* Englewood Cliffs, N.J.: Prentice-Hall.

Blaxter, N. 1983. The causes of disease: women talking. *Social Science and Medicine* **17**:59–69.

BMA. 1986. *Alternative Therapy.* Oxford: Oxford University Press.

BMA. 1993. *Complementary Medicine: New approaches to Good Practice.* Oxford: Oxford University Press.

Boisset, M and Fitzcharles, M-A. 1994. Alternative medicine use by rheumatology patients in a universal health care setting. *Journal of Rheumatology* **21**(1):148–52.

Bone, ME, Wilkinson, DJ, Young, JR, McNeil, J and Charlton, S. 1990. Ginger root— a new antiemetic. *Anaesthesia* **45**:669–71.

Borglum-Jensen, L, Melsen, B and Borglum-Jensen, S. 1979. Effect of acupuncture on headache measured by reduction in number of attacks and use of drugs. *Scandinavian Journal of Dental Research* **87**:373–80.

Bourke, I and Goodare, H. 1991. Bristol Cancer Help Centre. *Lancet* **338**:1401.

Bowen, R, Genn, C, Lupton, G, Payne, S, Sheehan, M and Western, J. 1977. New patients to alternative care. Committee of Inquiry on Chiropractice, Osteopathy, Homeopathy and Naturopathy, Parliamentary Paper 102.

Brannon, L and Feist, J. 1992. *Health psychology: An introduction to behavior and health.* Belmont, CA: Wadsworth Publishing Co.

Briskman, L. 1987. Doctors and witchdoctors: which doctors are which? *British Medical Journal* 295:1108–10.

Brunarski, DJ. 1984. Clinical trials of spinal manipulation: a critical appraisal and review of the literature. *Journal of Manipulative Physiological Therapy* 7(4):243–9.

Buckalew, LW and Ross, S. 1981. Relationship of perceptual characteristics to efficacy of placebos. *Psychological Reports* 49:955–61.

Budd, C, Fisher, B, Parrinder, D and Price, L. 1990. A model of cooperation between complementary and allopathic medicine in a primary care setting. *British Journal of General Practice* 40(338):376–8.

Bullock, ML, Culliton, PD and Olander, RT. 1989. Controlled trial of acupuncture for severe recidivist alcoholism. *Lancet* (i):1435–9.

Burton, AK. 1990. Complementary and allopathic cooperation. *British Journal of General Practice* November:478.

Calnan, M. 1987. *Health and Illness: The Lay Perspective.* London: Tavistock.

Cant, S and Calnan, M. 1991. On the margins of the medical market place? An exploratory study of alternative practitioners' perceptions. *Sociology of Health and Illness* 13:39–57.

Canter, D and Booker, CK. 1987. Multiple consultations as a basis for classifying patients' use of conventional and unconventional medicine. *Complementary Medical Research* 2(2):141–60.

Canter, D and Nanke, L. 1989. Individual variation and symptomatology: A homeopathic perspective. *British Homeopathy Research Group Communications* 1:43–91.

Canter, D and Nanke, L. 1991. Psychological aspects of complementary medicine. Social aspects of complementary medicine. Staffordshire: University of Keele.

Canter, D and Nanke, L. 1993. Emerging priorities in complementary medical research. In: Lewith, GT and Aldridge, D, eds. *Clinical Research Methodology for Complementary Therapies.* London: Hodder and Stoughton.

Carne, S. 1961. The action of chorionic gonadotrophin in the obese. *Lancet* ii: 1282–4.

Cassileth, BR. 1986. Unorthodox cancer medicine. *Cancer Investigation* 4(6):591–8.

Cassileth, BR. 1989. The social implications of questionable cancer therapies. *Cancer* 63(7):1247–50.

Cassileth, BR, Lusk, EJ, Strouse, TB and Bodenheimer, BJ. 1984. Contemporary unorthodox treatments in cancer medicine. *Annals of Internal Medicine* 101(1): 105–12.

Chan, TYK, Chan, AYW and Critchley, AJH. 1992. Hospital admissions due to adverse reactions to Chinese herbal medicines. *Journal of Tropical Medicine and Hygiene* 95:296–8.

Chassein, MR, Brook, RM, Park, RE, Keesey, J, Fink, A and Kossof, J. 1986. Variations in the use of medical and surgical services by the medicare population. *New England Journal of Medicine* 314:285–90.

Chatfield, C. 1985. *The Analyses of Time Series.* London: Chapman and Hall.

Chilvers, C, Bagenal, F and Harris, E. 1991. Bristol Cancer Help Centre. *Lancet* 338:1402.

Chilvers, CED, Easton, DF, Bagenal, FS, Harris, E and McElwain, TJ. 1990. Bristol Cancer Help Centre. *Lancet* 336:1186–8.

Chrisman, N. 1977. The health seeking process: An approach to the natural history of illness. *Culture, Medicine and Psychiatry* 1:351–77.

Christensen, PA, Laursen, LC and Taudorf, E. 1984. Acupuncture and bronchial asthma. *Allergy* **39**:379–85.

Chung, S-H and Dickenson, A. 1980. Pain, enkephalin and acupuncture. *Nature* **283**:243–4.

Clement-Jones, VL, Tomlin, S, Rees, LH, McLouglin, L, Besser, GM and Wen, HL. 1980. Increased beta-endorphin but not met-enkephalin levels in human cerebrospinal fluid after acupuncture for recurrent pain. *Lancet* **ii**:946–8.

Coan, RM, Wang, G, Ku, SL, Chan, YC, Ozer, FT and Coan, PL. 1980. The acupuncture treatment of low back pain: a randomized controlled study. *American Journal of Chinese Medicine* **8**:181–9.

Coan, RM, Wong, G and Coan, PL. 1982. The acupuncture treatment of neck pain: a randomized controlled study. *American Journal of Chinese Medicine* **9**:326–32.

Cobb, LA, Thomas, GI and Dillard, DH. 1959. An evaluation of internal-mammary-artery ligation by a double blind technique. *New England Journal of Medicine* **260**:1115–18.

Cohen, LH, Sargent, MM and Sechrest, LB. 1986. Use of psychotherapy research by professional psychologists. *American Psychology* **41**(2):198–206.

Cole, P. 1975. Acupuncture and pulse diagnosis in Great Britain [PhD thesis]: University of Surrey.

Colquhoun, D. 1990. Re-analysis of clinical trials of homeopathic treatment in fibrositis. *Lancet* **336**(8712):441–2.

Cook, M and Ferner, RE. 1993. Adverse drug reactions: who is to know? *British Medical Journal* **307**:480–1.

Cosh, J and Sikora, K. 1989. Conventional and complementary treatment for cancer. *British Medical Journal* **298**(6682):1200–1.

Curtis, P. 1988. Spinal manipulation: does it work? *Occupational Medicine* **3**(1): 31–44.

D'Arcy, PF. 1991. Adverse reactions and interactions with herbal medicines. Part 1—Adverse reactions. *Adverse Drug Reactions Toxicological Reviews* **10**(4): 189–208.

D'Arcy, PF. 1993. Adverse reactions and interactions with herbal medicines. Part 2—Drug interactions. *Adverse Drug Reactions and Toxicological Reviews* **12**(3): 147–62.

Danielson, KJ, Stewart, DE and Lippert, GP. 1988. Unconventional cancer remedies. *Cancer Medical Association Journal* **138**(11):1005–11.

Darlington, LG, Ramsey, NW and Mansfield JR. 1986. Placebo-controlled, blind study of dietary manipulation in rheumatoid arthritis. *Lancet* **1**(8475):236–8.

Davenas, E, Beauvais, F, Amara, J, Oberbaum, M, Robinson, B, Miadonna, A et al. 1988. Human basophil degranulation triggered by very dilute antiserum against IgE. *Nature* **333**:816–18.

Deluze, C, Bosia, L, Zirbs, A, Chantraine, A and Vischer, TL. 1992. Electro-acupuncture in fibromyalgia: results of a controlled trial. *British Medical Journal* **305**(6864):1249–52.

Dennison, JAG. 1989. Conventional and complementary treatment for cancer. *British Medical Journal* **298**:1583.

Derogatis, LR. 1986. Psychosocial adjustment to illness scale (PA 15). *Journal of Psychosomatic Research* **30**(1):77–91.

Derogatis, LR and Melisaratos, N. 1983. The brief symptom inventory: An introductory report. *Psychological Medicine* **13**:595–605.

DHSS. 1991. *Hospital inpatients enquiry summary tables*. London: HMSO.

DiFabio, RP. 1986. Clinical assessment of manipulation and mobilization of the lumbar spine. *Physical Therapy* **66**:51.

Dimond, EG, Kittle, CF and Cockett, JE. 1960. Comparison of internal mammary-artery ligation and sham operation for angina pectoris. *American Journal of Cardiology* **4**:483–6.

Ditto, PH, Moore, KA, Hilton, JL and Kalish, JR. 1995. Beliefs about physicians: their role in health care utilization, satisfaction and compliance. *Basic and Applied Social Psychology* **17**(1–2):23–48.

Dolan, G, Jones, AP, Blumsohn, A, Reilly, JT and Brown MJ. 1991. Lead poisoning due to Asian ethnic treatment for impotence. *Journal of the Royal Society of Medicine* **84**:630–1.

Donnelly, WJ, Spykerboer, JE and Thong, YH. 1985. Are patients who use alternative medicine dissatisfied with orthodox medicine? *Medical Journal of Australia* **142**(10):539–41.

Downer, SM, Cody, MM, McLuskey, P, Wilson, PD, Arnott, SJ, Lister, TA and Slevin, ML. 1994. Pursuit and practice of complementary therapies by cancer patients receiving conventional treatment. *British Medical Journal* **309**:86–9.

Dowson, D, Lewith, GT and Machin, D. 1985. The effects of acupuncture versus placebo in the treatment of headache. *Pain* **21**:35–42.

Easterbrook, PJ, Berlin, JA, Gopalan, R and Matthews, DR. 1991. Publication bias in clinical research. *Lancet* **337**(8746).

Eddy, DM. 1994. Clinical decision making: from theory to practice. Principles for making difficult decisions in difficult times. *Journal of the American Medical Association* **271**(22):1792–8.

Einarson, TR. 1993. Drug-related hospital admissions. *Annals of Pharmacotherapy* **27**:832–40.

Eisele, JW and Reay, DT. 1980. Deaths related to coffee enemas. *Journal of the American Medical Association* **244**(14):1608–9.

Eisenberg, D, Kessler, RC and Foster, C. 1993. Unconventional medicine in the United States. *New England Journal of Medicine* **328**:246–52.

Elliott-Binns, CP. 1973. An analysis of lay medicine. *Journal of the Royal College of General Practitioners* **23**:255–64.

Elliott-Binns, CP. 1986. An analysis of lay medicine: fifteen years later. *Journal of the Royal College of General Practitioners* **36**:542–4.

Evans, FJ. 1974. The placebo response in pain reduction. *Advances in Neurology* **4**:289–96.

Evans, FJ. 1985. Expectancy, therapeutic instructions and the placebo response. In: White, L, Tursky, B and Schwartz, GE, eds. *Placebo, Theory, Research, and Mechanisms*. New York: Guilford Press.

Eysenck, HJ. 1952. The effects of psychotherapy: an evaluation. *Journal of Consulting Psychology* **16**:319–24.

Eysenck, HJ. 1983. Personality as a fundamental concept in scientific psychology. *Australian Journal of Psychology* **35**(3):289–304.

Fallowfield, L. 1990. *The Quality of Life: The Missing Measurement in Health Care*. London: Souvenir Press.

Fawzy, FI, Fawzy, NW, Hyun, CS, Elashoff, R, Guthrie, D, Fahey, JL and Morton, DC. 1993. Malignant melanoma. *Archives of General Psychiatry* **50**:681–9.

Feldman, PE. 1956. The personal element in psychiatric research. *American Journal of Psychiatry* **113**:52–4.

Ferley, JP, Poutignat, N, Azzopardi, Y, Charrel, M and Zmirou, D. 1987. Évaluation en médecine ambulatoire de l'activité d'un complexe homéopathique dans la prévention de la grippe et des syndromes grippaux. *Immunologie Médecine* **20**: 22–8.

Ferley, JP, Zmirou, D, d'Adhemar, D and Balducci, F. 1989. A controlled evaluation of a homoeopathic preparation in the treatment of influenza-like syndromes. *British Journal of Clinical Pharmacology* **27**:329–35.

Fernandez, E and Turk, DC. 1989. The utility of cognitive coping strategies for altering pain perception: a meta-analysis. *Pain* **38**(2):123–35.

Festinger, L. 1957. *A Theory of Cognitive Dissonance*. Stanford: Stanford University Press.

Filshie, J and Redman, D. 1985. Acupuncture and malignant pain problems. *European Society of Clinical Oncology* **11**(4):389–94.

Finnigan, M. 1991a. The Centre for the Study of Complementary Medicine: An attempt to understand its popularity through psychological, demographic and operational criteria. *Complementary Medical Research* **5**:83–8.

Finnigan, M. 1991b. Complementary medicine: Attitudes and expectations, a scale for evaluation. *Complementary Medical Research* **5**:75–82.

Fisher, P. 1993. Research into the homoeopathic treatment of rheumatological disease: why and how? In: Lewith, GA and Aldridge, D, eds. *Clinical Research Methodology for Complementary Therapies*. London: Hodder and Stoughton.

Fisher, P and Ward, A. 1994. Complementary medicine in Europe. *British Medical Journal* **309**:107–11.

Fisher, RA and MacKenzie, WA. 1923. Studies in crop variation. II. The manurial response of different potato varieties. *Agricultural Science* **13**:311–20.

Fisher, RA. 1926. The arrangement of field experiments. *Journal of the Ministry of Agriculture* **33**:503–13.

Fitter, M and Blackwell, R. 1993. Are acupuncturists interested in research? A survey of registered acupuncturists in the UK. Submitted for publication.

Fitzpatrick, R. 1984. Lay concepts of illness. In: Fitzpatrick, R, Hirlon, J, Newman, S, Scambler, G and Thompson, J, eds. *The Experience of Illness*. London: Tavistock.

Fox, EJ and Melzack, R. 1976. Transcutaneous nerve stimulation and acupuncture: comparison of treatment for low back pain. *Pain* **2**:141–8.

Freer, CB. 1985. What kind of alternative is alternative medicine? [editorial]. *Journal of the Royal College of General Practitioners* **35**(279):459–60.

Friedman, M, Thoresen, CE, Gill, JJ, Ulmer, D, Powell, LH, Price, VA et al. 1986. Alteration of Type A behavior and its effect on cardiac recurrences in post myocardial infarction patients: summary results of the Recurrent Coronary Prevention Project. *American Heart Journal* **112**:653–65.

Fulder, S. 1984. *The Handbook of Complementary Medicine*. London: Hodder and Stoughton.

Fulder, SJ and Munro, RE. 1985. Complementary medicine in the United Kingdom: patients, practitioners, and consultations. *Lancet* **2**(8454):542–5.

Furnham, A. 1988. *Lay Theories: Everyday Understanding of Problems in the Social Sciences*. Oxford: Pergamon Press.

Furnham, A. 1993. Attitudes to alternative medicine: a study of the perception of those studying orthodox medicine. *Complementary Therapies in Medicine* **1**: 120–6.

Furnham, A and Bhagrath, R. 1993. A comparison of health beliefs and behaviours of clients of orthodox and complementary medicine. *British Journal of Clinical Psychology* **32**:237–46.

Furnham, A and Forey, J. 1994. The attitudes, behaviours, and beliefs of patients of traditional vs complementary (alternative) medicine. *Journal of Clinical Psychology* **50**:458–69.

Furnham, A and Kirkcaldy, B. 1996. The medical beliefs and behaviours of orthodox and complementary medicine clients. *British Journal of Clinical Psychology* **35**: 49–62.

Furnham, A and Smith, C. 1988. Choosing alternative medicine: A comparison of the beliefs of patients visiting a general practitioner and a homoeopath. *Social Science and Medicine* **26**:685–9.

Furnham, A and Steele, H. 1993. Measuring locus of control: a critique of general, children's, health and work-related locus of control questionnaires. *British Journal of Psychology* **84**(4):443–79.

Furnham, A, Vincent, C and Wood, R. 1995. The health beliefs and behaviours of three groups of complementary medicine and a general practice group of patients. *Journal of Alternative and Complementary Medicine* **1**:347–59.

Gallachi, G. 1981. Acupuncture for cervical and lumbar syndrome. *Scheiz Med Wschr* **111**:1360–6.

Gaw, AC, Chang, LW and Shaw, LC. 1975. Efficacy of acupuncture on osteoarthritic pain: a double blind controlled trial. *New England Journal of Medicine* **293**:375–8.

Gibson, RG and Gibson, SLM. 1988. Controversy continues [letter]. *Nature* **335**:200.

Gilovich, T. 1991. *How Do We Know What Isn't So*. New York: Free Press.

GMC. 1992. *Professional Conduct and Discipline: Fitness to Practise*. London: GMC.

Godfrey, CM and Morgan, P. 1978. A controlled trial of the theory of acupuncture in musculoskeletal pain. *Journal of Rheumatology* **5**:121–4.

Goldstein, MS, Sutherland, C, Jaffe, DT and Wilson, J. 1988. Holistic physicians and family practitioners: similarities, differences and implications for health policy. *Social Science and Medicine* **26**(8):853–61.

Goodare, H and Smith, R. 1995. The rights of patients in research. *British Medical Journal* **310**:1277–8.

Goodwin, JS, Goodwin, JM and Vogel, JM. 1979. Knowledge and use of placebo by house officers and nurses. *Annals of Internal Medicine* **91**:106–10.

Gray, G and Flynn, P. 1981. A survey of placebo use in general hospital. *General Hospital Psychiatry* **3**:199–203.

Gray, D. 1985. The treatment strategies of arthritis sufferers. *Social Science and Medicine* **21**(5):507–15.

GRECHO UI, ARC, GREPA. 1989. Évaluation de deux produits homéopathiques sur la reprise du transit après chirurgie digestive. Un essai contrôlé multi-centrique. *Presse Méd* **18**:59–62.

Greenblatt, RM, Hollander, H, McMaster, JR and Henke, CJ. 1991. Polypharmacy among patients attending an AIDS clinic: utilization of prescribed, unorthodox, and investigational treatments. *Journal of Acquired Immune Deficiency Syndrome* **4**(2):136–43.

Greenland, S, Reisbord, LS, Haldeman, S and Buerger, AA. 1980. Controlled clinical trials of manipulation: a review and a proposal. *Journal of Occupational Medicine* **22**:670.

Greer, S. 1991. Psychological response to cancer and survival. *Psychological Medicine* **21**:43–9.

Grenfell, R, Briggs, AH and Holland, WC. 1961. A double-blind study of the treatment of hypertension. *Journal of the American Medical Association* **176**:124–67.

Grisso, JA. 1993. Making comparisons. *Lancet* **342**(8746):157–60.

Grunbaum, A. 1981. The placebo concept. *Behaviour Research and Therapy* **19**: 157–67.

Gunn, CC, Milbrandt, WE, Little, AS and Mason, KE. 1980. Dry needling of muscle motor points for chronic low back pain. *Spine* **5**:279–91.

Hand, R. 1989. Alternative therapies used by patients with AIDS. *New England Journal of Medicine* **320**(10):672–3.

Hansen, PA. 1991. A suggested medical curriculum for learning about complementary medicine. *Journal of the Royal Society of Medicine* **84**(1):702–3.

Hashish, I, Feinman, C and Harvey, W. 1988. Reduction of postoperative pain and swelling by ultrasound: a placebo effect. *Pain* **83**:303–11.

Hayes, RJ, Smith, PG and Carpenter, L. 1990. Bristol Cancer Help Centre. *Lancet* **336**:1185.

Helman, C. 1990. *Culture, Health and Illness* (2nd edn). Oxford: Butterworth-Heineman.

Henry, P, Baille, H, Dartigues, JF and Jogeix, M. 1985. Headache and acupuncture. In: Pfaffenrath, V, Lundberg, PO and Sjaastad, O, eds. *Updating in Headache*. Berlin: Springer Verlag.

Heron, J. 1986. Critique of conventional research methodology. *Complementary Medical Research* **1**:12–22.

Hewer, W. 1983. The relationship between the alternative practitioner and his patient. A review. *Psychotherapy and Psychosomatics* **40**(1–4):172–80.

Hiatt, HH, Barnes, BA, Brennan, TA, Laird, MM, Lawthers, HG, Lempe, LL et al. 1989. A study of medical injury and medical malpractice: an overview. *New England Journal of Medicine* **321**:480.

Hill, C and Doyon, F. 1990. Review of randomized trials of homeopathy. *Revue Epidemiologie Santé Publique* **38**(2):139–47.

Himmel, W, Schulte, M and Kochen, MM. 1993. Complementary medicine: Are patients' expectations being met by their general practitioners? *British Journal of General Practice* **43**(371):232–5.

Holohan, TV. 1987. Referral by default. The medical community and unorthodox therapy. *Journal of the American Medical Association* **257**(12):1641–2.

Horwitz, RI, Viscoli, CM, Bermkan, L, Donaldson, RM, Horowitz, SM et al. 1990. Treatment adherence and risk of death after a myocardial infarction. *Lancet* **336**:542–5.

Howarth, E and Schokman-Gates, KL. 1981. Self report multiple mood instruments. *British Journal of Psychology* **72**:421–41.

Hunt, L, Jordan, B and Irwin, S. 1989. Views of what's wrong: Diagnosis and patients' concepts of illness. *Social Science and Medicine* **28**:945–6.

Hunt, SM, McEwen, J and McKenna, SP. 1985. Measuring health status: A new tool for clinicians and epidemiologists. *Journal of the Royal College of General Practitioners* **35**:185–8.

Hunt, SM, McKenna, SP, McEwen, J, Williams, J and Papp, E. 1981. The Nottingham health profile: Subjective health status and medical consultations. *Social Science and Medicine* **15a**:221–9.

Huxtable, RJ. 1992. The myth of beneficent nature: the risks of herbal preparations. *Annals of Internal Medicine* **117**(2):165–6.

Illich, I. 1976. *Limits to Medicine*. Harmondsworth: Pelican Books.

Inglis, B. 1964. *Fringe Medicine*. London: Faber and Faber.

Inglis, B. 1985. Alternative medicine: is there a need for registration? *Lancet* **1**(8420):95–6.

Jayson, MIV. 1986. A limited role for manipulation. *British Medical Journal* **293**:1454–5.

Jobst, K, Chen, JH, McPherson, K, Arrowsmith, J, Brown, V et al. 1986. Controlled trial of acupuncture for disabling breathlessness. *Lancet* **2**:1416–19.

Johnson, ES, Kadam, NP, Hylands, DM and Hylands, PJ. 1985. Efficacy of feverfew as a prophylactic treatment of migraine. *British Medical Journal* **291**:569–73.

Kazdin, AE. 1984. Statistical analyses for single case experimental designs. In: Barlow, DH and Hersen, M, eds. *Single Case Experimental Designs*. New York: Pergamon.

Kazdin, AE. 1986. Research designs and methodology. In: Garfield, SL and Bergin, AE, eds. *Handbook of Psychotherapy and Behavior Change*. New York: Wiley.

King, J. 1983. Health beliefs in the consultation. In: Pendleton, D and Hasler, J, eds. *Doctor-patient Communication*. London: Academic Press.

King, K, Shaw, J, Bochner, F and Brooks, PM. 1985. Therapeutics. Alternative medicine. *Medical Journal of Australia* **142**:547–51.

Kleijnen, J and Knipschild, P. 1992. Ginkgo biloba. *Lancet* **340**:1136–9.

Kleijnen, J, Knipschild, P and ter Riet, G. 1991. Clinical trials of homeopathy. *British Medical Journal* **302**:316–23.

Kleijnen, J, ter Riet, G and Knipschild, P. 1989. Vitamin C and the common cold; a review of a megadose of literature. *Ned Tijdschr Geneeskd* **124**:418–23.

Kleijnen, J, ter Riet, G and Knipschild, P. 1991. Acupuncture and asthma: a review of controlled trials. *Thorax* **46**(11):799–802.

Kleinman, A. 1980. *Patients and Healers in the Context of Culture*. Berkeley: University of California Press.

Knipschild, P. 1988. Looking for gall bladder disease in the patient's iris. *British Medical Journal* **297**(6663):1578–81.

Knipschild, P, Kleijnen, J and ter Riet, G. 1990. Belief in the efficacy of alternative medicine among general practitioners in The Netherlands. *Social Science and Medicine* **31**(5):625–6.

Koes, BW, Assendelft, WJJ, van der Heijden, GJMG, Bouter, LM and Knipschild, PG. 1991. Spinal manipulation and mobilisation for back and neck pain: a blinded review. *British Medical Journal* **303**:1298–303.

Kramer, MS and Shapiro, SH. 1984. Scientific challenges in the application of randomized trials. *Journal of the American Medical Association* **252**(19):2739–45.

Laitinen, J. 1976. Acupuncture and transcutaneous nerve stimulation in the treatment of chronic sacro-lumbalgia and ischialgia. *American Journal of Chinese Medicine* **4**:169–75.

Lammes, FB. 1988. Miraculous cures in gynaecology. *European Journal of Obstetric and Gynaecological Reproduction Biology* **29**(3):191–5.

Langley, GB, Sheppeard, H, Johnson, M and Wigley, RD. 1984. The analgesic effects of transcutaneous nerve stimulation and placebo in chronic patients. *Rheumatology* **2**:1–5.

Lau, R and Ware, J. 1981. Refinements in the measurement of health-specific locus-of-control beliefs. *Medical Care* **19**:1147–58.

Leape, LL, Brennan, TA and Laird, NM. 1991. The nature of adverse events and negligence in hospitalized patients. *Iatrogenics* **1**:17.

Lee, PK, Andersen, PW, Modell, JH and Saga, SA. 1975. Treatment of chronic pain with acupuncture. *Journal of the Americal Medical Association* **232**:1133–5.

Lee, KP, Carlins, WG, McCormack, GF and Albers, GW. 1995. Neurologic complications following chiropractic manipulation: A survey of California neurologists. *Neurology* **45**:1213–15.

Lerner, IJ. 1987. Cancer quackery. *Psychiatric Medicine* **5**(4):419–29.

Levin, JS and Coreil, J. 1986. 'New age' healing in the U.S. *Social Science and Medicine* **23**(9):889–97.

Levy, SM and Wise, BD. 1987. Psychosocial risk factors, natural immunity, and cancer progression: Implications for intervention. *Current Psychology Research and Reviews* **6**(3):229–43.

Lewith, GT. 1988. Undifferentiated illness: some suggestions for approaching the polysymptomatic patient [editorial]. *Journal of the Royal Society of Medicine* **81**(10):563–5.

Lewith, GT and Aldridge, DA. 1991. *Complementary Medicine and the European Community*. Saffron Walden: C.W. Daniel.

Lewith, GT and Aldridge, D. 1993. *Clinical Research Methodology for Complementary Therapies*. London: Hodder and Stoughton.

Lewith, GT and Kenyon, JN. 1984. Physiological and psychological explanations for the mechanism of acupuncture as a treatment for chronic pain. *Social Science and Medicine* **19**(12):1367–78.

Lewith, GT and Lewith, NR. 1983. *Modern Chinese Acupuncture*. Wellingborough: Thorsons.

Lewith, GT and Machin, D. 1983. On the evaluation of the clinical effects of acupuncture. *Pain* **16**:111–27.

Lewith, G and Vincent, C. 1995. Evaluation of the clinical effects of acupuncture. *Pain Forum* **4**(1):1–11.

Lewith, GT, Field, J and Machin, D. 1983. Acupuncture compared with placebo in post-herpetic pain. *Pain* **16**:361–8.

Ley, P. 1989. Improving patients' understanding, recall, satisfaction and compliance. In: Broome, AK, ed. *Health Psychology*. London: Chapman and Hall.

Macdonald, AJR. 1989. Acupuncture analgesia and therapy. In: Wall, PD and Melzack, R, eds. *Textbook of Pain*. 2nd edn. London: Churchill Livingstone.

Macdonald, AJR, Macrae, KD, Master, BR and Rubin, AP. 1983. Superficial acupuncture in the relief of chronic low back pain. *Annals of the Royal College of Surgeons of England* **65**:44–6.

MacGregor, FB, Abernethy, VE, Dahabra, S, Cobden, I and Hayes, PC. 1989. Hepatotoxicity of herbal remedies. *British Medical Journal* **299**(6708):1156–7.

Maddox, J. 1988. Waves caused by extreme dilution. *Nature* **335**:760–3.

Maguire, P. 1981. Doctor-patient skills. In: Argyle, LM, ed. *Social Skills and Health*. London: Methuen.

Maguire, P. 1990. Can communication skills be taught? *British Journal of Hospital Medicine* **43**:215–16.

Maguire, P, Fairbairn, S and Fletcher, C. 1986. Consultation skills of young doctors. *British Medical Journal* **292**:1573–8.

Mansell, P and Reckless, JP. 1991. Garlic [editorial]. *British Medical Journal* **303**(6799):379–80.

Margetts, BM, Beilin, LJ, Vandongen, R and Armstrong, BK. 1986. Vegetarian diet in mild hypertension: a randomised controlled trial. *British Medical Journal* **293**:1468–71.

Marshall, RJ and Gee, R. 1990. The use of alternative therapies by Auckland general practitioners. *New Zealand Medical Journal* **103**(889):213–15.

Mayaux, MJ, Guihard-Moscato, ML, Schwartz, D, Benveniste, J, Coquin, Y, Crapanne, JB et al. 1988. Controlled clinical trial of homoeopathy in postoperative ileus. *Lancet* **1**:528–9.

McGinnis, LS. 1991. Alternative therapies 1990. An overview. *Cancer* **67**(6 Suppl):1788–92.

McGourty, H. 1993. *How to Evaluate Complementary Therapies*. Liverpool: Liverpool Public Health Observatory.

McManus, IC, Vincent, CA, Thom, S and Kidd, J. 1993. Teaching communication skills to clinical students. *British Medical Journal* **306**:1322–7.

Meade, TW, Dyer, S, Browne, W, Townsend, J and Frank, AO. 1990. Low back pain of mechanical origin: randomised comparison of chiropractic and hospital outpatient treatment. *British Medical Journal* **300**:1431–7.

Medeiros, DM, Bock, MA, Ortiz, M, Raab, C, Read, M, Schutz, HG et al. 1989. Vitamin and mineral supplementation practices of adults in seven western states. *Journal of the American Diet Association* **89**(3):383–6.

Mendelson, G, Selwood, TS, Kranz, H, Kidson, MA and Scott, DS. 1983. Acupuncture treatment of chronic back pain: a double blind placebo controlled trial. *American Journal of Medicine* **74**:49–55.

Menges, L. 1994. Regular and alternative medicine: the state of affairs in the Netherlands. *Social Science and Medicine* **39**:871–3.

Meserole, L. 1996. Western herbalism. In: Micozzi, MS, ed. *Fundamentals of Complementary and Alternative Medicine*. New York: Churchill Livingstone.

Micozzi, MS, ed. 1996. *Fundamentals of Complementary and Alternative Medicine*. New York: Churchill Livingstone.

Mills, S. 1993a. Herbal medicines: research strategies. In: Lewith, GT and Aldridge, D, eds. *Clinical Research Methodology for Complementary Therapies*. London: Hodder and Stoughton.

Mills, SY. 1993b. The 4th International Congress on phytotherapy 10–13 September 1992. *Complementary Therapies in Medicine* **1**:105–6.

Mills, SY and Fulder, S. 1984. Herbalism. In: Fulder, S, ed. *The Handbook of Complementary Medicine*. London: Coronet Books.

Mittman, P. 1990. Randomized, double-blind study of freeze-dried *Urtica dioica* in the treatment of allergic rhinitis. *Planta Medica* **56**:44–7.

Monckton, J. 1993. Research: The way forward. 10th Anniversary Colloquium of the Research Council for Complementary Medicine. Royal Society of Medicine, London: Research Council for Complementary Medicine.

Montbriand, MJ and Laing, GP. 1991. Alternative health care as a control strategy. *Journal of Advanced Nursing* **16**(3):325–32.

Moore, J, Phipps, K, Marcer, D and Lewith, G. 1985. Why do people seek treatment by alternative medicine? *British Medical Journal* **290**(6461):28–9.

Morrow-Bradley, C and Elliott, RE. 1986. Utilization of psychotherapy research by practising psychotherapists. *American Psychology* **41**(2):188–97.

Moss, F. 1992. Quality in health care. *Quality in Health Care* **1**(1):1–3.

Murphy, JJ, Heptinstall, S and Mitchell, JRA. 1988. Randomised double-blind placebo-controlled trial of feverfew in migraine prevention. *Lancet* **ii**:189–92.

Murray, J and Shepherd, S. 1988. Alternative or additional medicine? A new dilemma for the doctor. *Journal of the Royal College of General Practitioners* **38**(316): 511–14.

Murray, RH and Rubel, AJ. 1992. Physicians and healers—unwitting partners in health care. *New England Journal of Medicine* **326**(1):61.

Murray, J and Shepherd, S. 1993. Alternative or additional medicine? An exploratory study in general practice. *Social Science and Medicine* **37**:938–88.

Nanda, R, James, R, Smith, H, Dudley, CRK and Jewell, DP. 1989. Food intolerance and the irritable bowel syndrome. *Gut* **30**:1099–104.

Newman-Turner, R. 1990a. *Naturopathic Medicine* (new ed.). Wellingborough: Thorsons.

Newman-Turner, R. 1990b. Self-medication and alternative prescribing. *Practitioner* **234**(1482):117–20.

Norheim, AJ and Fonnebo, V. 1995. Adverse effects of acupuncture. *Lancet* **345**: 1576.

O'Connor, J and Bensky, D. 1981. *Acupuncture: A Comprehensive Text.* Shanghai College of Traditional Chinese Medicine. Chicago, IL: Eastland Press.

Ong, L, de Haes, J and Lammes, F. 1995. Doctor-patient communication. A review of the literature. *Social Science and Medicine* **40**:903–18.

Ornish, D, Brown, SE, Scherwitz, LW and Billings, JH. 1990. Can lifestyle changes reverse coronary heart disease? *Lancet* **336**:129–33.

Panush, RS, Carter, RL, Katz, P, et al. 1983. Diet therapy for rheumatoid arthritis. *Arthritis and Rheumatism* **26**:462–71.

Patel, M, Gutzwiller, F, Paccaud, F and Marazzi, A. 1989. A meta-analysis of acupuncture for chronic pain. *International Journal of Epidemiology* **18**(4):900–6.

Patijn, J. 1991. Complications in manual medicine: a review of the literature. *Journal of Manual Medicine* **6**:89–92.

Pattrick, M, Heptinstall, S and Doherty, M. 1989. Feverfew in rheumatoid arthritis: a double blind, placebo controlled study. *Annals of the Rheumatic Diseases* **48**:547–9.

Pendleton, D and Hasler, J, eds. 1983. *Doctor-patient Communication.* London: Academic Press.

Perkin, MR, Pearcy, RM and Fraser, JS. 1994. A comparison of the attitudes shown by general practitioners, hospital doctors and medical students towards alternative medicine. *Journal of the Royal Society of Medicine* **87**(9):523–5.

Petrie, J and Hazelman, B. 1985. Credibility of placebo transcutaneous nerve stimulation and acupuncture. *Clinical and Experimental Rheumatology* **3**:151–3.

Petsko, GA. 1988. Unreproducible results. *Nature* **335**:109.

Pfifferling, JH. 1980. A cultural prescription for mediocentrism. In: Eisenberg, L and Kleinman, A, eds. *Relevance of Social Science for Medicine.* Dordrecht: Reidel.

Pietroni, PC. 1986. Alternative medicine. *Practitioner* **230**(1422):1053–4.

Pietroni, P. 1987. Holistic medicine: new lessons to be learned. *Practitioner* **231**(1437):1386–90.

Pocock, SJ. 1985. Current issues in the design and interpretation of clinical trials. *British Medical Journal* **290**:39–42.

Pocock, SJ. 1993. *Clinical Trials.* Chichester: Wiley.

Pollock, AV. 1989. The rise and fall of the random controlled trial in surgery. *Theoretical Surgery* **4**:163–70.

Prance, SE, Dresser, A, Wood, C, Fleming, J, Aldridge, D and Pietroni, P. 1988. Research on traditional Chinese acupuncture—science or myth: a review. *Journal of the Royal Society of Medicine* **81**:588–90.

Price, DD, Rafii, A, Watkins, LR and Buckingham, B. 1984. A psychophysical analysis of acupuncture analgesia. *Pain* **19**:27–42.

Rampes, H and James, R. 1995. Complications of acupuncture. *Acupuncture in Medicine* **13**(1):26–33.

Rasmussen, N and Morgall, J. 1990. The use of alternative treatment in the Danish adult population. *Complementary Medical Research* **4**:16–22.

Reilly, DT. 1983. Young doctors' views on alternative medicine. *British Medical Journal* **287**(6388):337–9.

Reilly, DT, Taylor, MA, McSharry, C and Aitchison, T. 1986. Is homoeopathy a placebo response? *Lancet* **2**:881–6.

Richards, T. 1990. Death from complementary medicine. *British Medical Journal* **301**:510–1.

Richardson, PH and Vincent, CA. 1986. Acupuncture for the treatment of pain: a review of evaluative research. *Pain* **24**:15–40.

Richardson, P. 1989. Placebos: their effectiveness and mode of action. In: Broome, AK, ed. *Health Psychology: Processes and Applications*. London: Chapman and Hall.

Richardson, JC, Shelton, DR, Krailo, M and Levine, AM. 1990. The effect of compliance with treatment on survival among patients wth hematologic malignancies. *Journal of Clinical Oncology* **8**(2):356–64.

Richardson, PH. 1994. Placebo effects in pain management. *Pain Reviews* **1**:15–32.

Richardson, P. 1995. Placebos: their effectiveness and modes of action. In: Broome, AK, ed. *Health Psychology: Processes and Applications*. London: Chapman and Hall.

Robinson, E and Whitfield, M. 1987. Participation of patients during general practice consultation. *Family Practice* **4**:5–10.

Rosen, L. 1974. Acupuncture and Chinese medical practices. *Volta Review* **76**:340–50.

Ross, M and Olson, JM. 1982. Placebo effects in medical research and practice. In: Eiser, JR, ed. *Social Psychology and Behavioural Medicine*. Chichester: Wiley.

Rouse, IL, Berlin, LJ, Armstrong, BK and Vandongen, R. 1983. Blood pressure lowering effect of a vegetarian diet: controlled trial in normotensive subjects. *Lancet* **1**(8314–5):5–10.

Sacks, HS, Berrier, J, Reitman, D and Ancona, BVA. 1987. Meta-analyses of randomized controlled trials. *New England Journal of Medicine* **316**(8):450–5.

Saks, M, ed. 1992. *Alternative Medicine in Britain*. Oxford: Oxford University Press.

Salmon, JW, ed. 1985. *Alternative Medicine: Popular and Policy Perspectives*. London: Tavistock Publications.

Scofield, AM. 1984. Experimental research in homoeopathy: a critical review. *British Homoeopathic Journal* **73**(July–October):161–80, 211–26.

Shapiro, AK. 1960. A contribution to a history of the placebo effect. *Behavioral Science* **5**:398–430.

Shapiro, AK and Morris, LA. 1978. The placebo effect in medical and psychological therapies. In: Bergin, AE and Garfield, S, eds. *Handbook of Psychotherapy and Behavioral Change* (vol. 2). New York: Wiley.

Shapiro, DA. 1981. Comparative credibility of treatment rationales: three tests of expectancy theory. *British Journal of Clinical Psychology* **20**:111–22.

Sharma, U. 1992. *Complementary Medicine Today: Practitioners and Patients*. London: Routledge.

Sheard, TAB. 1990. Bristol Cancer Help Centre. *Lancet* **336**:1185–6.

Sheehan, MP, Rustin, MHA, Atherton, DJ, Buckley, C, Harris, DJ, Bristoff, J. et al. 1992. Efficacy of traditional Chinese herbal therapy in adult atopic dermatitis. *Lancet* **340**:13–17.

Silagy, C and Neil, A. 1994a. Garlic as a lipid lowering agent—a meta-analysis. *Journal of the Royal College of Physicians* **28**(1):39–45.

Silagy, CA and Neil, HA. 1994b. A meta-analysis of the effect of garlic on blood pressure. *Journal of Hypertension* **12**(4):463–8.

Simanowitz, A. 1985. Standards, attitudes and accountability in the medical profession. *Lancet* **2**:546–7.

Skolstan, L, Larson, L and Linstrom, FD. 1979. Effects of fasting and lactovegetarian diet on rheumatoid arthritis. *Scandinavian Journal of Rheumatology* **8**:249–55.

Skrabanek, P and McCormick, JS. 1987. General practitioners and alternative medicine [letter]. *Journal of the Royal College of General Practitioners* **37**(298):224–5.

Skrabanek, P. 1988. Paranormal health claims. *Experientia* **44**(4):303–9.

Sloane, RB. 1975. Organic brain syndrome. In: Birren, JE and Sloane, RB, eds. *Handbook of Mental Health and Aging*. Englewood Cliffs, NJ: Prentice-Hall.

Smart, HL, Mayberry, JF and Atkinson, M. 1986. Alternative medicine consultations and remedies in patients with the irritable bowel syndrome. *Gut* **27**:826–8.

Smith, R. 1978. And all that. *British Journal of Medicine* **298**:1297–1300.

Smith, R. 1991. Where is the wisdom . . .? *British Medical Journal* **303**(6806):798–9.

Smith, R. 1994. Charity Commission censures British cancer charities. *British Medical Journal* **308**:155–6.

Smith, T. 1983. Alternative medicine [editorial]. *British Medical Journal* **287**(6388):307–8.

Sobell, DS. 1979. *Ways of Health*. New York: Harcourt Brace.

Sontag, S. 1983. *Illness as a Metaphor*. Harmondsworth: Penguin Books.

Spiegel, D, Bloom, JR, Kraemer, HC and Gottheil, E. 1989. Effect of psychological treatment on survival of patients with metastatic breast cancer. *Lancet* **2**:888–91.

Stamler, R, Stamler, J, Grimm, R, Gosch, FC et al. 1987. Nutritional therapy for high blood pressure. Final report of a four-year randomized controlled trial—the Hypertension Control Program. *Journal of the American Medical Association* **257**(11):1484–91.

Stanton-Rogers, W. 1991. *Explaining Health and Illness: An Exploration of Diversity*. London: Wheatsheaf.

Stanway, A. 1986. *Alternative Medicine: A Guide to Natural Therapies*. Harmondsworth: Penguin Books.

Strickland, B. 1978. Internal-external expectancies and health related behaviours. *Journal of Consulting and Clinical Psychology* **46**:1192–221.

Sutherland, S. 1992. *Irrationality*. London: Constable.

Tashkin, DP, Bresler, DP and Kroening, RJ. 1977. Comparison of real and simulated acupuncture and isoproterenol in metacholine induced asthma. *Annals of Allergy* **39**:379–87.

Tashkin, DP, Kroening, RJ and Bresler, DP. 1985. A controlled trial of real and simulated acupuncture in the management of chronic asthma. *Journal of Allergy and Clinical Immunology* **76**:855–64.

Tate, P. 1983. Doctors' style. In: Pendleton, D and Hasler, J, eds. *Doctor-patient Communication*. London: Academic Press.

Tavola, T, Gala, C, Conte, G and Invernizzi, G. 1992. Traditional Chinese acupuncture in tension-type headache: a controlled study. *Pain* **48**(3):325–9.

Taylor, R. 1985. Alternative medicine and the medical encounter in Britain and the United States. In: Salmon, W, ed. *Alternative Medicine: Popular Policy and Perspectives*. London: Tavistock.

Ter Riet, G, Kleijnen, J and Knipschild, P. 1990a. Acupuncture and chronic pain: a criteria based meta-analysis. *Journal of Clinical Epidemiology* **11**:1191–9.

Ter Riet, G, Kleijnen, J and Knipschild, P. 1990b. A meta-analysis of studies into the effect of acupuncture on addiction. *British Journal of General Practice* **40**: 379–82.

Terrett, AGT. 1995. Misuse of the literature by medical authors in discussing spinal manipulative therapy injury. *Journal of Manipulative and Physiological Therapeutics* **18**(4):203–10.

Thomas, KJ, Carr, J, Westlake, L and Williams, BT. 1991. Use of non-orthodox and conventional health care in Great Britain. *British Medical Journal* **302**(6770): 207–10.

Tonkin, RD. 1987. Role of research in the rapprochement between conventional medicine and complementary therapies: discussion paper. *Journal of the Royal Society of Medicine* **80**(6):361–3.

Totman, R. 1987. *The Social Causes of Illness* 2nd edn. London: Souvenir Press.

Tsutani, K. 1993. The evaluation of herbal medicines: an east Asian perspective. In: Lewith, GT and Aldridge, D, eds. *Clinical Research Methodology for Complementary Therapies*. London: Hodder and Stoughton.

Turner, S and Mills, S. 1993. A double-blind clinical trial on a herbal remedy for premenstrual syndrome: a case study. *Complementary Therapies in Medicine* 1: 73–7.

Ullman, D. 1991. *Discovering Homeopathy*. Berkeley: North Atlantic Books.

Vaskilampi, T. 1990. The role of alternative medicine: The Finnish experience. *Complementary Medical Research* 4:23–7.

Vecchio, PC. 1994. Attitudes to alternative medicine by rheumatology outpatient attenders. *Journal of Rheumatology* 21(1):145–7.

Verhoef, MJ, Sutherland, LR and Brkich, L. 1990. Use of alternative medicine by patients attending a gastroenterology clinic. *Canadian Medical Association Journal* 142(2):121–5.

Verhoef, M and Sutherland, L. 1995. General practitioners' assessment of and interest in alternative medicine in Canada. *Social Science and Medicine* 41:511–15.

Vincent, CA. 1989a. The methodology of controlled trials of acupuncture. *Acupuncture in Medicine* 6:9–13.

Vincent, CA. 1989b. A controlled trial of the treatment of migraine by acupuncture. *Clinical Journal of Pain* 5:305–12.

Vincent, CA. 1990a. The treatment of tension headache by acupuncture: a controlled single case design with time series analysis. *Journal of Psychosomatic Research* 34(5):553–61.

Vincent, CA. 1990b. Credibility assessment in trials of acupuncture. *Complementary Medical Research* 4(1):8–11.

Vincent, CA. 1992. Acupuncture research. *Complementary Medical Research* 6(i):21–4.

Vincent, CA. 1993. Acupuncture as a treatment for chronic pain. In: Lewith, GT and Aldridge, D, eds. *Clinical Research Methodology for Complementary Therapies*. London: Hodder and Stoughton.

Vincent, CA. 1997. *Complementary Medicine. Cambridge Handbook of Psychology in Medicine*. Cambridge: Cambridge University Press. In press.

Vincent, CA. 1997. Perceived efficacy of complementary and orthodox medicine. A replication. *Complementary Therapies in Medicine*. In press.

Vincent, CA and Chapman, CR. 1989. Pain measurement in trials of acupuncture. *Acupuncture in Medicine* 6:14–19.

Vincent, CA and Furnham, A. 1994. The perceived efficacy of complementary and orthodox medicine: preliminary findings and the development of a questionnaire. *Complementary Therapies in Medicine* 2:128–34.

Vincent, C and Furnham, A. 1996. Why do patients turn to complementary medicine? An empirical study. *British Journal of Clinical Psychology* 35:37–48.

Vincent, CA and Furnham, AF. 1997. The perceived efficacy of complementary and orthodox medicine. *Complementary Therapies in Medicine*. In press.

Vincent, C and Lewith, G. 1995. Placebo controls for acupuncture studies. *Journal of the Royal Society of Medicine* 88:199–202.

Vincent, CA and Mole, P. 1989. Acupuncturists and research. *Complementary Medical Research* 3(3):25–30.

Vincent, CA and Richardson, PH. 1986. The evaluation of therapeutic acupuncture: concepts and methods. *Pain* 24:1–13.

Vincent, CA and Richardson, PH. 1987. Acupuncture for some common disorders: a review of evaluative research. *Journal of the Royal College of General Practitioners* **37**:77–81.

Vincent, C, Furnham, A and Willsmore, M. 1995. The perceived efficacy of complementary and orthodox medicine in complementary and general practice patients. *Health Education Research* **10**:395–405.

Visser, GJ and Peters, L. 1990. Alternative medicine and general practitioners in The Netherlands: towards acceptance and integration. *Family Practice* **7**(3):227–32.

Visser, GJ, Peters, L and Rasker, JJ. 1992. Rheumatologists and their patients who seek alternative care: An agreement to disagree. *British Journal of Rheumatology* **31**:485–90.

Volgyesi, FA. 1954. School for patients, hypnosis therapy, and psychoprophylaxis. *British Journal of Medical Hypnotism* **5**:8.

Voudouris, NJ, Peck, CL and Coleman, G. 1990. The role of conditioning and verbal expectancy in the placebo response. *Pain* **43**:121–8.

Wadsworth, M, Butterfield, W and Blaney, R. 1971. *Health and Sickness: The Choice of Treatment*. London: Tavistock.

Warden, J. 1993. Model for GMC? *British Medical Journal* **306**:608.

Wardwell, WI. 1994. Alternative medicine in the United States. *Social Science and Medicine* **38**(8):1061–8.

Warshafsky, S, Kamer, RS and Sivak, SL. 1993. Effect of garlic on total serum cholesterol. A meta-analysis. *Annals of Internal Medicine* **119**(7 pt 1):599–605.

Weinman, J and Johnston, M. 1988. Stressful medical procedures: An analysis of the effects of psychological interventions and of the stressfulness of the procedures. In: Maes, S, Spielberger, CD, Defares, PB and Sarason, IG, eds. *Topics in Health Psychology*. Chichester: Wiley.

Weir, MW. 1993. Bristol Cancer Help Centre: success and setbacks but the journey continues. *Complementary Therapies in Medicine* **1**(1):42–5.

Wharton, R and Lewith, G. 1986. Complementary medicine and the general practitioner. *British Medical Journal* **292**(6534):1498–500.

White, L, Tursky, B and Schwartz, GE. 1985. Placebos in perspective. In: White, L, Tursky, B and Schwartz, GE, eds. *Placebo: Theory, Research, and Mechanism*. New York: Guilford Press.

Whorton, JC. 1989. The first holistic revolution: Alternative medicine in the nineteenth century. In: Stalker, D and Glymour, C, eds. *Examining Holistic Medicine*. New York: Prometheus Books.

Wickramasekera, I. 1985. A conditioned response model of the placebo effect: predictions from the model. In: White, L, Tursky, B and Schwartz, GE, eds. *Placebo: Theory, Research and Mechanisms*. New York: Guilford Press.

Wiegant, FAC, Kramers, CW and van Wijk, R. 1993. The importance of patient selection. In: Lewith, GT and Aldridge, D, eds. *Clinical Research Methodology for Complementary Therapies*. London: Hodder and Stoughton.

Wikler, D. 1985. Holistic medicine: concepts of personal responsibility for health. In: Stalker, D and Glymour, C, eds. *Examining Holistic Medicine*. Buffalo, New York: Prometheus Books.

Williams, SJ and Calnan, M. 1991. Key determinants of consumer satisfaction with general practice. *Family Practice* **8**(3):237–42.

Williamson, JW, Goldschmidt, PG and Colton, T. 1986. The quality of medical literature: an analysis of validation assessments. In: Bautar, JC and Mostellar, R, eds. *Medical Use of Statistics*. Waltham, Mass.: NEJM Books.

Winship, KA. 1991. Toxicity of comfrey. *Adverse Drug Reactions and Toxicological Reviews* **10**:47–59.

Worsley, JR. 1973. *Is Acupuncture for You?* New York: Harper and Row.

Wright, SG. 1995. Bringing the heart back into nursing. *Complementary Therapies in Nursing and Midwifery* **1**(1):15–20.

Zang, J. 1990. Immediate anti-asthmatic effect of acupuncture in 192 cases of bronchial asthma. *Journal of Traditional Chinese Medicine* **10**:89–93.

Zimbardo, PG. 1969. *The Cognitive Control of Motivation.* Illinois: Scott, Foresman.

Index

Index compiled by Caroline Sheard